VEGANISSIMO A to Z

A Comprehensive Guide to Identifying and
Avoiding Ingredients of Animal Origin in
Everyday Products

Reuben Proctor and Lars Thomsen

THE EXPERIMENT
NEW YORK

Veganissimo A to Z:
A Comprehensive Guide to Identifying and Avoiding Ingredients of Animal Origin in Everyday Products
Canadian edition
Copyright © 2012, 2013 Reuben Proctor and Lars Thomsen

The Experiment, LLC
260 Fifth Avenue
New York, NY 10001–6408
www.theexperimentpublishing.com

Many of the designations used by manufacturers and sellers to distinguish their products are claimed as trademarks. Where those designations appear in this book and The Experiment was aware of a trademark claim, the designations have been capitalized.

The Experiment's books are available at special discounts when purchased in bulk for premiums and sales promotions as well as for fundraising or educational use. For details, contact us at info@theexperimentpublishing.com.

The purpose of this book is to provide information regarding animal ingredients in consumer goods and everyday products. Its contents are the product of painstaking research, and all statements are made to the best of our knowledge and in good faith. They do not, however, constitute either legal or health advice. No liability can be assumed for potential adverse situations that might be seen to be the result of using this book.

ISBN 978-1-61519-069-0
Ebook ISBN 978-1-61519-167-3

Cover design by Daniel Rembert
Interior design by Nicole Hollatz and Reuben Proctor
Thanks to Emiko Badillo for her help with this Canadian edition.
Manufactured in the United States of America
Distributed by Thomas Allen & Son Ltd.
First published February 2013
10 9 8 7 6 5 4 3 2 1

This book is printed on
recycled paper that includes
30% post-consumer waste.

Contents

Introduction   v
About Using This Book   xi

Part 1: Ingredients A to Z   1–234

Part 2: Product Labelling   235–263
Food   238
Supplements/Natural health products   245
Pharmaceutical drugs   246
Cosmetics   247
Household cleaning products   250
Textiles   251
Footwear   255
Seals, logos and labels   256

Part 3: Vegan Alternatives to Animal Ingredients   265–288
Food   268
Dietary supplements   277
Pharmaceutical drugs   278
"Pet" food   279
Cosmetics   280
Household cleaning products • Clothing and accessories   281
Footwear   282
Brooms and brushes • Interior decoration and household items   283
Sport and leisure   284
Arts and crafts   285
Photography and printing • Musical instruments   286
Electronics and technology   287
Closing remarks   288

Part 4: References and Resources   289–301
Glossary   291
Bibliography   295
Online resources   298
Canadian legislation   300

Introduction

In today's world, "products" obtained from animals are more or less ubiquitous. Sometimes they are easy to recognize, for instance meat, milk, eggs, leather or wool. More often, however, they are not immediately visible, but "hidden" in industrially processed substances, the names of which we often do not understand, and sometimes cannot even pronounce.

Animal substances are also used in many industrial processes most people are unaware of—even products that do not contain animal substances may have been produced using them.

Animal products are usually made behind closed doors. We are not meant to look behind the scenes, because then we would see what most people still successfully block out: that these products are made from sentient beings who are bred, held captive, killed and exploited by us humans by the millions, as if they were lifeless automatons.

We want this book to help people look behind the closed doors and recognize where our commodities come from and at whose expense they are made.

We would like this book to be a guide for those who have just become aware of the abuse inflicted on animals by our industrial society, as well as those who would like to deepen their current knowledge regarding animal ingredients. It is in the interests of all consumers to find out more about the contents of food, cosmetics, clothing, etc.

It was important for us during the writing of this book that you, the reader, not only be easily able to recognize and avoid substances that are definitely or potentially animal but also to find their vegan alternatives.

We hope that we have been able to demonstrate not only which products are off-limits from the point of view of ethically motivated veganism, but also that there are many possibilities for living a fulfilled life that is not marked by asceticism. It is in fact not only possible but also liberating—both for us in a figurative sense and also quite literally for the animals that are still the slaves of our society.

With this book in your hand, you can now consciously look for new options. They do exist, you just have to discover them.

About this English-language edition

Veganissimo A to Z: A Comprehensive Guide to Identifying and Avoiding Ingredients of Animal Origin in Everyday Products was originally researched and written with German-speaking countries in mind. However, much of what can be said about animal ingredients there also applies to other countries. What may differ most noticeably is the availability of vegan alternatives to animal products.

In light of the differences between Canada and the European single market, this edition differs somewhat from the original German version. However, there are some similarities between the Canadian and European markets, and we trust that readers in Canada will find this book as relevant and helpful as we believe our German-speaking readers have. That said, we would be glad to receive any feedback that will help us to improve future editions.

Development

Since the first German edition of *Veganissimo A to Z* seventeen years ago, there have been a number of changes in the field of ingredients and additives, some for the better, some for the worse. Labelling has improved overall and the number of explicitly vegan products is constantly increasing; on the other hand—partly because of those very improvements in labelling—seemingly vegan products turn out not to be vegan after all. Or producers "improve" their formulas, for instance adding lactose or clarified butter to previously vegan products. The production of ingredients has also partly changed: Newer, cheaper and more advanced production methods continue to be developed, with the result that substances previously obtained from animals are now obtained from partly or entirely vegetable, microbiological or synthetic sources. On the other hand, the advance of biotechnology and genetic engineering means that animals once again or for the first time become potential "suppliers" of certain ingredients or active agents.

Some entries in the last edition of *Veganissimo A to Z* turned out to be inaccurate or outdated. We are very grateful for letters from our readers, which helped us to identify and correct such entries.

In short: It became necessary to completely revise *Veganissimo A to Z* and adapt it to the changed circumstances. It was also important to us to continue to develop *Veganissimo A to Z*, increasing its breadth and depth.

Goal and contents of this book

This edition of *Veganissimo A to Z* is based on the standardized labelling of foods and cosmetics as defined by Canadian law, as well as standard reference works on food chemistry and cosmetics. However, this book is not exhaustive, and in the light of the sheer number of ingredients and additives that are available, approved and actually used, this is in fact hardly possible.

This book is not meant to be a scientific reference, but rather a practical aid in the jungle of confusing and often incomprehensible product labelling.

All information on individual ingredients is the result of painstaking research, but we cannot guarantee that all statements made in this book are correct, nor can we assume any responsibility for any problems that may arise with regard to the information in this book. In uncertain cases, only the producer of a specific ingredient can provide clarity regarding its source.

The subject of this book is ingredients and additives that derive from animals or may do so. For completeness' sake and to avoid misunderstanding, we have also included substances that occur naturally in animal tissues, body fluids or secretions, etc., but can also be obtained for human use from vegetable sources, microbial cultures or synthetic sources. We have especially listed all important and ubiquitous nutrients (especially amino acids, fatty acids and vitamins) regardless of their actual sources. We have also listed substances that are not of animal origin but might be confused with animal substances.

We hope that this will provide more clarity, with regard to both specific ingredients and the part they play in our commodities in general.

For reasons of space, we have completely omitted those substances that are obviously vegetable or synthetic and that cannot be confused with animal substances.

Due to the multitude of ingredients and additives, and the complexity of the chemical relationships between many of these substances, it was a considerable challenge keeping the book within a sensible scale that would not demand too much of consumers. We have aimed to achieve the greatest possible comprehensibility and clarity. Nonetheless, we must point out that you will not always immediately find the complete answer you are looking for, and will often need to follow cross-references to other substances. This was unfortunately not always avoidable and shows how interconnected different substances can often be.

The scope of the new edition also made it necessary to concentrate on essential details, i.e., the characteristics that most easily identify whether an ingredient is of animal origin and how it is used. We are aware that this approach can lead to statements which may be chemically imprecise or oversimplified. It was nonetheless more important for us to identify the origins of substances as far as possible rather than to publish a chemistry textbook.

Alternatives to animal substances

A further consequence of the size of the new edition was the need to find a new way of dealing with the question of alternatives to animal ingredients, especially with cosmetic ingredients. It would have required an inappropriate amount of space to name alternatives to each single substance, or would have resulted in information that would not have been particularly helpful, such as dozens of entries with identical references to the same vegetable alternatives.

We therefore decided to forgo naming alternatives within the A to Z entries themselves and have instead dedicated a separate chapter to the subject of alternatives. This allowed us to address the most important fundamental questions and will also, we hope, help to make your buying decisions as easy and confident as possible.

Animal testing

Many different products—especially those intended to be used as cosmetics or household products (e.g. detergents)—may be tested on animals in order to ascertain their safety for humans.

Unfortunately, Canadian law does not prohibit testing cosmetic products on animals, but on the other hand it does not require animal tests, either. It remains the responsibility of the manufacturers to decide whether such tests are necessary to substantiate the safety of their products.

This means that any cosmetic product may have been tested on living animals, either as individual ingredients or as the final product—or even both. Unless the producer decides to disclose such information, there is no way of knowing whether this is in fact the case. This is why logos stating that a product has not been tested on animals are especially important (see pages 256–263).

Animal tests with finished cosmetic products and their ingredients have been banned in the European Union since 2009. Unfortunately, animal tests are still legally required for other chemicals under the EU REACH Regulation (Registration, Evaluation, Authorisation and Restriction of Chemicals). This includes tests for preservatives, dyes, food additives, household chemicals and detergents.

For further information on cruelty-free products, see *www.leapingbunny.org*.

Genetic engineering

In a few places we name genetically engineered or modified substances as possible alternatives to animal ingredients or additives. In these cases, substances from microorganisms such as yeasts or bacteria are involved. This does not imply a statement on genetic engineering as such, but is rather a question of supplying complete information. Whether a vegan lifestyle necessarily means rejecting genetic engineering is a decision you must make for yourself.

Cosmetic ingredients

Cosmetics labelling can be confusing. On the one hand it is comprehensive, as virtually all ingredients must be named; on the other hand the ingredients are generally listed according to their INCI names (INCI = *International Nomenclature of Cosmetic Ingredients*). Certain defined ingredients may instead be listed using their English or French common names, but often the ingredients lists can nonetheless be hard to understand. This book contains all the INCI names we consider relevant with regard to potentially animal ingredients, as well as their synonyms wherever these might be helpful.

Food additives

Some food additives are recognizably from animal sources, but some can also be of animal origin without it being obvious. This can make it difficult to judge whether products are vegan or not, and the fact that food additives must not always be declared does not help, either. On pages 241–243, we have summarized the general situation with regard to food additives and trust that this will go some way towards clarifying matters.

Although food additives do not have numbers assigned to them in Canada, you might see them on products imported from Europe ("E numbers"). For this reason, we have also included them where these are relevant as synonyms.

Health and ecological considerations

For reasons of space, we have concentrated on whether or not individual substances are vegan and not addressed health and ecological considerations regarding individual substances; as we see it, a substance that is not vegan is for that reason alone out of the question, regardless of other important and proper health or ecological considerations. We assume that you have already taken such considerations into account and are reading this book because you have decided on, or are interested in, a vegan way of life.

Final remarks on the subject of vocabulary

Commonplace terms such as *product, production, source material*, etc. are not entirely avoidable. What is concealed behind these terms, and is often forgotten only too quickly, is the merciless exploitation of sentient beings and the resulting suffering caused to them in the process. With the help of language, living individuals are declared things, objects. With our language we define not only ourselves but also our dealings with our environment.

And a request

This A to Z reference can never be exhaustive. Nonetheless, we aim to keep it as comprehensive, up-to-date and correct as possible. We would therefore be especially grateful for information on ingredients not yet included and alternatives to them, as well as constructive criticism of the existing entries. Please send correspondence to: *feedback@veganissimo-a-to-z.com*

Reuben Proctor and Lars Thomsen, January 2013

In order to make the somewhat dry subject a little more accessible, the entries in the ingredients list have the following structure:

Name

(Alternative names)

Source (animal, vegetable, synthetic, etc.). Description, where appropriate with a ► *cross reference*. Sources, functions, production, processing and uses.

Some substances have many chemical variants with names that differ only in the numbers contained, e.g. *Laneth-9 Acetate* and *Laneth-10 Acetate*. When such substances also have the same uses, rather than name all the variants, we have replaced the numbers with *n*, e.g. *Laneth-n Acetate*. In other cases where distinct substances have such similar uses that a joint entry is warranted, the substance names appear on consecutive lines or on the same line separated by periods, e.g. *Dog Fur. Dog Leather.* Where slashes appear in an entry name, e.g. *Lactobacillus/Skeletonema Ferment*, the slashes are part of the complete name for that substance.

The icons next to the names show the possible sources of a substance (with common/primary sources in orange and less common/partial sources in grey):

- vegetable *(includes mushrooms in this book)*
- animal *(both from living and killed animals)*
- synthetic *(derived from petroleum)*
- mineral *(rocks, metals)*
- microbiological *(e.g. yeast cultures, bacteria)*

A Key to the Icons appears on the next page and on the inner front and back covers for easy reference. Substances with several icons have several possible sources. We decided not to use the category *chemical*, as it does not in fact say anything about the source: A chemical substance may just as easily have been produced using animal materials as vegetable ones.

The complexity of modern chemical processing means that it is not always possible to know which source was used for a specific product, unless the product carries a certified logo (see pages 256–263). Slashes in the source description indicate that the production of a substance requires raw materials in multiple categories, e.g. *can be vegetable/synthetic or animal* describes a substance that is either *both* vegetable and synthetic in origin, or animal in origin.

Key to the Icons

 always or often vegetable
 sometimes or rarely vegetable

 always or often animal
sometimes or rarely animal

 always or often synthetic
sometimes or rarely synthetic

always or often mineral
sometimes or rarely mineral

 always or often microbiological
 sometimes or rarely microbiological

VEGANISSIMO A to Z

Part 1

Ingredients A to Z

Including:

- *Food ingredients*
- *Food additives*
- *Dietary supplements*
- *Drugs*
- *Cosmetic ingredients*
- *Household cleaning products*
- *Textiles, apparel, accessories*
- *Technical appliances*

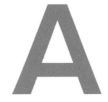

Acetic Acid Esters of Mono- and Diglycerides of Fatty Acids
(E 472a)
Can be vegetable or animal. Reaction product of acetic acid with ► *glycerides* of ► *fatty acids.* Emulsifiers, carriers and glazing agents in foods.

Acetyl Cysteine
(ACC)
From living or killed animals, can also be microbiological or synthetic. A ► *cysteine* derivative. Active ingredient in mucolytic medication. Antioxidant in cosmetics. Ingredient in some dietetic foods.

Acetyl Glucosamine
From killed animals. ► *Glucosamine* compound. Skin conditioner in cosmetics.

Acetyl Glutamic Acid
Mostly vegetable/synthetic, can also be animal. ► *Glutamic acid* compound. Skin conditioner in cosmetics.

Acetyl Glutamine
Mostly vegetable/synthetic, can also be animal. Chemically altered ► *glutamine.* Industrial production by fermentation of ► *glutamic acid.* Skin conditioner in cosmetics.

Acetyl Tyrosine
Mostly vegetable/synthetic, can also be animal. ► *Tyrosine* compound. Tanning agent in cosmetics.

Acetylated Glycol Stearate
Can be animal or vegetable. Chemically altered ► *stearic acid.* Emulsifier and emollient in cosmetics.

Acetylated Hydrogenated Lanolin
From living or killed animals. Chemically altered ► *lanolin.* Emollient in cosmetics.

Acetylated Hydrogenated Lard Glyceride(s)
From killed animals. Chemically altered ► *lard.* Emollient in cosmetics.

Acetylated Hydrogenated Tallow Glyceride(s)
From killed animals. Chemically altered ► *tallow.* Emollient and emulsifier in cosmetics.

Acetylated Lanolin
(Lanolin acetate)
From living or killed animals. Chemically altered ► *lanolin*. Antistatic, emollient and emulsifier in cosmetics.

Acetylated Lanolin Alcohol
From living or killed animals. Chemically altered ► *lanolin alcohol*. Antistatic, emollient and emulsifier in cosmetics.

Acetylated Lanolin Ricinoleate
From living or killed animals. Chemically altered ► *lanolin*. Antistatic and emollient in cosmetics.

Acetylated Lard Glyceride
From killed animals. Chemically altered ► *lard*. Emollient in cosmetics.

Acetylated Sucrose Distearate
Can be vegetable or animal. Compound of ► *sugar* and ► *stearic acid*. Emollient in cosmetics.

Acetylmethionyl Methylsilanol Elastinate
From killed animals. Chemically altered ► *elastin*. Antistatic, skin and hair conditioner in cosmetics.

Acrylates/Ceteth-20 Itaconate Copolymer
Acrylates/Ceteth-20 Methacrylate Copolymer
Mostly vegetable/synthetic, can also be partly animal. Polymer compounds of ► *cetyl alcohol*. Viscosity controlling agents in cosmetics.

Acrylates/Steareth-20 Itaconate Copolymer
Acrylates/Steareth-20 Methacrylate Copolymer
Acrylates/Steareth-50 Acrylate Copolymer
Can be vegetable/synthetic or animal/synthetic. Polymer compounds of ► *stearyl alcohol*. Film forming and viscosity controlling agents in cosmetics.

Acrylates/Vinyl Isodecanoate Crosspolymer
Mostly vegetable/synthetic, can also be partly animal. Polymer compound of ► *capric acid*. Film forming and viscosity controlling agent in cosmetics.

Activated Carbon
(Activated charcoal. Carbo animalis [animal charcoal]. Carbo medicinalis [medicinal charcoal]. Carbo vegetabilis [vegetable charcoal. E 153])
Vegetable, synthetic or from killed animals. Fine-grained, porous carbon with a large internal surface area. Obtained by charring carbon-rich substances, such as wood, nutshells, coffee beans, blood, bones, lignite, coal or petroleum. Medicinal charcoal is derived solely from plant matter. Used for extracting undesired or harmful substances such as colours, flavours or odours, for instance in chemical and pharmaceutical industries, water and sewage treatment, and ventilation/air conditioning; for purifying and bleaching foods, e.g. starch or ► *sugar*; for fining/clarifying wine, beer and fruit juice.

In cigarette filters. In some shoe inlays. Used for treating poisoning and diarrhea, and for cleansing wounds.

Adenosine
Adenosine Cyclic Phosphate
Adenosine Phosphate
Adenosine Triphosphate

(Adenosine monophosphate [AMP]. Adenosine diphosphate [ADP]. Adenosine triphosphate [ATP])
Synthetic. Compounds of adenine (constituent of ► *DNA* and ► *RNA*) that play an important part in the energy balance of all living cells. Skin conditioners in cosmetics.

Adeps Bovis
From killed animals. ► *Tallow*, from cattle. Emollient in cosmetics.

Adeps Cervidae ► Deer Tallow

Adeps Lanae ► Lanolin

Adeps Solidus ► Hard Fat

Adeps Suillus
From killed animals. Purified ► *lard.* Emollient in cosmetics.

Adipic Acid
(E 355)
Synthetic. An organic acid. Occurs naturally in beets. Industrial production from petroleum derivatives. Buffering agent in cosmetics. Source for additional cosmetic substances, e.g. in conjunction with ► *fatty acids.* Acidity regulator in foods.

Adrenalin
(Epinephrin. Suprarenin®)
Synthetic. Stress hormone and neurotransmitter produced in animals' adrenal glands. Industrial synthesis from ► *phenylalanine.* Emergency medication (for cardiac arrest or allergic reactions) or for constricting blood vessels (for instance, in association with local anesthesia and to reduce bleeding).

ALA ► Linolenic Acid

Alanine
(Aminopropanoic acid)
Can be microbiological or synthetic. Nonessential ► *amino acid.* Occurs naturally in almost all ► *proteins.* Antistatic in cosmetics. In dietetic foods. In intravenous drips. Can be used to create sweet-sour flavour in vinegar and for synthesizing ► *vitamin B$_6$.*

Alanine Glutamate
Mostly vegetable/synthetic, can theoretically also be animal. Compound of ► *glutamic acid* and ► *alanine.* Skin conditioner in cosmetics.

Alanine/Histidine/Lysine Polypeptide Copper HCl
Mostly vegetable/synthetic, can also be animal. Copper compound of ► *alanine*, ► *histidine* and ► *lysine.* Skin conditioner in cosmetics.

Albumen
(Egg white)
From living or killed animals. Clear, liquid ► *protein* in birds' eggs surrounding the yolk. Obtained from captive birds (e.g. chickens) or gathered from wild birds' nests. In foods, e.g. as a binding agent in baked goods. For fining/clarifying wine and other beverages. In nutritional supplements. Film forming agent in cosmetics. In adhesives and as a fixative for textile colurs. Fertilizer. Leather care substance. Additive in animal food.

Albumin
From living or killed animals. General term for soluble ► *proteins* that coagulate under heat. Several vital functions as serum albumin in mammal ► *blood.* Main constituent of egg white (► *albumen*). Also in ► *milk*, muscle and plant seeds. Often isolated from cattle blood. Binding agent in adhesives, e.g. plywood glue. Bovine albumin is used in laboratory diagnostics and as a nutrient solution for cell cultures. Certain intravenous solutions contain human albumin.

Alcloxa
Aldioxa
Synthetic, can theoretically also be animal. Aluminum salts of ► *allantoin.* Antimicrobial, astringent and soothing substances in cosmetics (e.g. in deodorants, antiperspirants, shaving products and childcare products).

Aleuritic Acid
From living and killed animals. Variant of ► *palmitic acid.* Main constituent of ► *shellac.* Obtained by saponification of shellac resin. Used in perfumes (e.g. musk scent). Skin conditioner in cosmetics.

Alkylglycerols
From killed animals. Hydrocarbon lipid compounds. Occur naturally in ► *marine oils*, especially shark liver oil (► *squali iecur oil*), as well as in bone marrow and breast milk. Obtained from shark liver oil or cattle bone marrow. Used in cosmetics and nutritional supplements (e.g. as immunostimulant), and as complementary cancer therapy. See also ► *batyl alcohol*, ► *chimyl alcohol*.

Allantoin
Synthetic, can theoretically also be animal. Degradation product of ► *uric acid.* Part of the ► *protein* metabolism of most mammals. Also in many plants, such as comfrey, black salsify, horse chestnut. Traditionally extracted from cows' urine or comfrey extract. For economic reasons, industrially produced allantoin is always synthetic. Soothing agent and plasticizer in cosmetics.

Allantoin Acetyl Methionine
Synthetic, can theoretically also be animal. Compound of ► *allantoin* and ► *methionine.* Skin protecting substance in cosmetics.

Allantoin Ascorbate
Synthetic, can theoretically also be animal. Compound of ► *allantoin* and ascorbic acid (► *vitamin C*). Soothing agent and skin protective substance in cosmetics.

Allantoin Biotin
Synthetic, can theoretically also be animal. Compound of ► *allantoin* and ► *biotin*. Soothing agent, antiseborrheic and skin protective substance in cosmetics.

Allantoin Calcium Pantothenate
Synthetic, can theoretically also be animal. Compound of ► *allantoin* and ► *pantothenic acid*. Soothing agent and skin protective substance in cosmetics.

Allantoin Glycyrrhetinic Acid
Allantoin (Poly)Galacturonic Acid
Allantoin PABA
Synthetic, can theoretically also be animal. Compounds of ► *allantoin* and plant-derived acids. Soothing agent and skin protecting substances in cosmetics. Allantoin PABA is used as a UV absorber.

Allyl Caproate
(Allyl hexanoate)
Can be vegetable or partly animal. Hydrocarbon compound of ► *caproic acid*. Emollient in cosmetics.

Allyl Stearate/VA Copolymer
Can be vegetable or animal. Hydrocarbon polymer compound of ► *stearic acid*. Film forming agent in cosmetics.

Alpaca
(Alpaca wool)
From living animals. The ► *wool* of alpacas, a South American camelid species, used in clothing/textiles. Not yet common in North America, but on the rise, with alpacas now being bred in Canada and the United States.

Alpha-Linolenic Acid ► *Linolenic Acid*

Alpha-Tocopherol ► *Vitamin E*

Aluminum Caprylate
Mostly mineral/vegetable, can also be animal. Aluminum salt of ► *caprylic acid*. Emulsion stabilizer, opacifier and viscosity controlling agent in cosmetics.

Aluminum Capryloyl Hydrolyzed Collagen
From killed animals. Chemically altered ► *collagen*. Cosmetic hair and skin conditioner.

Aluminum Dicetyl Phosphate
Mostly mineral/vegetable, can also be animal. Aluminum salt of ► *cetyl alcohol*. Emulsion stabilizer in cosmetics.

Aluminum Distearate
Aluminum Isostearate
Aluminum Isostearates/Stearates
Can be mineral/vegetable or animal. Aluminum salts of ► *stearic acid*. Emulsion stabilizer, opacifier and viscosity controlling agent in cosmetics.

Aluminum Hydrogenated Tallow Glutamate
From killed animals. Chemically altered ► *tallow.* Surfactant in cosmetics.

Aluminum Isostearates/Laurates/Palmitates
Can be mineral/vegetable or animal. Aluminum salts of ► *stearic acid,* ► *lauric acid* and ► *palmitic acid.* Emulsion stabilizer, opacifier, viscosity controlling agent in cosmetics.

Aluminum Isostearates/Laurates/Stearates
Can be mineral/vegetable or animal. Aluminum salts of ► *stearic acid* and ► *lauric acid.* Emulsion stabilizer, opacifier and viscosity controlling agent in cosmetics.

Aluminum Isostearates/Myristates
Can be mineral/vegetable or animal. Aluminum salts of ► *stearic acid* and ► *myristic acid.* Emulsion stabilizer, opacifier and viscosity controlling agent in cosmetics.

Aluminum Isostearates/Palmitates
Can be mineral/vegetable or animal. Aluminum salts of ► *stearic acid* and ► *palmitic acid.* Emulsion stabilizer, opacifier and viscosity controlling agent in cosmetics.

Aluminum Myristates/Palmitates
Can be mineral/vegetable or partly animal. Aluminum salts of ► *myristic acid* and ► *palmitic acid.* Emulsion stabilizer, opacifier and viscosity controlling agent in cosmetics.

Aluminum Lactate
Mostly mineral/vegetable/microbiological, can also be animal. Aluminum salt of ► *lactic acid.* Skin protective substance, astringent and antiperspirant in cosmetics.

Aluminum Lanolate
From living or killed animals. Aluminum salt of wool fatty acids (► *lanolin*). Emulsifier and surfactant in cosmetics.

Aluminum Stearate
Can be mineral/vegetable or animal. Aluminum salt of ► *stearic acid.* Colourant and anti-caking agent in cosmetics. Used in industrial lubricants and the production of plastics and lacquers.

Aluminum Stearates
Can be mineral/vegetable or animal. Mixed ► *aluminum distearate* and ► *aluminum tristearate.* Emollient, emulsion stabilizer, opacifier and viscosity controlling agent in cosmetics.

Aluminum Tristearate
Can be mineral/vegetable or animal. Aluminum salt of ► *stearic acid.* Emollient, emulsion stabilizer, opacifier and viscosity controlling agent in cosmetics.

Aluminum Undecylenoyl Collagen Amino Acids
From killed animals. Chemically altered ► *amino acids* from ► *collagen.* Hair and skin conditioner in cosmetics.

Aluminum/Magnesium Hydroxide Stearate
Can be mineral/vegetable or animal. Aluminum and magnesium salt of ► *stearic acid.* Emulsifier and stabilizer in cosmetics.

Ambergris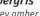
(Grey amber)
From living or killed animals. Grey, waxy substance produced in the digestive tract of sperm whales. Ambergris is excreted by the whales and can be collected from beaches, but is also extracted from slaughtered whales. Medicinal use as a tonic, digestive aid and for treating abdominal cramps. Used as an ► *aphrodisiac*. Also in ► *homeopathic medicines*. Used in earlier times as a fixative in perfumes, now used in very few "high-end" perfumes.

Amino Acids
Can be vegetable or animal. ► *Protein* building blocks, occurring naturally in all organisms. Diverse uses in cosmetics, foods and nutritional supplements. For further information regarding amino acids and their derivatives, see the respective entries in this ingredients list.

The 20 most important amino acids are: ► *alanine*, ► *arginine[*]*, ► *asparagine*, ► *aspartic acid*, ► *cysteine*, ► *glutamine*, ► *glutamic acid*, ► *glycine*, ► *histidine[*]*, ► *isoleucine**, ► *leucine**, ► *lysine**, ► *methionine**, ► *phenylalanine**, ► *proline*, ► *serine*, ► *threonine**, ► *tryptophan**, ► *tyrosine*, ► *valine**.

* = essential amino acids, cannot be produced by the body and must be supplied in the diet.
[*] = semiessential amino acids, must be supplied/supplemented in certain life phases (e.g. infancy, pregnancy).

Amino Acids Complex
Can be vegetable or animal. Combination of various ► *amino acids*. In nutritional supplements and cosmetics.

Aminosuccinic Acid ► Aspartic Acid

Aminobutyric Acid
(Gamma-aminobutyric acid. Aminobutyrate)
Synthetic, can theoretically also be animal. Important neurotransmitter, derivative of ► *glutamic acid*. Occurs naturally in mammalian central nervous systems. Industrial production from glutamic acid with the aid of microorganisms. Hair conditioner in cosmetics. In antiaging creams. In nutritional supplements. Additive in animal food.

Aminoacetic Acid ► Glycine

Aminopropanoic Acid ► Alanine

Aminopropyl Laurylglutamine
Mostly vegetable, can also be animal. Compound of ► *glutamine* and ► *lauryl alcohol*. Antistatic, surfactant and hair conditioner in cosmetics.

Ammonia Caramel ► Caramel Colouring

Ammonium Capryleth Sulfate
Ammonium Capryleth-3 Sulfate
Can be vegetable/synthetic or partly animal. Compounds of ammonium salts, ► *PEG* and ► *caprylic acid*. Surfactants, foaming agents and cleansing substances in cosmetics.

Ammonium Carbonate
(Baker's ammonia. E 503. Salt of hartshorn)
Mineral. Ammonium salts of carbonic acid. Leavening/raising agent in flat baked goods (e.g. gingerbread, biscuits). Buffering agent in cosmetics. Historically obtained by dry distillation of organic matter such as antlers (hence "hartshorn"), bone, horn, leather, hooves, etc. Is now chemically derived from mineral substances.

Ammonium Caseinate
From living animals (► milk). Ammonium salt of ► *casein*. Antistatic in cosmetics.

Ammonium Cocoyl Sarcosinate
Can be from killed animals or vegetable/synthetic. Ammonium salt of ► *sarcosine* and coconut derivatives. Surfactant, foaming agent and cleansing agent in cosmetics.

Ammonium Glutamate ► *Glutamates*

Ammonium Hydrolyzed Collagen
From killed animals. Chemically altered ► *collagen*. Antistatic, hair and skin conditioner in cosmetics.

Ammonium Isostearate
Can be vegetable or animal. Ammonium salt of ► *stearic acid*. Emulsifier and surfactant in cosmetics.

Ammonium Lactate
Can be vegetable or partly animal. Ammonium salt of ► *lactic acid*. Skin protecting substance in cosmetics. Additive in animal food.

Ammonium Lauroyl Sarcosinate
Can be from killed animals or vegetable/synthetic. Ammonium salt of ► *lauric acid* and ► *sarcosine*. Antistatic, surfactant, foaming agent and cleansing agent in cosmetics.

Ammonium Oleate
Can be vegetable or animal. Ammonium salt of ► *oleic acid*. Emulsifier, surfactant and cleansing agent in cosmetics.

Ammonium Phosphatides
(E 442. Mixed ammonium salts of phosphorylated glycerides)
Can be mineral/animal or mineral/vegetable. Chemically altered ► *fatty acids*. Emulsifier and stabilizer in confectionery (cocoa and chocolate products).

Ammonium Stearate
Can be mineral/vegetable or animal. Ammonium salt of ► *stearic acid*. Emulsifier, surfactant and cleansing agent in cosmetics. In textile coatings.

Ammonium Tallate
Vegetable. Ammonium salt of ► *tallol* fatty acids. Emulsifier and surfactant in cosmetics.

Amniotic Fluid
From living or killed animals. Fluid that surrounds mammalian fetuses in the placenta. Mostly obtained from cows. Used as a humectant and skin conditioner in cosmetics.

AMPD-Isostearoyl Hydrolyzed Collagen
AMPD-Rosin Hydrolyzed Collagen
AMP-Isostearoyl Hydrolyzed Collagen

From killed animals. Various forms of chemically altered ► *collagen.* Emulsifiers, hair and skin conditioners in cosmetics.

AMP-Isostearoyl Gelatin/Keratin Amino Acids/
Lysine Hydroxypropyltrimonium Chloride

From killed animals. Chemical complex of ► *stearic acid,* ► *gelatin,* ► *keratin* and ► *lysine.* Surfactant, hair and skin conditioner in cosmetics.

Amphoteric Surfactants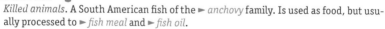
(Zwitterionic surfactants)

Mostly vegetable, can also be animal. Collective term for ► *surfactants* that possess both a positively and a negatively charged hydrophilic group. Derived from ► *fatty acids,* primarily from coconut fat or other vegetable fats. In cosmetics, especially shampoos (declaration according to the respective INCI denominations, usually with "betaine" as part of the name).

Amylase
(E 1100)

Mostly vegetable, can also be from killed animals. Digestive ► *enzyme* that breaks down starch into sugar. Industrial production via fermentation of vegetable matter. Is also obtained from pancreases of slaughtered pigs. Skin protective substance in cosmetics. Active ingredient in medicines. Baking aid. Used in laundry detergents in order to improve the cleansing effect. Used also in the production of starch, and in malt used for brewing ► *beer* and distilling ethanol. In fabric surface treatment in the textile industry.

Anchoveta
Killed animals. A South American fish of the ► *anchovy* family. Is used as food, but usually processed to ► *fish meal* and ► *fish oil.*

Anchovy
Killed animals. Small Atlantic ► *fish,* from industrial fishing. Usually preserved in oil and/or salt and used as side dish or garnish for salads, pizzas, etc., or as a flavour intensifier, especially in condiment sauces such as Worcester sauce or sambal nasi goreng.

Angora
(Angora wool. Angora fibre)

From living or killed animals. ► *Wool* of angora rabbits (the wool of angora goats is known as ► *mohair*). The hair is either shorn or plucked. In some countries (for instance Germany, but not Canada) plucking is banned by animal welfare legislation and the wool is only shorn. Used as knitting yarn, in clothing, blankets, doll hair, etc.

Anhydrous Lanolin ► Lanolin, Anhydrous

Animal Tissue Extract
From killed animals. Extract from animal body tissues. Skin conditioner in cosmetics.

A

Anionic Surfactants
Can be animal, vegetable or synthetic. Collective term for ► *surfactants* that possess a negatively charged hydrophilic group. Obtained from animal or vegetable ► *fats* or petroleum products. In laundry detergents, household cleaning agents, dish soap, etc.

Aorta Extract
From killed animals. Extract from animal arteries. Skin conditioner in cosmetics.

Aphrodisiac
Can be animal or vegetable. Substance that supposedly heightens sexual desire or prowess. Often derived from killed animals, e.g. ► *ambergris*, ► *oysters*, ► *castoreum* and ► *Spanish fly*. The efficacy is usually not medically verifiable and often believed in due to the appearance (usually similarity to sexual organs, e.g. animals' horns) or the origin of the substance (sexual organs of supposedly virile animals, e.g. tiger penises).

Apis Mellifera. Apis Mellifica
(Honey bee)
Killed animals. Whole ► *bees*, processed in ► *homeopathic medicines*, for instance for treating insect stings and various inflammations.

Apisinum ► Bee Venom

Apitoxin ► Bee Venom

Arachideth-20
Mostly vegetable, can also be from killed animals. ► *PEG* compound of ► *arachidyl alcohol*. Surfactant in cosmetics.

Arachidic Acid
(Icosanoic acid. Eicosanoic acid)
Mostly vegetable, can also be from killed animals. Saturated ► *fatty acid*. Occurs naturally in many vegetable oils (especially peanut oil) and some animal ► *fats*. Industrial extraction mainly from peanut oil, but also from ► *arachidonic acid* (in animal fats).

Arachidonic Acid
Can be from killed animals or microbiological. Unsaturated ► *fatty acid*. Occurs naturally only in animal fats. Obtained from internal organs of killed animals, but also using fungal cultures. Emollient in cosmetics. In bodybuilding nutritional supplements.

Arachidyl Alcohol
Mostly vegetable, can also be from killed animals. A ► *fatty alcohol* obtained from ► *arachidic acid*. Emollient in cosmetics.

Arginine
Can be vegetable or animal. Semiessential ► *amino acid*. Occurs naturally in almost all animal and plant tissues. Antistatic in cosmetics. In nutritional supplements.

Arginine Aspartate
Can be vegetable or animal. Compound of ► *arginine* and ► *aspartic acid*. Hair and skin conditioner in cosmetics.

Arginine Glutamate
Can be vegetable or animal. Compound of ► *arginine* and ► *glutamic acid*. Hair and skin conditioner in cosmetics.

Arginine HCl
Can be vegetable or animal. Compound of ► *arginine*. Skin conditioner in cosmetics.

Arginine Hexyldecyl Phosphate
Can be vegetable or animal. Compound of ► *arginine* and ► *decyl alcohol*. Emollient in cosmetics.

Arginine PCA
Can be vegetable or animal. Compound of ► *arginine* and ► *proline*. Humectant in cosmetics.

Arginine/Lysine Polypeptide
Can be vegetable or animal. Compound of ► *arginine* and ► *lysine*. Skin conditioner in cosmetics.

Artemia Extract
From killed animals. Extract from body tissue of brine shrimps (*Artemia salina*). Skin conditioner in cosmetics.

Artificial Honey ► *Inverted Sugar Cream*

Ascorbic Acid ► *Vitamin C*

Ascorbic Acid Polypeptide
Can be vegetable or animal. Reaction product of ascorbic acid (► *vitamin C*) with peptides (► *protein* building blocks). Skin protective substance in cosmetics.

Ascorbyl (Di)Palmitate ► *Fatty Acid Esters of Ascorbic Acid*

Ascorbyl Stearate ► *Fatty Acid Esters of Ascorbic Acid*

Asparagic Acid. Asparaginic Acid ► *Aspartic Acid*

Asparagine
Synthetic/vegetable. Nonessential ► *amino acid*, derivative of ► *aspartic acid*. Occurs naturally in plants (especially pulses, asparagus) and animal tissues. Industrially produced from aspartic acid. Antistatic in cosmetics. In nutritional supplements.

Aspartic Acid
(Aminosuccinic acid. Asparagic acid. Asparginic acid)
Microbiological/vegetable. Nonessential ► *amino acid*. Occurs naturally in vegetable and animal tissues. Industrial production from plant sources via biotechnological processes (microorganisms). In cosmetic creams and ointments. In nutritional supplements.

Aspic
From killed animals. Foods glazed with or set in ► *gelatin*, such as ► *fish* or ► *meat*, but also vegetables.

Atelocollagen ► *Collagen*

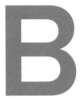

B

Backferment 🌱 🐄
(German for "baking ferment")
Of both vegetable and animal origin. Special sourdough (fermentation product of cereals, water, ► *lactic acid bacteria* and yeasts) based on ► *honey*. Raising agent in bread (especially organic or whole food bread). Standard sourdough is made without honey.

Badger Hair 🐄
From killed animals. ► *Hair* of European badgers. From factory farms, mostly in China, which also deliver badger meat for the Asian market. Used in brushes (most shaving brushes have badger hair bristles).

Baker's Honey 🐄
From living animals. ► *Honey* that does not meet the standards (especially taste) for direct consumption, but is allowed as an ingredient in cooked or baked foods.

Bakery Margarine. Baking Margarine 🌱 🐄
Can be vegetable or vegetable/from killed animals. Special composition of ► *fats*, water and emulsifiers used to improve the quality of baked goods, especially yeast-risen pastry. Can contain a high percentage of animal fats (e.g. ► *tallow*).

Baking Aids 🌱 🐄 ⚗ 💎
Can be vegetable, animal, microbiological or mineral. Collective term for substances or mixtures used to improve processing and results of baked goods. Covers a variety of substances (e.g. acidifiers, enzymes, emulsifiers), including ► *amylase*, ► *cystine*, ► *lecithin*, ► *lactic acid*, ► *milk powder*, ► *mono- and diglycerides of fatty acids*, ► *protease*, ► *stearoyl lactylic acid* and ► *whey powder*. Used in all kinds of baked goods. Not always subject to mandatory food labelling.

Bassia Latifolia Butter ► *Illipé Butter*

Batilol ► *Batyl Alcohol*

Batroxobin 🐄
(Defibrase. Reptilase)
From living or killed animals. ► *Enzymes* from snake venom. Used in laboratory diagnostics (blood work), as well as for treating blood clotting disorders.

Batyl Alcohol
(Batilol)
From killed animals. A fatty hydrocarbon compound found in liver oils of marine animals, bone marrow and breast milk. Extracted from shark or ray liver oil, or yellow bone marrow of cattle. Emollient and emulsifier in cosmetics. Used to treat leukopenia (decreased white blood cells), for instance as a result of radiation, as well as cancer.

Batyl Isostearate
Batyl Stearate
From killed animals. Compounds of ► *batyl alcohol* and ► *stearic acid*. Emollients in cosmetics.

Beeswax Acid
From living animals. ► *Fatty acids* from ► *beeswax*. Stabilizer in cosmetics.

Beeswax PEG-8 Esters
From living animals. Chemically altered ► *beeswax*. Emulsifier in cosmetics.

Behenyl Beeswax
From living animals. Chemically altered ► *beeswax*. Viscosity controlling agent in cosmetics.

Behenyl Isostearate
Can be animal or vegetable. Compound of ► *stearic acid* with ► *fatty alcohols*. Emollient in cosmetics.

Behenyl/Isostearyl Beeswax
From living or killed animals. Compound of ► *beeswax* and ► *fatty alcohols*. Emollient, emulsifier and film forming agent in cosmetics.

Benzyl Hyaluronate
From killed animals. Compound of ► *hyaluronic acid*. Skin conditioner and humectant in cosmetics.

Benzylidene Camphor Hydrolyzed Collagen Sulfonamide
From killed animals. Chemically altered ► *collagen*. Hair conditioner and skin protecting substance in cosmetics.

Benzyltrimonium Hydrolyzed Collagen
From killed animals. Chemically altered ► *collagen*. Antistatic, hair and skin conditioner in cosmetics.

Beta-Carotene ► *Carotene*

Betaine
Can be vegetable or synthetic. Ammonium compound, found naturally in plants (especially beets) as well as in animal tissues. Obtained from beet molasses or synthetically from petroleum derivatives. Antistatic and viscosity controlling agent in cosmetics. In combination with other substances, such as various ► *fatty acids*, also part of other cosmetic ingredients.

Beaver (Hair) ► *Hair*

Bees

Denomination for a multitude of insect species. In everyday usage, "bee" usually refers to the European honey bee (*Apis mellifera*), which produces a number of substances economically significant for humans: ► *bee venom*, ► *beeswax*, ► *honey*, ► *pollen*, ► *propolis* and ► *royal jelly*. These are usually obtained by beekeepers from hives kept in apiaries, but also by removal from the hives of wild bees. Whole bees are also used in the preparation of ► *homeopathic medicines*.

Bee Pollen ► *Pollen*

Bee Venom

(Apisinum. Apitoxin. Honey bee venom. Bee poison)
From living or killed animals. The venom of the honey bee. Obtained by provoking the bees with electric current, so that they feel threatened and sting the glass or plastic sheet beneath them, thus delivering the venom. In the process they can lose their sting and die. Used in medication for treating rheumatic or arthritic disorders, as well as for hyposensitization therapy in the case of a venom allergy. Used in ► *homeopathic medicines*.

Beer

Vegetable/microbiological, may contain animal substances. Alcoholic beverage brewed from water, hops and malt. Beer brewed according to the German *Reinheitsgebot* ("Purity Law") may contain no additives. The *Reinheitsgebot* is no longer in force as legislation, but is often still adhered to as a sign of quality and purity, and although beer brewed according to German law need not comply with the *Reinheitsgebot*, it may only be labelled and sold as such if it does. Otherwise only the following additives are allowed in German beer labelled and sold without reference to the *Reinheitsgebot*: ► *caramel colouring*, ► *lactic acid*, propylene glycol alginate, ascorbic acid (► *vitamin C*), sodium ascorbate, citric acid and gum arabic. Beer not brewed according to German law (e.g. in other European countries or North America) can additionally have been fined with ► *isinglass*, ► *activated carbon*, ► *gelatin* or ► *albumen*. Used as a refreshment beverage and as an addictive drug. Also as hair and skin conditioner in cosmetics.

Beeswax

(Cera alba [white/bleached wax]. Cera flava [yellow/unbleached wax]. E 901)
From living or killed animals. A ► *wax* secreted by ► *bees* and used for building their honeycombs, in which the larvae are reared and ► *honey* and ► *pollen* are stored. Obtained by humans by being cut out of beehives. Used in the form of unbleached yellow wax (cera flava) or bleached white wax (cera alba). Emollient, emulsifier and film forming agent in cosmetics. Bulking agent, glazing agent and anticaking agent in foods. Also in candles, oil pastels, crayons and modelling wax). In polishes, waterproofing and all kinds of coating (e.g. furniture polish, floor care products, wood treatment, sport equipment wax and car polish, also in shoe polish, textile impregnation and paper). Industrial material, e.g. in foundries and for creating casts and moulds. Can be used for glazing coffee, but this practice is rare.

Biotin
(Vitamin H. Vitamin B₇)

Can be vegetable, synthetic or animal. Water-soluble ► *vitamin* that plays an important part in cell growth and metabolism. Occurs naturally in differing amounts in many foods, notably in yeast, liver, kidney, egg yolk, soybeans, nuts and cereals. Is typically manufactured by synthesis from petroleum products, but can also be derived from ► *cysteine*. Hair and skin conditioner in shampoos and cosmetic creams. Food supplement, for instance in the case of hair loss. Active agent in medication for treating skin disorders.

Bis-Diglyceryl Polyacyladipate-n
Can be vegetable or animal. Reaction products of ► *adipic acid*, ► *caprylic acid*, ► *capric acid* and ► *stearic acid*. Emollients in cosmetics.

Bivalves
(Shellfish)

From killed animals. Aquatic molluscs (invertebrate animals) with a hard outer shell consisting of two halves and mainly comprising calcium carbonate. Bivalve animals are generally referred to generically simply as "shellfish"; the outer shells are known as "seashells." Bivalves are collected from the seabed or the foreshore, but most often "farmed" and "harvested" in banks or beds. Used as food, e.g. ► *oysters*, mussels, cockles. Green-lipped mussel extract is used as a dietary supplement and for treating rheumatic complaints and joint disorders. Mussel extract, mussel shells and pearls are used as cosmetic ingredients (► *conchiorin powder*, ► *hydrolyzed pearl*, ► *margarita powder*, ► *mytilus extract*, ► *ostrea shell extract*, ► *ostrea shell powder*). Oyster shells are used for preparing ► *homeopathic medicines* (► *calcium carbonicum*). The outer shells of bivalves are used as jewellery, decoration and accessories (► *pearls*, ► *mother of pearl*), and also as decoration or in decorative objects (e.g. ► *capiz*). Used in many different regions of the world as tools, musical instruments and cultic or religious objects or symbols. The flesh of bivalves is also regarded by some as an ► *aphrodisiac*.

Blasting Gelatin ► Gelignite

Blood
From killed animals. Opaque, red body fluid that circulates in the cardiovascular system of vertebrate animals and is responsible for transporting respiratory gases, degradation products, hormones, antibodies, etc. within the body. Comprises a liquid fraction (► *plasma*) and cells (corpuscles). Is usually obtained from slaughtered cattle and pigs. Main ingredient in some foods, e.g. black pudding. An often purported use of blood as an unlabelled ingredient in chocolate products is clearly an urban myth, since that would be uneconomical to start off with and is not permitted by Canadian law anyway. Blood proteins (► *serum albumin*, ► *serum proteins*) are, however, used in cosmetics, and as binding agents in some foods and adhesives, e.g. ► *albumin* from bovine blood in plywood. Clotting factors from bovine blood were used medicinally in earlier times, but have now been replaced by synthetic clotting factors. A blood replacement product based on bovine blood (Hemopure®) is currently being tested in Europe. Hemopure®

has also already been used for doping in athletics. Bovine blood is used in veterinary transfusion therapy (Oxyglobin®) for dogs. ▸ *Blood meal* is used as a plant fertilizer.

Blood Meal

From killed animals. Dried, ground mammal ▸ *blood* from slaughterhouse waste. Used as organic supplementary fertilizer in organic farming. This is no longer allowed by some organic farming associations (e.g. Demeter) due to the fear of triggering Creutzfeldt-Jakob disease. Canadian law does however still permit its use in organic farming, if it is sterilized. Blood meal is also used a biological plant protection product (Certosan®).

Blood Plasma

Can be from killed animals or living humans. The liquid fraction of ▸ *blood*. Comprises ▸ *serum* and clotting factors. Bovine plasma is used as a source of serum and proteins (▸ *deproteinized serum*, ▸ *hydrolyzed serum protein*, ▸ *serum albumin*, ▸ *serum protein*). Plasma from human donors is used in medical transfusion solutions.

Blood Plasma Proteins ▸ *Serum Proteins*

Blood Protein

From killed animals. Various animal ▸ *blood* proteins (▸ *albumin*, ▸ *serum proteins*).

Bombyx Extract

From killed animals. Extract from crushed ▸ *silk* worms. Skin conditioner in cosmetics.

Bombyx Lipida

From killed animals. Lipids from crushed ▸ *silk* worms. Skin conditioner in cosmetics.

Bone

From killed animals. Hard connective tissue in animals. Collectively, the single bones form the skeleton. The tasks of bones include providing the body with structure and cohesiveness, and protecting internal organs. In the long bones the ▸ *bone marrow* also produces ▸ *blood*. The bone tissue consists mostly of mineral salts, as well as ▸ *proteins* (mainly ▸ *collagen*) and water. Bone is used as a raw material, for instance for crafting jewellery and decorative objects, buttons and handles of all kinds and in musical instruments. Bones fulfil ritual religious or cultic functions in a variety of different cultural circles. ▸ *Bone ash*, ▸ *bone char*, ▸ *bone meal*, ▸ *glue* and ▸ *collagen* are obtained from the bone tissue, ▸ *bone marrow* is obtained from the long bones.

Bone Ash

(Spodium)

From killed animals. Fine mineral residue from the complete burning of ▸ *bone*. Important constituent of ▸ *bone china*. In fertilizers and some polishing agents. Can be used as a source of ▸ *calcium phosphate*. Traditionally used as medicine.

Bone Char ▸ *Activated Carbon*

Bone China

From killed animals. Porcelain with a high proportion of calcined ▸ *bone ash*. Notable for its strength, superior whiteness and translucency. Is generally regarded as the finest and most precious porcelain. In fine, often thin-walled, tableware (typically tea sets).

Bone Glue ► *Glue*

Bone Marrow

From killed animals. Soft tissue in the interior of ► *bone*. Comprises hematopoietic cells (red marrow, responsible for the creation of blood cells) and fat cells (yellow marrow). Obtained from the bones of killed animals (mostly cattle). Source of cosmetic ingredients (► *marrow extract*). Ingredient in some foods (e.g. marrow dumplings).

Bone Meal

From killed animals. Ground ► *bone* of mammals. Supplementary fertilizer in organic farming, constituent in some chemical fertilizers and source of calcium in animal husbandry. Sometimes used as abrasive in animal dental care. Bone meal is no longer used as a dietary supplement for humans but can be used in animal feed. Can also be used in some cement products.

Bonito Flakes. Bonito Powder

(Katsuobushi)

From killed animals. Dried, smoked and shaved bonito (a kind of tuna). Used as a condiment and soup ingredient, especially in Japanese cuisine.

Bouillon ► *Broth*

Brain Extract

From killed animals. Extract from mammals' brains. Skin protecting substance in cosmetics.

Brevoortia Oil

From killed animals. Oil of the Atlantic menhaden (a fish of the herring family). Plasticizer and solvent in cosmetics.

Bristles

From living or killed animals. Stiff ► *hair*, especially from domestic or wild pigs, also from goats and other mammals. Used in brooms and ► *brushes*.

Brooms ► *Brushes*

Broth

(Bouillon. Stock)

Can be from killed animals or vegetable. Liquid in which ► *meats*, or alternatively vegetables, have been cooked. The strained liquid is referred to as stock; the liquid with the cooked foods is known as broth or bouillon. Used as a basis for soups and sauces, as well as cooking fluid for other foods. Ingredient in ready-to-serve foods. Also available dried, as powder or cubes.

Brushes

Can be animal or synthetic. Tool for applying paints, inks, surface treatment, etc., as well as for cleaning surfaces. Brushes consist of a handle or stem, to which bundled (often animal) ► *hair* or ► *bristles* are attached. Large painting brushes normally contain pig bristles (also known as "China bristles" or "natural bristles"). Fine brushes for artwork, conservation/restoration or for applying cosmetics contain hair from martens, weasels, squirrels, sables, cows' ears, badgers, skunks, goats or beavers. Shaving brushes usually contain badger hair. Brushes can also have synthetic fibres instead of animal hairs, for instance nylon. Brooms are large brushes used for cleaning larger surfaces and can also have animal bristles, although synthetic bristles are more common.

Bubulum Oil ► Neatsfoot Oil

Buckskin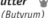
From killed animals. Soft ► *leather* made from the skin of deer or other wild animals, can also be from sheepskin treated to resemble real buckskin. In outer garments, footwear, accessories (e.g. handbags), furniture. Can be confused with ► *suede* or ► *nubuck*.

Bufo
(Bufo bufo. Rana bufo. Bufo rana)
From living or killed animals. Poison of the common or European toad. In ► *homeopathic medicines*.

Butanoic Acid ► Butyric Acid

Butoxy Chitosan
From killed animals. Chemically altered ► *chitosan*. Film forming and viscosity controlling agent in cosmetics.

Butter
(Butyrum)
From living and killed animals (► *milk*). ► *Fat* from ► *cream*. Contains at least 80% ► *butterfat*, water, ► *proteins* and carbohydrates. Obtained primarily from the ► *milk* of cattle and buffaloes, but also the milk of sheep or goats. Used as spreadable fat, for frying and as an ingredient in cooked and baked foods. Emollient in cosmetics (► *goat butter*). Some vegetable fats are also referred to as "butter," e.g. ► *illipé butter*, ► *cocoa butter*, ► *kokum butter*, shea butter (► *Butyrospermum parkii butter*) and ► *Shorea robusta butter*.

Butterfat
From living and killed animals (► *milk*). The sum of the ► *lipids* contained in ► *milk*, comprising many ► *fatty acids*, especially ► *palmitic acid*, ► *oleic acid*, ► *myristic acid* and ► *stearic acid*. The separation of butterfat from ► *milk proteins* and ► *whey* produces ► *cream*, ► *butter* or ► *clarified butter*, depending on the degree of purity.

Buttermilk
From living and killed animals (► *milk*). Fermented liquid fraction of ► *milk*, also a byproduct of ► *butter* production. Used as a beverage. Skin conditioner in cosmetics.

Butyl Isostearate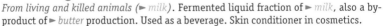
Can be synthetic/vegetable or animal. Hydrocarbon compound of ► *stearic acid*. Emollient in cosmetics.

Butyl Lactate
Can be synthetic/vegetable or partly animal. Hydrocarbon compound of ► *lactic acid*. Solvent in cosmetics.

Butyl Stearate
Can be synthetic/vegetable or animal. Hydrocarbon compound of ► *stearic acid*. Emollient in cosmetics.

Butylene Glycol Dicaprylate/Dicaprate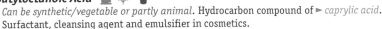
Can be synthetic/vegetable or partly animal. Hydrocarbon compound of ► *capric acid* and ► *caprylic acid*. Emollient in cosmetics.

Butylglucoside Caprate
Can be synthetic/vegetable or partly animal. Hydrocarbon compound of ► *capric acid*. Surfactant, cleansing agent and emulsifier in cosmetics.

Butyloctanoic Acid
Can be synthetic/vegetable or partly animal. Hydrocarbon compound of ► *caprylic acid*. Surfactant, cleansing agent and emulsifier in cosmetics.

Butyloctanol
Can be synthetic/vegetable or partly animal. Hydrocarbon compound of ► *capryl alcohol*. Humectant in cosmetics.

Butyloctyl Beeswax
From living animals. Hydrocarbon compound of ► *beeswax*. Emollient in cosmetics.

Butyric Acid
(Butanoic acid)
Mostly synthetic, can also be animal or vegetable. A ► *fatty acid* that occurs in animal and vegetable fats, also in fermentation processes (e.g. rancid ► *butter*). Industrial production primarily from petroleum products, but also by bacterial fermentation of saccharides, e.g. ► *lactose*. In compounds used as skin protective substances or skin conditioners in cosmetics. Ingredient in some medication. Used for making weatherproof plastics.

Butyris Lac Powder
From living and killed animals (► *milk*). Dried ► *buttermilk*. Hair and skin conditioner in cosmetics.

Butyrospermum Parkii Butter
(Karité butter. Shea butter)
Vegetable. Fat from the fruit of the shea tree (also known as karité). Not to be confused with ► *butter* of animal origin. Skin conditioner and emollient in cosmetics. Also used as partial substitute for ► *cocoa butter* (cocoa butter equivalent) in chocolate products.

Butyrospermum Parkii Butter Extract
Vegetable. Extract of shea butter (► *Butyrospermum parkii butter*). Emollient in cosmetics.

Butyrospermum Parkii Butter Unsaponifiables
Vegetable. Non-saponifiable fraction of shea butter (► *Butyrospermum parkii butter*). Emollient in cosmetics.

Butyrum ► *Butter*

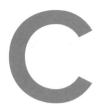

C10-18 Triglycerides
Can be vegetable or animal. Mixed ► *triglycerides*. Emollient and solvent in cosmetics.

C10-30 Cholesterol/Lanosterol Esters
From killed or living animals. ► *Fatty acid* compound of ► *cholesterol* and ► *lanosterol*. Emulsifier in cosmetics.

C11-15 Pareth-n Stearate
Can be vegetable or animal. Compounds of ► *stearic acid*. Emollients in cosmetics.

C12-15 Pareth-9 Hydrogenated Tallowate
From killed animals. Hydrogenated ► *fatty acids* from ► *tallow*. Emulsifier and surfactant in cosmetics.

C12-18 Acid Triglyceride
Can be vegetable or animal. Mixed ► *triglycerides*. Emulsifier in cosmetics.

C12-20 Acid PEG-8 Ester
Can be vegetable/synthetic or animal. ► *PEG* compound of ► *fatty acids*. Emulsifier in cosmetics.

C14-16 Glycol Palmitate
Mostly vegetable, can also be animal. ► *Palmitic acid* compound. Emulsifier in cosmetics.

C18-20 Glycol Isostearate
Can be vegetable/synthetic or animal. ► *Glycol* compound of ► *stearic acid*. Emulsifier in cosmetics.

C18-36 Acid Glycol Ester
Can be vegetable/synthetic or animal. ► *Glycol* compound of ► *fatty acids*. Emollient in cosmetics.

C18-36 Acid Triglyceride
Can be vegetable or animal. Mixed ► *triglycerides*. Emollient in cosmetics.

C18-38 Alkyl C24-54 Acid Ester
Can be vegetable/synthetic or animal. Chemically altered ► *fatty acids*. Viscosity controlling agent in cosmetics.

C18-38 Alkyl Hydroxystearoyl Stearate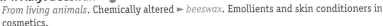
C20-30 Glycol Isostearate
Can be vegetable or animal. Compounds of ► *stearic acid.* Emollients in cosmetics.

Cn-n Acid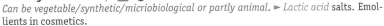
Can be vegetable or animal. Various mixtures of ► *fatty acids.* Emulsifiers in cosmetics.

Cn-n Alkyl Beeswax
From living animals. Chemically altered ► *beeswax.* Emollients and skin conditioners in cosmetics.

Cn-n Alkyl Lactate
Can be vegetable/synthetic/micriobiological or partly animal. ► *Lactic acid* salts. Emollients in cosmetics.

Cn-n Alkyl Stearate
Can be vegetable/synthetic or animal. ► *Stearic acid* salts. Skin conditioners in cosmetics.

Calcitonin
(Thyreocalcitonin)
From killed animals or microbiological. ► *Hormone* that influences blood calcium levels and bone mineral metabolism. Obtained genetically from ► *DNA* or salmon glands. In medication for treating elevated calcium levels, osteoporosis and other bone disorders.

Calcitriol ► *Vitamin D*

Calcium Carbonicum (Hahnemanni)
(Calcarea carbonica [Hahnemanni])
From killed animals. Calcium carbonate used in ► *homeopathic medicines.* Made from ► *mother of pearl* from ► *oyster* shells ground with ► *lactose.*

Calcium Caseinate
Animal. Calcium salt of ► *casein.* Skin protective substance in cosmetics.

Calcium Diglutamate
(E 623. Calcium glutamate)
Microbiological/vegetable, can theoretically also be animal. Calcium salt of ► *glutamic acid.* Flavour enhancer in foods (also see ► *glutamates*).

Calcium Guanylate
(E 629)
Microbiological. Calcium salt of ► *guanylic acid.* Flavour enhancer in foods.

Calcium Inosinate
(E 633)
Microbiological. Calcium salt of ► *inosinic acid.* Flavour enhancer in foods.

Calcium Lactate
(E 327)
Can be vegetable/microbiological or partly animal. Calcium salt of ► *lactic acid.* Skin protective substance in cosmetics. Acidity regulator and humectant in foods.

Calcium Phosphate
(E 341. Tricalcium phosphate)
Mostly mineral, can also be from killed animals. Calcium salt of phosphoric acid. Occurs naturally in rock, is also a major constituent of animal bones and teeth. Mostly obtained from minerals, but also from ► *bone*. Raising agent, acidity regulator and anticaking agent in foods. In calcium-enriched foods and food supplements. Abrasive, opacifier and anticaking agent in cosmetics. Used as surgical bone replacement. Major constituent in ► *bone china*.

Calcium-5'-Ribonucleotides
(E 634)
Can be vegetable or animal. Calcium salts of ► *guanylic acid* and ► *inosinic acid*. Obtained from animal or plant cells. Flavour enhancer in foods.

Calcium Stearate
Can be vegetable or animal. Calcium salt of ► *stearic acid*. Colourant and anticaking agent in cosmetics.

Calcium Stearoyl Lactylate
(E482)
Can be vegetable/microbiological or animal. Calcium salt of ► *stearoyl lactylic acid*. Does not occcur naturally, but is produced via chemical reactions of ► *stearic acid*, ► *lactic acid* and ► *polylactic acid*. Emulsifier, stabilizer and thickener in certain foods, especially baked goods. Emulsifier in cosmetics.

Calcium Tartarate. Calcium Tartrate
(E 354)
Vegetable/microbiological, animal substances may be involved in processing. Calcium salt of ► *tartaric acid*. Raising agent, complexing agent, acidifier and acidity regulator in foods. Skin conditioner in cosmetics.

Calf Blood Extract
From killed animals. Extract from calves' ► *blood*. Skin conditioner in cosmetics.

Calf Skin Extract
From killed animals. Extract from calfskin. Refatting substance in cosmetics.

Calf Skin Hydrolysate
From killed animals. Chemically altered calfskin. Skin conditioner in cosmetics.

Camel Hair
From living animals. The ► *hair* of camels. Consists of two hair types, the coarse outer hair and the soft undercoat. Camel hair is not shorn, but collected in the moulting season in spring. The outer hair is used in robust textiles (e.g. carpets), whereas the undercoat is used for soft textiles (clothing, accessories, blankets, etc.).

Cantharis Vesicatoria
From killed animals. Preparation of ► *Spanish fly*. Used for making ► *homeopathic medicines*.

Canthaxanthin

(E 161g. CI 40850)
Synthetic, can theoretically be animal. Red pigment that occurs naturally in crabs, salmon, flamingo feathers and chanterelle mushrooms. Is produced synthetically in the modern day. Colouring agent in foods, cosmetics, and fish and bird feed.

Capiz

(Placuna placenta. Windowpane shells)
From killed animals. A ► *bivalve* species native to Southeast Asia. The cleaned shells of the killed animals are processed to translucent discs of ► *mother of pearl*. Used in the Philippines as traditional windowpanes, worldwide in decorative objects (lampshades, vases, lanterns, jewellery, etc.).

Caprae Butyrum ► *Goat Butter*

Caprae Lac ► *Goat Milk*

Capramide DEA

Mostly vegetable, can also be animal. Derivative of ► *capric acid*. Antistatic, viscosity controlling agent, foam booster and hair conditioner in cosmetics. Industrial use as a viscosity controlling agent and foam booster.

Capric Acid

(Decanoic acid. Decanoate)
Mostly vegetable, can also be animal. A saturated ► *fatty acid*. Occurs naturally in coconut fat and animal fats, e.g. ► *goat butter*. Industrial production from vegetable fats (e.g. coconut), but can also be from animal fats. Emulsifier in cosmetics and in perfumes. In slow-release psychotropic drugs (depot injections). Source of ► *triglycerides*, also diverse indutrial uses, e.g. in plastics, lubricants, colourants.

Capric Alcohol ► *Decyl Alcohol*

Caproic Acid

(Hexanoic acid)
Mostly vegetable, can also be animal. A saturated ► *fatty acid*. Occurs naturally in coconut fat and animal fats, especially ► *milk* or ► *butter*. Industrial production from vegetable fats (e.g. coconut), but can also be obtained from animal fats. Emulsifier in cosmetics. Used in the production of fruit flavours.

Caproyl Ethyl Glucoside

Can be vegetable or partly animal. Saccharide alcohol compound of ► *capric acid*. Surfactant and cleansing agent in cosmetics.

Caproyl Sphingosine

Can be from killed animals or vegetable/microbiological. Compound of ► *capric acid* and ► *sphingosine*. Hair and skin conditioner in cosmetics.

Capryl Hydroxyethyl Imidazoline

Mostly vegetable/synthetic, can also be partly animal. Nitrogen carbon compound of ► *caprylic acid*. Antistatic and hair conditioner in cosmetics.

Capryl/Capramidopropyl Betaine

Mostly vegetable, can also be animal. Compound of ► *caprylic acid*. Antistatic, hair and skin conditioner, surfactant, cleansing agent, foam booster and viscosity controlling agent in cosmetics.

Capryleth-4

Mostly synthetic, can also be partly vegetable/animal. ► *PEG* compound of ► *caprylic alcohol*. Surfactant and emulsifier in cosmetics.

Capryleth-n Carboxylic Acid

Mostly synthetic, can also be partly vegetable/animal. ► *PEG* compounds of ► *caprylic alcohol*. Emulsifiers in cosmetics.

Caprylic Acid

(Octanoic acid)

Mostly vegetable, can also be animal. A saturated ► *fatty acid*. Occurs naturally in coconut fat and animal fats, especially ► *butterfat*. Industrial production from vegetable fats (e.g. coconut), but also from animal fats. Emulsifier in cosmetics. In food supplements. Active agent against bacterial and fungal infections. In insect repellants.

Caprylic Alcohol

(Octyl alcohol. Octanol)

Mostly synthetic, can also be vegetable or animal. ► *Fatty alcohol* of ► *caprylic acid*. Derived mostly from petroleum products, but can also be obtained from vegetable and animal fats. Viscosity controlling agent in cosmetics.

Caprylic/Capric Glycerides

Mostly vegetable, can also be partly animal. Mixed ► *glycerides* of ► *capric acid* and ► *caprylic acid*. Emollient and emulsifier in cosmetics.

Caprylic/Capric Triglyceride

Mostly vegetable, can also be partly animal. Mixed ► *triglycerides* of ► *capric acid* and ► *caprylic acid*. Emollient and solvent in cosmetics.

Caprylic/Capric Triglyceride PEG-4 Esters

Mostly vegetable, can also be partly animal. ► *PEG* compound of ► *triglycerides* of ► *capric acid* and ► *caprylic acid*. Emulsifier in cosmetics.

Caprylic/Capric/Lauric Triglyceride

Mostly vegetable, can also be partly animal. ► *Triglycerides* of ► *capric acid*, ► *caprylic acid* and ► *lauric acid*. Emollient and solvent in cosmetics.

Caprylic/Capric/Linoleic Triglyceride

Mostly vegetable, can also be partly animal. Mixed ► *triglycerides* of ► *capric acid*, ► *caprylic acid* and ► *linoleic acid*. Emollient in cosmetics.

Caprylic/Capric/Myristic/Stearic Triglyceride

Can be vegetable or animal. Mixed ► *triglycerides* of ► *capric acid*, ► *caprylic acid*, ► *myristic acid* and ► *stearic acid*. Used as an emollient and skin protective substance in cosmetics.

Caprylic/Capric/Stearic Triglyceride 🌱 🐮
Can be vegetable or animal. Mixed ► *triglycerides* of ► *capric acid*, ► *caprylic acid* and ► *stearic acid*. Emollient and solvent in cosmetics.

Caprylic/Capric/Succinic Triglyceride 🌱 🐮
Mostly vegetable, can also be partly animal. Mixed ► *triglycerides* of ► *capric acid*, ► *caprylic acid* and ► *succinic acid*. Emollient and solvent in cosmetics.

Capryloyl Collagen Amino Acids 🐮
From killed animals. Chemically altered ► *collagen*. Antistatic and hair conditioner in cosmetics.

Capryloyl Glycine 🐮 🌱 🧪
Can be from killed animals or vegetable/synthetic. Compound of ► *caprylic acid* and ► *glycine*. Cleansing substance in cosmetics.

Capryloyl Hydrolyzed Collagen 🐮
From killed animals. Chemically altered ► *collagen*. Antistatic and hair conditioner in cosmetics.

Capryloyl Hydrolyzed Keratin 🐮
From killed or living animals. Chemically altered ► *keratin*. Antistatic and hair conditioner in cosmetics.

Capryloyl Keratin Amino Acids 🐮
From killed or living animals. Chemically altered ► *amino acids* from ► *keratin*. Antistatic and hair conditioner in cosmetics.

Capryloyl Pea Amino Acids 🌱 🐮
Mostly vegetable, can also be partly animal. Compound of ► *amino acids* from peas and ► *caprylic acid*. Hair and skin conditioner in cosmetics.

Capryloyl Quinoa Amino Acids 🌱 🐮
Mostly vegetable, can also be partly animal. Compound of ► *amino acids* from quinoa and ► *caprylic acid*. Hair and skin conditioner in cosmetics.

Capryloyl Salicylic Acid 🌱 🧪 🐮
Mostly vegetable/synthetic, can also be partly animal. Compound of salicylic acid with ► *caprylic acid*. Skin conditioner in cosmetics.

Capryloyl Silk Amino Acids 🐮
From killed animals. Compound of ► *amino acids* from ► *silk* with ► *caprylic acid*. Hair conditioner, surfactant and cleansing agent in cosmetics.

Caprylyl Butyrate 🌱 🧪 🐮
Mostly vegetable/synthetic, can also be animal. Compound of ► *caprylic acid* and ► *butyric acid*. Solvent in cosmetics.

Caprylyl Glycol 🧪 🌱 🐮
Mostly synthetic, can also be vegetable or animal. Compound of ► *caprylic alcohol* and ► *glycol*. Emollient, humectant and hair conditioner in cosmetics.

Caprylyl Hydroxyethyl Imidazoline
Mostly vegetable/synthetic, can also be partly animal. Compound of ► *caprylic acid* and an alkaloid. Antistatic and hair conditioner in cosmetics.

Caprylyl Pyrrolidone
Mostly vegetable/synthetic, can also be partly animal. Compound of ► *caprylic acid* and synthetic pyrrolidone. Surfactant, cleansing agent and foaming agent in cosmetics.

Caprylyl/Capryl Glucoside
Mostly vegetable, can also be partly animal. A ► *sugar surfactant* and compound of ► *caprylic acid*. Surfactant, cleansing agent and foaming agent in cosmetics.

Captopril
Vegetable/microbiological, can theoretically be partly animal. Most important of the ACE inhibitors (pharmaceutical drugs that lower blood pressure). Originally synthesized on the basis of ► *proteins* found in snake venom. Is now biochemically produced from ► *proline*, which in turn is derived from ► *glutamic acid*. In medication for treating high blood pressure.

Caramel
Vegetable, may have been processed with animal substances. ► *Sugar* that has been melted by means of strong heat, darkening its colour to brown and altering its flavour. Flavouring in confectionery. Also used as ► *caramel colouring* in foods and confectionery.

Caramel Colouring
(E 150)
Vegetable, may have been processed with animal substances. Food colour made from dark ► *caramel* with the aid of various reaction accelerants. There is plain caramel (E 150a, made using caustic soda), caustic sulfite caramel (E 150b), ammonia caramel (E 150c) and sulfite ammonia caramel (E 150d). Used for instance in beverages, sauces, vinegars and desserts.

Carbamide ► *Urea*

Carbo Animalis *(Animal Charcoal)* ► *Activated Carbon*

Carbo Medicinalis *(Medicinal Charcoal)* ► *Activated Carbon*

Carbocystein
(Carbocistein. Carboxymethylcystein)
Can be synthetic or from killed animals. A derivative of ► *cysteine*. Antiseborrheic and skin conditioner in cosmetics. Active agent in mucolytic medicines.

Carboxybutyl Chitosan
From killed animals. A derivative of ► *chitosan*. Film forming agent, hair and skin conditioner and viscosity controlling agent in cosmetics.

Carboxyethyl Aminobutyric Acid
Synthetic, can theoretically also be animal. A derivative of ► *aminobutyric acid*. Skin conditioner in cosmetics.

Carboxymethyl Chitin
Carboxymethyl Chitosan
From killed animals. Derivatives of ► *chitin* or ► *chitosan*. Gelling agent in cosmetics.

Carboxymethyl Chitosan Succinamide
From killed animals. Derivative of ► *chitosan*. Film forming agent and humectant in cosmetics.

Carboxymethyl Isostearamidopropyl Morpholine
Can be synthetic/vegetable or animal. A hydrocarbon compound of ► *stearic acid*. Surfactant and foaming agent in cosmetics.

Carmine
(Carminic acid. CI 75470. Cochineal. Crimson lake. E 120)
From killed animals. Red dye from crushed female cochineal scale insects. More than 150 000 insects may be required for 1 kg of the dye. Used as a colourant in cosmetics and foods (e.g. in confectionery and red beverages), paints and textile dyes. Also used as a colourant in laboratory diagnostics (microbiology, genetic engineering).

Carminic Acid ► Carmine

Carnitine
(L-carnitine)
Can be synthetic, vegetable or animal. Vitamin-like substance with an important function in the metabolism of animal and plant cells. Is synthesized in the body from ► *methionine* and ► *lysine*. Is especially present in muscle tissue, occurs in plants only in low concentrations. Industrially produced L-carnitine is mostly obtained by biotechnological means. Cleansing substance and foam booster in cosmetics. In nutritional supplements and "energy drinks," among other things for the purpose of enhancing performance and weight loss (scientifically disputed). Although a balanced vegan diet delivers much less carnitine than a diet that includes meat, the body's autonomous production is sufficient, so dietary supplementation is not necessary.

Carnosine
Can be vegetable, animal or synthetic. A ► *protein* compound comprising the amino acids ► *alanine* and ► *histidine*. Occurs in higher concentration in muscle and brain tissue. Is used as a nutritional supplement, as well as for the complementary treatment of autism or epilepsy.

Carotene
(Beta-carotene. E 160. CI 75130. CI 40800. Provitamin A)
Can be vegetable or synthetic. Denomination for a group of yellow to red natural pigments. The most important of these is beta-carotene, a precursor of ► *vitamin A*. Carotenes occur naturally in many plants but also in animal tissues. Industrially produced carotene is extracted from dried vegetable material (e.g. carrots). Colourant in cosmetics and foods (e.g. margarine). Used in the industrial production of ► *vitamin A*.

Cartilago Suis ► Organ Extracts

Casein

From living and killed animals (► milk). ► *Proteins* in ► *milk*, main constituent of ► *cheese*. The proteins are separated from the other milk constituents by biological, mechanical or chemical means. Ingredient in foods (either as pure casein or as cheese) and cosmetics (either as pure casein or chemically altered). In adhesives (e.g. in some wood glues).

Caseinate

From living and killed animals (► milk). Chemically altered ► *casein*, especially as sodium caseinate or calcium caseinate. Functional product in foods, e.g. for imitation cheese, as a binding agent, foam mass or in biodegradable food packaging. Also used as protein enrichment in medicinal products and protein-rich food supplements.

Cashgora

From living or killed animals. The ► *wool* of cashgora goats (hybrid of ► *cashmere* and ► *angora* goats). In textiles (clothing, accessories, blankets, etc.).

Cashmere. Cashmere Wool

From living or killed animals. The ► *wool* of cashmere goats. In textiles (clothing, accessories, blankets, etc.).

Castoreum

From living or killed animals. A fatty secretion from the "castor sacs" of beavers, used for grooming and marking territory. The castor sacs used to be cut out of the killed animals and dried. Castoreum is now usually obtained on beaver farms by burying containers in the ground, on which the beavers rub off the castoreum. Used earlier as a medicine against many diseases, now only in ► *homeopathic medicines*. In some perfumes and fragrances (e.g. incense sticks), flavouring in some cigarettes.

Cat Fur

From killed animals. The skin of domestic cats. Traditionally used as blankets for the purpose of relieving rheumatic ailments, also in clothing. The import and trade of cat furs is banned in the European Union and the United States, but so far not in Canada.

Catgut

From killed animals. ► *Gut strings* (e.g. from sheep), used especially as suture material for surgical wound closure that dissolves in the body during wound healing. The name is misleading, insofar as the gut used is not actually from cats. Genuine catgut is no longer commonly used in developed countries, having been supplanted by synthetic suture materials.

Cationic Surfactants

Can be synthetic/animal or synthetic/vegetable. ► *Surfactants* with a positively charged hydrophilic group. Obtained from processed animal or vegetable fats. In laundry detergents, fabric softeners and disinfectants/antiseptics (such as in mouthwash, lozenges, etc.). Examples: ► *cetrimonium bromide*, ► *cetylpyridinium chloride*.

Caustic Sulfite Caramel ► *Caramel Colouring*

Caviar
(Sturgeon roe)
From living or killed animals. Salted roe (ripe, unlaid fish eggs) from sturgeon species such as Beluga, Ossiotr and Sevruga, in particular from the Black and Caspian Seas. The roe is cut out of the female sturgeons, who then may be sewn up again in order to produce more roe. "German caviar" is imitation caviar made from salted, coloured and seasoned lumpfish roe. "Red caviar" is made from salmon roe.

Cephalins
(Phosphatidylethanolamine)
From killed and living animals. ► *Lipids* that occur naturally in biological cell membranes, especially in nerve tissue and ► *eggs*. Obtained from the cell membranes of killed animals (e.g. cattle, goats) or from eggs. Skin conditioner in cosmetics.

Cera Alba ► *Beeswax*

Cera Flava ► *Beeswax*

Cera Microcristallina ► *Microcrystalline Wax*

Ceralan
From living or killed animals. The name "Ceralan" does not denote a single specific substance, being used for the product Ceralan™ (► *lanolin alcohol*), manufactured by the U.S. chemical company Lubrizol, as well as for ► *polyglyceryl-3 beeswax* and a Finnish skin care brand with the main ingredient ► *ceramide*.

Ceramides
Mostly from killed animals, can also be vegetable. Denomination for a group of ► *lipid* molecules, comprising ► *sphingosine* and a ► *fatty acid*. Occurs naturally only in animal tissues, especially in brain matter and nerve sheaths. Obtained from killed animals, but also derived biotechnologically from vegetable fats. Hair and skin conditioner in cosmetics.

Cerebrum Suis ► *Organ Extracts*

Ceresin
(Ceresin wax. Cerin)
Mineral/from killed animals. Waxy resin product. Produced from mineral resins using copious amounts of ► *animal charcoal*. In candles. In wax paper. Antistatic, binding agent, emulsifier and hair conditioner in cosmetics.

Cerotic Acic
(Hexacosanoic acid)
Can be animal, vegetable or mineral. A solid ► *fatty acid* in ► *waxes*. Important constituent of ► *beeswax*, also in carnauba wax (vegetable) and ► *montan wax* (mineral). Viscosity controlling agent in cosmetics.

Ceteareth-25 Carboxylic Acid
Can be vegetable/synthetic or animal. ► *PEG* compound of ► *cetostearyl alcohol*. Surfactant and cleansing agent in cosmetics.

Ceteareth-60 Myristyl Glycol 🐄 🌱 🐄

Can be synthetic/vegetable or animal. ► *PEG* compound of ► *cetyl alcohol*, ► *stearyl alcohol* and myristyl alcohol (obtained from ► *myristic acid*). Surfactant and emulsifier in cosmetics.

C

Ceteareth-n 🐄 🌱 🐄

Can be synthetic/vegetable or animal. ► *PEG* compounds of ► *cetostearyl alcohol* with phosphoric acid salts. Emulsifiers in cosmetics.

Ceteareth-n Phosphate 🐄 🌱 🐄

Can be synthetic/vegetable or animal. ► *PEG* compounds of ► *cetostearyl alcohol* with phosphoric acid salts. Surfactants and cleansing substances in cosmetics.

Cetearyl Alcohol ► *Cetostearyl Alcohol*

Cetearyl Behenate 🐄 🌱 🐄

Can be synthetic/vegetable or animal. Compound of ► *cetostearyl alcohol* and behenic acid. Emollient and skin protecting substance in cosmetics.

Cetearyl Candelillate 🐄 🌱 🐄

Can be synthetic/vegetable or animal. Compound of ► *cetostearyl alcohol* with vegetable wax. Emollient and skin protecting substance in cosmetics.

Cetearyl Dimethicone/Vinyl Dimethicone Crosspolymer 🐄 🌱 🐄

Can be synthetic/vegetable or animal. Synthetic polymer compound of ► *cetostearyl alcohol*. Film forming agent, hair and skin conditioner, and viscosity controlling agent in cosmetics.

Cetearyl Ethylhexanoate 🐄 🌱 🐄

Can be synthetic/vegetable or animal. Compound of ► *cetostearyl alcohol* and ► *caproic acid*. Emollient in cosmetics.

Cetearyl Glucoside 🐄 🌱 🐄

Can be synthetic/vegetable or animal. Compound of ► *cetostearyl alcohol* and saccharides. Emulsifier in cosmetics.

Cetearyl Isononanoate 🐄 🌱 🐄

Can be synthetic/vegetable or animal. Compound of vegetable nonanoic acid with ► *cetostearyl alcohol*. Emollient in cosmetics.

Cetearyl Methicone 🐄 🌱 🐄

Can be synthetic/vegetable or animal. Polymer compound of ► *cetostearyl alcohol*. Skin conditioner in cosmetics.

Cetearyl Octanoate 🐄 🌱 🐄

Can be synthetic/vegetable or animal. Compound of ► *cetostearyl alcohol* and ► *caprylic acid*. Emollient and refatting substance in cosmetics.

Cetearyl Palmitate 🐄 🌱 🐄

Can be synthetic/vegetable or animal. Compound of ► *cetostearyl alcohol* and ► *palmitic acid*. Emollient in cosmetics.

Cetearyl Stearate 🌱 ⬛ 🐄
Can be vegetable/synthetic or animal. Compound of ► *cetostearyl alcohol* and ► *stearic acid.* Skin conditioner and skin protecting substance in cosmetics.

Ceteth-8 Phosphate 🌱 ⬛ 🐄
Mostly vegetable/synthetic, can theoretically also be animal. Compound of phosphoric acid salt and ► *cetyl alcohol.* Emulsifier in cosmetics.

Ceteth-10 Phosphate 🌱 ⬛ 🐄
Mostly vegetable/synthetic, can theoretically also be animal. Compound of phosphoric acid salt and ► *cetyl alcohol.* Surfactant and cleansing agent in cosmetics.

Ceteth-n 🌱 ⬛ 🐄
Mostly vegetable/synthetic, can theoretically also be animal. ► *PEG* compounds of ► *cetyl alcohol.* Emulsifiers and surfactants in cosmetics.

Cetoleth-n 🌱 ⬛ 🐄
Can be vegetable/synthetic or animal. Compounds of ► *cetyl alcohol* and ► *oleyl alcohol.* Emulsifiers, surfactants and cleansing substances in cosmetics.

Cetostearyl Alcohol 🌱 ⬛ 🐄
(Cetearyl alcohol. Cetylstearyl alcohol)
Can be vegetable/synthetic or animal. Mixed ► *fatty alcohols,* mainly ► *cetyl alcohol* and ► *stearyl alcohol.* Emollient, emulsifier, emulsion stabilizer, opacifier and viscosity controlling agent in cosmetics, and medicinal ointments and creams. The *German Pharmacopeia* lists it as a substitute for ► *spermaceti.*

Cetrimide ► *Cetrimonium Bromide*

Cetrimonium Bromide 🌱 ⬛ 🐄
(Cetrimide. Cetyltrimethylammonium bromide [CTAB])
Can be vegetable/synthetic or partly animal. ► *Quaternary ammonium compound* with ► *cetyl alcohol.* Can be derived from animal ► *fats.* Preservative in cosmetics. Active agent in topical antiseptics. ► *Cationic surfactant* in laundry detergents.

Cetrimonium Chloride ⬛ 🐄
(Cetyltrimethylammonium chloride [CTAC])
Synthetic, can also be partly animal. ► *Quaternary ammonium compound.* Can be derived from animal ► *fats.* Is used for the same purposes as ► *cetrimonium bromide.*

Cetrimonium Methosulfate ⬛ 🐄
Cetrimonium Saccharinate
Synthetic, can be partly animal. ► *Quaternary ammonium compounds.* Can be derived from animal ► *fats.* Antistatics, hair conditioners and antimicrobial substances in cosmetics.

Cetrimonium Tosylate ⬛ 🐄
Synthetic, can be partly animal. ► *Quaternary ammonium compound.* Can be derived from animal ► *fats.* Antimicrobial substance, antistatic, emulsifier, surfactant and hair conditioner in cosmetics.

Cetyl Acetate

Synthetic, can theoretically be partly animal. Compound of acetic acid and ► *cetyl alcohol*. Emollient in cosmetics.

Cetyl Acetyl Ricinoleate

Mostly vegetable/synthetic, can theoretically also be partly animal. Compound of ► *cetyl alcohol*, acetic acid and ricinoleic acid(from castor oil). Emollient in cosmetics.

Cetyl Alcohol

(Hexadecanol. Palmityl alcohol)
Mostly vegetable/synthetic, can theoretically also be animal. A ► *fatty alcohol*. Originally extracted from the ► *spermaceti* of hunted sperm whales (*cetus* = Latin for "whale"). Today, cetyl alcohol is a product of the petroleum industry or is obtained from palm or coconut oils. Emollient, emulsifier, opacifier and viscosity controlling agent in cosmetics.

Cetyl Betaine

Mostly vegetable/synthetic, can theoretically also be partly animal. Compound of ► *cetyl alcohol* and ► *betaine*. Antistatic, surfactant, hair conditioner, cleansing agent and foam booster in cosmetics.

Cetyl C12-15-Pareth-9 Carboxylate

Mostly vegetable/synthetic, can theoretically also be partly animal. Polymer compound of ► *cetyl alcohol*. Emollient in cosmetics.

Cetyl Caprylate

Mostly vegetable/synthetic, can also be animal. Compound of ► *cetyl alcohol* and ► *caprylic acid*. Emollient in cosmetics.

Cetyl Dimethicone

Mostly vegetable/synthetic, can theoretically also be partly animal. Silicone compound of ► *cetyl alcohol*. Emollient in cosmetics.

Cetyl Dimethicone Copolyol

Mostly vegetable/synthetic, can theoretically also be partly animal. Silicone compound of ► *cetyl alcohol*. Emulsifier in cosmetics.

Cetyl Esters

Mostly vegetable/synthetic, can also be partly animal. Reaction product of mixed acids and alcohols that imitates the composition of ► *spermaceti*. Comprises mainly myristyl alcohol (from ► *myristic acid*), ► *cetyl alcohol*, ► *palmityl alcohol*, ► *myristic acid* and ► *palmitic acid*. Emollient in cosmetics.

Cetyl Ethylhexanoate

Mostly vegetable/synthetic, can also be partly animal. Compound of ► *cetyl alcohol* and ► *caproic acid*. Emollient in cosmetics.

Cetyl Glyceryl Ether

Mostly vegetable/synthetic, can also be partly animal. Compound of ► *cetyl alcohol* and ► *glycerol*. Skin conditioner and emollient in cosmetics.

Cetyl Glycol
Mostly vegetable/synthetic, can theoretically also be partly animal. ► *Glycol* compound of ► *cetyl alcohol.* Hair conditioner and emollient in cosmetics.

Cetyl Glycol Isostearate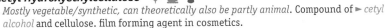
Can be vegetable/synthetic or animal. ► *Glycol* compound of ► *cetyl alcohol* and ► *stearic acid.* Emollient in cosmetics.

Cetyl Hydroxyethylcellulose
Mostly vegetable/synthetic, can theoretically also be partly animal. Compound of ► *cetyl alcohol* and cellulose. film forming agent in cosmetics.

Cetyl Isononanoate
Mostly vegetable/synthetic, can theoretically also be partly animal. Compound of ► *cetyl alcohol* and nonanoic acid (vegetable). Emollient in cosmetics.

Cetyl Lactate
Can be vegetable/microbiological/synthetic or animal. Compound of ► *cetyl alcohol* and ► *lactic acid.* Emollient in cosmetics.

Cetyl Laurate
Mostly vegetable/synthetic, can theoretically also be partly animal. Compound of ► *cetyl alcohol* and ► *lauric acid.* Emollient and viscosity controlling agent in cosmetics.

Cetyl Myristate
Mostly vegetable/synthetic, can also be animal. Compound of ► *cetyl alcohol* and ► *myristic acid.* Emollient in cosmetics.

Cetyl Oleate
Can be vegetable/synthetic or animal. Compound of ► *cetyl alcohol* and ► *oleic acid.* Emollient in cosmetics.

Cetyl Palmitate
Can be vegetable/synthetic or partly animal. Compound of ► *cetyl alcohol* and ► *palmitic acid.* Emollient in cosmetics.

Cetyl PCA
Mostly vegetable/synthetic, can theoretically also be partly animal. Compound of ► *cetyl alcohol* and ► *proline.* Skin conditioner in cosmetics.

Cetyl Phosphate
Mostly vegetable/synthetic, can theoretically also be partly animal. Compound of ► *cetyl alcohol* and phosphoric acid. Emulsifier in cosmetics.

Cetyl PPG-2 Isodeceth-8 Carboxylate
Mostly vegetable/synthetic, can also be partly animal. Polymer compound of ► *cetyl alcohol* and ► *decyl alcohol.* Skin conditioner and emollient in cosmetics.

Cetyl Pyrrolidonylmethyl Dimonium Chloride
Mostly vegetable/synthetic, can theoretically also be partly animal. Ammonium compound of ► *cetyl alcohol.* Antistatic and hair conditioner in cosmetics.

Cetyl Ricinoleate

Mostly vegetable/synthetic, can theoretically also be partly animal. Compound of ► *cetyl alcohol* and castor oil. Emollient in cosmetics.

Cetyl Ricinoleate Benzoate

Mostly vegetable/synthetic, can theoretically also be partly animal. Compound of ► *cetyl alcohol*, castor oil and benzoic acid (both vegetable). Skin conditioner in cosmetics.

Cetyl Stearate

Can be vegetable/synthetic or animal. Compound of ► *cetyl alcohol* and ► *stearic acid*. Emollient in cosmetics.

Cetyl Triethylammonium Dimethicone Copolyol Phthalate

Mostly vegetable/synthetic, can theoretically also be partly animal. Silicone ammonium salt compound with ► *cetyl alcohol*. Hair conditioner in cosmetics.

Cetylamine Hydrofluoride

Mostly vegetable/synthetic, can also be partly animal. Fluorine salt based on ammonia derivatives. Can be derived from animal fats. In oral care and antiplaque products.

Cetylarachidol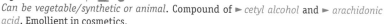

Can be vegetable/synthetic or animal. Compound of ► *cetyl alcohol* and ► *arachidonic acid*. Emollient in cosmetics.

Cetyl-PG Hydroxyethyl Decanamide

Mostly vegetable/synthetic, can also be partly animal. Compound of ► *cetyl alcohol*, ► *capric acid* and ammonia derivatives. Skin conditioner in cosmetics.

Cetyl-PG Hydroxyethyl Palmitamide

Mostly vegetable/synthetic, can also be partly animal. Compound of ► *cetyl alcohol*, ► *palmitic acid* and ammonia derivatives. Skin conditioner in cosmetics

Cetylpyridinium Chloride

Mostly vegetable/synthetic, can also be partly animal. ► *Quaternary ammonium compound* and ► *cationic surfactant*. Can be derived from animal fats. Antimicrobial/antiseptic substance (e.g. in dental care products), antistatic, deodorant, emulsifier, surfactant and hair conditioner in cosmetics.

Chamois

From killed animals. Soft ► *leather* made from the skin of chamois bucks, also goats, sheep and deer. Used as cleaning cloth, for instance chamois leather for windows.

Charcoal

Can be from killed animals, vegetable or mineral. Carbon residue produced by heating organic substances in the absence of oxygen (► *activated carbon*, ► *bone char*).

Cheese

From living and killed animals (► milk). Coagulated ► *casein*, separated from the other constituents of ► *milk* using ► *rennin*, ► *pepsin*, bacteria or moulds and further processed. Used as food or a food ingredient.

Chewable Mass 🔲 🌿 🐄

Mostly synthetic, can also be partly vegetable or animal. Mixture of substances used as a base for chewing gum. Consists mostly of synthetic waxes, may also contain ► *beeswax*, ► *fatty acids*, ► *shellac*, rubber or plant waxes.

Chimyl Alcohol 🐄

From killed animals. An ► *alkylglycerol*. Occurs naturally in the liver oils of marine animals as well as in bone marrow and breast milk. Is obtained from shark liver oil or bovine yellow bone marrow. Skin conditioner and emollient in cosmetics. In food supplements and as a complementary cancer treatment.

Chimyl Isostearate 🐄

From killed animals. Compound of ► *chimyl alcohol* and ► *stearic acid*. Emollient in cosmetics.

Chimyl Stearate 🐄

From killed animals. Compound of ► *chimyl alcohol* and ► *stearic acid*. Emulsifier in cosmetics.

China ► *Porcelain*

China Bristles 🐄

(Chungking bristles. Hog bristles. Pig bristles)
Mostly from killed animals. The ► *bristles* of domestic or wild pigs. In ► *brushes*.

Chitin 🐄 🌿

Mostly from killed animals, can also be vegetable. A polyaminosaccharide (sugar and ► *protein* compound). Occurs naturally in the exoskeletons of insects and crustaceans. Obtained industrially from the shells of crabs and shrimps. Can also be obtained from the cell walls of mushrooms, although this is less common. In hair mousse, skin care products, thickening agent and humectant in shampoos. Also see ► *chitosan*.

Chitin Glycolate 🐄

Mostly from killed animals. Compound of glycolic acid and ► *chitin*. Skin conditioner in cosmetics.

Chitosan 🐄 🌿

Mostly from killed animals, can also be vegetable. ► *Chitin* derivative. Obtained by chemically treating chitin with lye or ► *enzymes*. Film forming agent in cosmetics. Increasing medicinal use as a structural element for artificial blood vessels and skin, for wound dressing and in sutures. Inhibits bleeding and is antibacterial. Smoothing agent in paper manufacture and fibre treatment in the textile industry. Used for fining foods. Applications in environmental engineering, e.g. for water treatment. Used in agriculture as a yield optimizing organic agent.

Chitosan Ascorbate. Chitosan Formate. Chitosan Glycolate. 🐄 🌿
Chitosan Lactate. Chitosan PCA. Chitosan Salicylate. Chitosan Succinamide

Mostly from killed animals, can also be vegetable. Chemical compounds (especially salts) of ► *chitosan*. Antioxidants, film forming agents and skin conditioners in cosmetics.

Cholecalciferol ► Vitamin D₃

Cholecalciferol Polypeptide

From living/killed animals or synthetic/vegetable. ► *Protein* compound of ► *vitamin D₃*. Antistatic and hair conditioner in cosmetics.

Cholesterol

Mostly animal, can also be synthetic. Most important member of the group of ► *steroids*, vital for the structure and function of body cells as well as metabolism, hormonal balance and vitamin status. Occurs naturally in all animal cells, especially in fats and oils, nerve tissue, egg yolk and blood. Is obtained industrially from ► *lanolin* or animal spinal cord, in recent years also from nonanimal sources. Emulsifier, soothing agent and stabilizer in cosmetics, eye creams, shampoos, etc. Used as a source material for producing ► vitamin D₃. Industrial use as source material for ► *liquid crystals* (also see ► *cholesteryl acetate* and subsequent entries). The human body is able to meet its own cholesterol requirements, so external sources are not necessary and cholesterol is not used as an ingredient or additive in foods. On the contrary, an elevated blood cholesterol level is regarded as a health risk, and there is a large market for low-cholesterol and cholesterol-reducing foods and supplements. A vegan diet is typically cholesterol-free.

Cholesteryl Acetate

Mostly animal, can also be synthetic. ► *Liquid crystal* based on ► *cholesterol* and acetic acid. Skin conditioner and viscosity controlling agent in cosmetics. In liquid crystal screens and displays (LCDs), as well as thermosensitive pigments.

Cholesteryl Benzoate

Mostly animal, can also be synthetic. ► *Liquid crystal* based on ► *cholesterol* and benzoic acid. First liquid crystal to be discovered. In liquid crystal screens and displays (LCDs), as well as thermosensitive pigments.

Cholesteryl Butyrate

(Cholesteryl butanoate)
Mostly animal, can also be synthetic. ► *Liquid crystal* based on ► *cholesterol* and ► *butyric acid*. Skin conditioner in cosmetics. In liquid crystal screens and displays (LCDs), as well as thermosensitive pigments.

Cholesteryl Chloride

Mostly animal, can also be synthetic. ► *Liquid crystal* based on ► *cholesterol* and chlorine. Skin conditioner in cosmetics. In liquid crystal screens and displays (LCDs), as well as thermosensitive pigments.

Cholesteryl Dichlorobenzoate

Mostly animal, can also be synthetic. ► *Liquid crystal* based on ► *cholesterol* and hydrocarbons. Skin conditioner in cosmetics.

Cholesteryl Hydroxystearate

Can be animal or synthetic/vegetable. ► *Liquid crystal* based on ► *cholesterol* and ► *stearic acid*. Emollient, viscosity controlling agent in cosmetics.

Cholesteryl Isostearate
Can be animal or synthetic/vegetable. ► *Liquid crystal* based on ► *cholesterol* and ► *stearic acid.* Emollient and viscosity controlling agent in cosmetics.

Cholesteryl Isostearyl Carbonate
Can be animal or synthetic/vegetable. ► *Liquid crystal* based on ► *cholesterol* and ► *stearic acid.* Skin conditioner in cosmetics.

Cholesteryl Lanolate
From living or killed animals. ► *Liquid crystal* based on ► *cholesterol* and ► *fatty acids* from ► *lanolin.* Skin conditioner in cosmetics.

Cholesteryl Macadamiate
Can be animal or synthetic/vegetable. ► *Liquid crystal* based on ► *cholesterol* and ► *fatty acids* from macadamia nuts. Emollient in cosmetics.

Cholesteryl Nonanoate
Can be animal or synthetic/vegetable. ► *Liquid crystal* based on ► *cholesterol* and nonanoic acid (vegetable/synthetic). Emollient and emulsifier in cosmetics. In liquid crystal screens and displays (LCDs).

Cholesteryl Oleate
Can be animal or synthetic/vegetable. ► *Liquid crystal* based on ► *cholesterol* and ► *oleic acid.* Skin conditioner in cosmetics. In liquid crystal screens and displays (LCDs).

Cholesteryl Stearate
Can be animal or synthetic/vegetable. ► *Liquid crystal* based on ► *cholesterol* and ► *stearic acid.* Emollient and emulsifier in cosmetics. In liquid crystal screens and displays (LCDs), as well as thermosensitive pigments.

Cholesteryl/Behenyl/Octyldodecyl Lauroyl Glutamate
Can be animal or synthetic/vegetable. Mixed ► *fatty alcohols,* ► *cholesterol* and ► *glutamic acid.* Skin conditioner and skin protective substance in cosmetics.

Choleth-n
Mostly animal, can also be synthetic. ► *PEG* compounds of ► *cholesterol.* Surfactants and emulsifiers in cosmetics.

Choline
Mostly synthetic, can also be vegetable or animal. An amino alcohol related to B vitamins, present in many animals and plants. Main constituent of ► *lecithin* and acetylcholine (an important neurotransmitter), important for fat metabolism. Can be obtained from animal and vegetable sources. Is synthesized industrially from petroleum products. In nutritional supplements, animal food and veterinary medication for liver damage.

Chondroitin
(Chondroitin sulfate)
From killed animals. A ► *protein* and sugar compound. Important constituent of animal cartilage. Obtained from the connective tissue of killed animals. In nutritional supplements and alternative medicine for treating joint disorders.

Chymosin ► *Rennet*

CI 75170 ► *Guanine*

CI 75470 ► *Carmine*

CI 77267 ► *Bone Char*

Citric Acid Esters of Mono- and Diglycerides of Fatty Acids
(E 472c)
Can be vegetable or animal. Reaction product of citric acid and ► *fatty acids*. Emulsifier, complexing agent and carrier in foods.

Civet. Civet Musk
From living animals. Strong smelling secretion from the anal glands of civet cats. The musk is obtained by squeezing the glands, a stressful and often painful procedure for the animals. Civet cats are kept in cruel conditions in cages. Civet musk is used as a scent in expensive perfumes.

Civetone
From living or killed animals, can also be vegetable. A pheromone and main constituent of ► *civet musk*, closely related to ► *muscone*. One of the oldest known perfume ingredients. Obtained from civet musk or ► *aleuritic acid*. Can also be manufactured chemically from palm oil consitituents. Often used as a scent in perfumes, soaps and household chemicals.

Clarified Butter
(Ghee)
From living and killed animals (► milk). Purified ► *butterfat* with a fat content of about 99%, free of water and protein. Made by heating ► *butter* or ► *cream*. In many foods, e.g. chocolate, as a substitute for ► *cocoa butter*. Ghee, which is heated longer than other clarified butter, plays an important part in South Asian—especially Indian—foods.

Coated Leather
From killed animals. ► *Leather* in footwear where the (synthetic) surface coating applied to the leather does not exceed one third of the total thickness but is in excess of 0.15 millimetres.

Cobalamine ► *Vitamin B$_{12}$*

Cocamidopropyl Dimethylamine Hydrolyzed Collagen
Cocamidopropyl Dimethylamino Hydroxypropyl Hydrolyzed Collagen
Cocamidopropyldimonium Hydroxypropyl Hydrolyzed Collagen
From killed animals. Compounds of coconut ► *fatty acids* and chemically altered ► *collagen*. Antistatics, surfactants and hair conditioners in cosmetics.

Cocamidopropyl Dimethylamine Lactate
Cocamidopropyl Morpholine Lactate
Mostly vegetable/microbiological, can also be partly animal. Compounds of coconut ► *fatty acids* and ► *lactic acid* salts. Surfactants in cosmetics.

Cocamidopropyl Dimethylammonium C8-16 Isoalkylsuccinyl Lactoglobulin Sulfonate 🐄

From living and killed animals (► milk). Compound of coconut ► *fatty acids* and ► *lactoglobulin* (milk protein). Antistatic, surfactant and hair conditioner in cosmetics.

Cocaminobutyric Acid 🌱 🧪 🐄

Mostly vegetable/synthetic, can also be partly animal. Compound of coconut derivatives and ► *butyric acid.* Emollient, surfactant and cleansing agent in cosmetics.

Coccus Cacti 🐄

Killed animals. Dried female scale insects. In ► *homeopathic medicines.*

Cochineal ► Carmine

Cochineal Red A 🧪

(E 124. Ponceau 4R)
Synthetic. Red food dye made from petroleum products. Cheap alternative to ► *carmine.*

Cocoa Butter 🌱

(Theobroma cacao butter)
Vegetable. Pale yellow fat from roasted cocoa beans. Not to be confused with ► *butter* of animal origin. Used as edible fat, especially in chocolate products and confectionery. Emollient in cosmetics. Carrier substance in some pharmaceutical products (e.g. in suppositories).

Cocoa Glaze ► Icing

Coco Hydrolyzed Animal Protein 🐄

From killed animals. Condensate of coconut ► *fatty acids* and unspecified animal ► *proteins.* Antistatic and surfactant in cosmetics.

Coco-Caprylate/Caprate 🌱 🐄

Mostly vegetable, can also be partly animal. Compound of coconut derivatives, ► *caprylic acid* and ► *capric acid.* Emollient in cosmetics.

Cocodimonium Hydroxypropyl Hydrolyzed Casein 🐄

From living and killed animals (► milk). Chemically altered ► *casein.* Antistatic and hair conditioner in cosmetics.

Cocodimonium Hydroxypropyl Hydrolyzed Collagen 🐄

From killed animals. Chemically altered ► *collagen.* Antistatic and hair conditioner in cosmetics.

Cocodimonium Hydroxypropyl Hydrolyzed Keratin 🐄

From killed or living animals. Chemically altered ► *keratin.* Antistatic and hair conditioner in cosmetics.

Cocodimonium Hydroxypropyl Hydrolyzed Silk 🐄
Cocodimonium Hydroxypropyl Silk Amino Acids

From killed animals. Chemically altered ► *silk* or ► *amino acids* from silk. Antistatics, hair and skin conditioners in cosmetics.

Cocoyl Glutamic Acid

Mostly vegetable/synthetic, can theoretically also be partly animal. Compound of coconut ► *fatty acids* and ► *glutamic acid*. Emollient, hair conditioner and cleansing agent in cosmetics.

Cocoyl Hydrolyzed Collagen

From killed animals. Chemically altered ► *collagen*. Antistatic, surfactant, hair conditioner and cleansing agent in cosmetics.

Cocoyl Hydrolyzed Keratin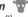

From killed or living animals. Chemically altered ► *keratin*. Antistatic, hair conditioner and cleansing agent in cosmetics.

Cocoyl Sarcosinamide DEA

From killed animals or synthetic. Compound of coconut ► *fatty acids* and ► *sarcosine* and the alcohol diethanolamine. Surfactant and foam booster in cosmetics.

Cocoyl Sarcosine

From killed animals or synthetic. Compound of coconut ► *fatty acids* and ► *sarcosine*. Surfactant and cleansing agent in cosmetics.

Cod Liver Oil ► *Fish Liver Oil*

Coenzyme A

(CoA)

Microbiological. A biologically active substance that binds to ► *enzymes*, influencing biochemical reactions, e.g. in energy and fat metabolism. Occurs naturally in all living cells, arising from ► *adenosine triphosphate*, ► *cysteine* and ► *pantothenic acid*. Industrially obtained from yeasts. Emollient and solvent in cosmetics. Chemical precursors are added to food supplements.

Coenzyme Q$_{10}$ ► *Ubiquinone*

Colecalciferol ► *Vitamin D$_3$*

Collagen

From killed animals. A fibrous ► *protein* with high longitudinal strength and minimal elasticity in the connective tissue of vertebrates. Various forms are present in bone, teeth, cartilage, ligaments, sinews and skin, making up about 30% of total body protein. Is obtained from "slaughterhouse waste," such as cartilage, sinews and skins of cattle and fish. Used as an active agent against wrinkles and a humectant in cosmetics. Processed collagen is also used as a cosmetic ingredient, especially ► *collagen amino acids*, and ► *hydrolyzed collagen* and its derivatives (listed here according to their standardized INCI names). Collagen is also used in cosmetic surgery in antiwrinkle injections. Collagenous tissue is also used as a source of ► *gelatin* and ► *glue*.

Collagen Amino Acids

From killed animals. ► *Amino acids* from ► *collagen*. Humectant in cosmetics.

Colon Suis ► *Organ Extracts*

Colostral Milk ► *Colostrum*

Colostrum

(Beestings. Colostral milk. First milk)

From living animals. Fluid produced by the mammary glands of mother mammals (in this case, cows) during the first days after the birth of their young and prior to the actual ► *milk*. Is obtained by milking the cow, which may lead to the calves being deprived of it. Skin protective substance in cosmetics. In food supplements that supposedly boost and enhance the immune system (not scientifically verified).

Colostrum Cream

From living animals. The fatty fraction of ► *colostrum*. Skin protecting substance in cosmetics.

Colostrum Serum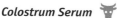

From living animals. The aqueous fraction of ► *colostrum*. Skin protecting substance in cosmetics.

Conchiorin Powder

From killed animals. Powder from the shells of pearl-producing ► *bivalves*. Abrasive in cosmetics.

Conjugated Estrogens ► *Estrogen*

Connective Tissue Extract

From killed animals. Extract from animal connective tissue (primarily from cattle or pigs). Moisturizer and skin conditioner in cosmetics.

Copper Acetyl Tyrosinate Methylsilanol

From killed or living animals. Copper compound of ► *tyrosine*. Humectant in cosmetics.

Cor Suis ► *Organ Extracts*

Coral

From dead animals. Hard, calcareous substance made up of the skeletons of polyps anchored to the sea floor, which gradually grow to form reefs. Coral is used by humans for making decorative objects and jewellery. Is also used as surgical bone replacement (implants). Can be obtained from both living or dead coral reefs.

Cordovan ► *Horse Leather*

Corticosteroids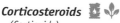

(Corticoids)

Synthetic/vegetable. Hormones that belong to the category of ► *steroids* and are synthesized from ► *cholesterol* in the adrenal glands of animals. They fulfill a number of important or even vital body functions in metabolism, fluid balance, and as sexual and stress hormones. The most important hormone is cortisol (hydrocortisone), and its derivative cortisone was the first corticosteroid to be discovered. In everyday usage, not only cortisone itself but also the other corticosteroids may be incorrectly referred to as "cortisone." A subgroup of the corticosteroids, the glucocorticoids (e.g. prednisone, prednisolone or dexamethasone), are used as active ingredients in a number of pharmaceutical drugs, especially for treating inflammatory, allergic, rheumatic and autoimmune diseases. The corticosteroids used in pharmaceutical drugs are derived from plant steroids.

Cortisone ► Corticosteroids

Cream
From living and killed animals (► milk). The fatty fraction of mammal ► milk. Obtained by mechanical separation of the milk. Used as food and food ingredient. Skin conditioner and skin protecting substance in cosmetics.

Cream of Tartar ► Potassium Bitartrate

Creatine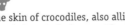
Can be vegetable/synthetic or from killed animals. An organic acid that plays a part in the energy supply of muscles and is synthesized in the body from ► *arginine*, ► *glycine* and ► *methionine*. Can be obtained from animal flesh, but is usually chemically derived, e.g. from cyanamide (synthetic) and ► *sodium sarcosinate*. Creatine is used as an ingredient in bodybuilding dietary supplements and occasionally also for treating muscle disorders.

Creatinine
Can be from killed animals or synthetic/vegetable. Degradation product of ► *creatine* in animal muscle tissue. Is eliminated from the body via urine excretion. Obtained industrially by chemical transformation of ► *creatine*. Skin conditioner in cosmetics.

Crimson Lake ► Carmine

Crocodile Leather
From killed animals. The skin of crocodiles, also alligators. In clothing and accessories (footwear, jackets, bags, belts, etc.). Comes either from wild animals (although most crocodile species are now protected), or crocodile or alligator farms.

Crustacea Extract
From killed animals. Extract from body fluids of ► *crustaceans*. Masking agent and skin conditioner in in cosmetics.

Crustaceans
Killed animals. Name for a large number of invertebrate animal species that belong to the arthropods, are mostly aquatic and possess ► *chitin* exoskeletons. Crustaceans include crabs, shrimps/prawns, crayfish and ► *lobsters*. The meat of crustaceans is used as food. The exoskeletons are used as a source of chitin.

CTAB ► Cetrimonium Bromide

CTAC ► Cetrimonium Chloride

Cutaneous Lysate
From killed animals. ► *Protein* extract from animal skins. Skin conditioner and moisturizer in cosmetics.

Cutis Suis ► *Organ Extracts*

Cuttlefish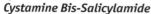

Killed animals. Order of cephalopods (marine invertebrates). Used as food, especially in the Mediterranean Basin, and for obtaining ► *sepia.*

Cyanocobalamin ► *Vitamin B₁₂*

Cystamine Bis-Lactamide
Cystamine Bis-Salicylamide

Can be from living or killed animals, microbiological or synthetic. ► *Cystine* derivative. Skin conditioner in cosmetics.

Cysteamine HCl

Can be from living or killed animals, microbiological or synthetic. ► *Cysteine* derivative. Antioxidant and reducing agent in cosmetics.

Cysteine

(L-cysteine. E920)

Can be from living or killed animals, microbiological or synthetic. An ► *amino acid.* Occurs naturally in keratinous animal tissue (e.g. ► *horn,* ► *hair,* feathers, sinews) as well as in ► *milk* and some plants. Obtained using hydrochloric acid from horn or hair (including human hair) or feathers, or via chemical treatment of ► *cystine.* Can also be fully synthesized or produced from ► *cystine* using genetically engineered bacteria. Used as flour treating agent in baked goods (not subject to mandatory labelling). In infant formulas and food supplements. Antioxidant, antistatic, reducing agent and hair conditioner in cosmetics. Used as ► *acetyl cysteine* or ► *carbocysteine* in mucolytic medication. Carbocysteine is also used in skin care products. In anabolics. Additive in animal feed.

Cysteine HCl

(Cysteine hydrochloride)

Can be from living or killed animals, microbiological or synthetic. ► *Cysteine* variant. Antioxidant and reducing agent in cosmetics.

Cystine

(E921. L-cystine)

Can be from living or killed animals, microbiological or synthetic. Oxidation product of ► *cysteine.* Occurs along with cysteine in keratinous tissues and some plants. Obtained with cysteine from keratinous tissues or biotechnologically. In nutritional supplements. Baking aid. Used for producing ► *acetyl cysteine* and ► *carbocysteine.* Antistatic and hair conditioner in cosmetics.

Cytochrome C

From killed animals or microbiological. ► *Protein* that plays an important part in the energy balance of cells. Is present in practically all organisms. Obtained primarily from heart tissue of tuna or mammals such as horses, pigs or cattle. Is also obtained from microbiological sources. Skin conditioner in cosmetics.

Dairy Products

(Milk products)

From living and killed animals (► *milk).* Products made from ► *milk,* including ► *butter,* ► *butterfat,* ► *buttermilk,* ► *casein,* ► *cheese,* ► *cream,* ► *whey* and ► *yogurt.*

DATEM ► *Mono- and Diacetyl Tartaric Acid Esters of Mono- and Diglycerides of Fatty Acids*

DEA-Ceteareth-2 Phosphate

Can be vegetable/synthetic or animal. Compound of ► *cetostearyl alcohol* and salts of phosporic acid with the alcohol diethanolamine. Emulsifier in cosmetics.

DEA-Cetyl Phosphate

Mostly vegetable/synthetic, can also be animal. Compound of ► *cetyl alcohol,* salts of phosporic acid and the alcohol diethanolamine. Surfactant and emulsifier in cosmetics.

DEA-Cetyl Sulfate

Mostly vegetable/synthetic, can also be animal. Compound of ► *cetyl alcohol,* sulphuric acid salts and the alcohol diethanolamine. Surfactant and emulsifier in cosmetics.

DEA-Hydrolyzed Lecithin

Mostly vegetable/synthetic, can also be animal. Compound of ► *lecithin* and the alcohol diethanolamine. Emulsifier in cosmetics.

DEA-Isostearate

Can be synthetic/vegetable or animal. Compound of ► *stearic acid* with the alcohol diethanolamine. Surfactant, cleansing agent and emulsifier in cosmetics.

DEA-Methyl Myristate Sulfonate
DEA-Myreth Sulfate

Vegetable/synthetic, can theoretically also be partly animal. Compounds of ► *myristic acid* with the alcohol diethanolamine. Surfactants, foaming agent and cleansing substances in cosmetics.

DEA-Myristate

Vegetable/synthetic, can theoretically also be partly animal. Compound of ► *myristic acid* with the alcohol diethanolamine. Surfactant and emulsifier in cosmetics.

DEA-Myristyl Sulfate

Vegetable/synthetic, can theoretically also be partly animal. Compound of myristyl alcohol (from ► *myristic acid*) with the alcohol diethanolamine. Surfactant, cleansing agent, foaming agent in cosmetics.

DEA-Oleth-n Phosphate

Mostly from killed animals, can also be vegetable. Compounds of ► *oleic acid* with the alcohol diethanolamine. Emulsifiers and surfactants in cosmetics.

Decanoate ► Capric Acid

Decanoic Acid ► Capric Acid

Decanol ► Decyl Alcohol

Decarboxy Carnosine HCl

Can be vegetable, animal or synthetic. Compound of ► *carnosine*. Antistatic and hair conditioner in cosmetics.

Deceth-7 Carboxylic Acid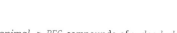

Mostly vegetable/synthetic, can also be animal. ► *PEG* compound of ► *decyl alcohol*. Surfactant and emulsifier in cosmetics.

Deceth-n

Mostly vegetable/synthetic, can also be animal. ► *PEG* compounds of ► *decyl alcohol*. Emulsifiers in cosmetics.

Deceth-n Phosphate

Mostly vegetable/synthetic, can also be animal. ► *PEG* compounds of ► *decyl alcohol* with phosphate salts. Surfactants and emulsifiers in cosmetics.

Decyl Alcohol

(Capric alcohol. Decanol)
Mostly vegetable/synthetic, can also be animal. ► *Fatty alcohol* of ► *capric acid*. Emollient and viscosity controlling agent in cosmetics.

Decyl Betaine

Mostly vegetable/synthetic, can also be partly animal. Compound of ► *decyl alcohol* and ► *betaine*. Antistatic, surfactant and foam booster in cosmetics.

Decyl Glucoside

Mostly vegetable/synthetic, can also be partly animal. ► *Sugar surfactant* and compound of ► *decyl alcohol*. Surfactant and emulsion stabilizer in cosmetics.

Decyl Isostearate

Can be vegetable/synthetic or animal. Compound of ► *decyl alcohol* and ► *stearic acid*. Emollient in cosmetics.

Decyl Mercaptomethylimidazole

Mostly vegetable/synthetic, can also be partly animal. Compound of ► *decyl alcohol* with an organic sulphur and hydrogen complex. Antioxidant in cosmetics.

Decyl Myristate

Mostly vegetable/synthetic, can also be partly animal. Compound of ► *decyl alcohol* and ► *myristic acid*. Emollient in cosmetics.

Decyl Oleate

Can be vegetable/synthetic or from killed animals. Compound of ► *decyl alcohol* and ► *oleic acid*. Emollient in cosmetics.

Decyl Polyglucose

Mostly vegetable/synthetic, can also be partly animal. Sugar compound of ► *decyl alcohol*. Surfactant and emulsion stabilizer in cosmetics.

Decyl Succinate

Mostly vegetable/synthetic, can also be partly animal. Salt of ► *succinic acid* and ► *decyl alcohol*. Emollient in cosmetics.

Deer Tallow

(Adeps cervidae)
From killed animals. ► *Tallow* from deer. In creams for especially stressed skin zones, used especially by athletes, in order to prevent sores, e.g. marathon runners and cyclists. Used as cork fat for wind instruments. Also in frost-protective products for car door seals. Traditional ingredient in soaps, candles and leather care products.

Defibrase ► Batroxobin

7-Dehydrocholesterol

(Provitamin D$_3$)
From living/killed animals or synthetic. A ► *steroid* and precursor of cholecalciferol (► *vitamin D$_3$*). Is synthesized in the bodies of living vertebrates from ► *cholesterol* and transformed into active vitamin D$_3$ under the influence of UV light (sunlight on the skin). Is also enzymatically transformed into cholesterol. Obtained from the skins of slaughtered cattle, sheep or pigs, or by chemical processing of cholesterol, e.g. from ► *lanolin*. Emulsion stabilizer and viscosity controlling agent in cosmetics.

Delta-Tocopherol ► Vitamin E

Deoxyribonuclease

(DNase)
From killed animals, can also be microbiological. An ► *enzyme* involved in breaking down nucleic acids (► *DNA*). Obtained from internal organs (e.g. pancreas, spleen) of killed animals (pigs, cattle). Can also be obtained from genetically altered microorganisms. Skin conditioner in cosmetics.

Deoxyribonucleic Acid ► DNA

Deproteinized Serum

From killed animals. Deproteinized ► *blood* extract. Skin conditioner in cosmetics.

Desamido Collagen

From killed animals. Chemically altered ► *collagen*. Film forming agent in cosmetics.

Dexpanthenol ▶ *Panthenol*

Dextrin Myristate
Vegetable/synthetic, can theoretically also be partly animal. Carbohydrate compound of ▶ *myristic acid.* Emulsifier in cosmetics.

Dextrin Palmitate
Mostly vegetable, can also be partly animal. Carbohydrate compound of ▶ *palmitic acid.* Emulsifier in cosmetics.

Dextrin Stearate
Can be vegetable or animal. Carbohydrate compound of ▶ *stearic acid.* Emulsifier in cosmetics.

DHA ▶ *Docosahexaenoic Acid*

Diacetin
(E 1517. Glyceryl diacetate)
Can be vegetable or from killed animals. Compound of acetic acid and ▶ *glycerol.* Solvent in cosmetics. Used for manufacturing food ▶ *flavourings.*

Diazolidinyl Urea
Synthetic. Polymer compound of ▶ *urea.* Preservative in cosmetics.

Dicapryl Adipate
Mostly vegetable/synthetic, can also be partly animal. Salt of ▶ *adipic acid* and ▶ *decyl alcohol.* Emollient, film forming agent and plasticizer in cosmetics.

Dicapryl Sodium Sulfosuccinate
Mostly vegetable/synthetic, can also be animal. Salt of ▶ *succinic acid* and ▶ *capryl alcohol.* Surfactant, emulsion stabilizer, hydrotrope and cleansing agent in cosmetics.

Dicapryl/Dicaprylyl Dimonium Chloride
Mostly vegetable/synthetic, can also be partly animal. Ammonium compound of ▶ *capryl alcohol* and ▶ *decyl alcohol.* Antistatic, emulsifier and hair conditioner in cosmetics.

Dicapryloyl Cystine
Mostly animal/vegetable, can also be microbiological or synthetic. Compound of ▶ *caprylic acid* and ▶ *cystine.* Antistatic and hair conditioner in cosmetics.

Dicaprylyl Ether
Mostly synthetic, can also be vegetable or animal. Compound of ▶ *capryl alcohol.* Solvent in cosmetics.

Dicaprylyl Maleate
Mostly synthetic, can also be partly vegetable or animal. Compound of maleic acid and ▶ *capryl alcohol.* Emollient and solvent in cosmetics.

Diceteareth-10 Phosphate
Mostly vegetable/synthetic, can also be partly animal. ▶ *PEG* compound of ▶ *cetostearyl alcohol.* Emulsifier in cosmetics.

Dicetyl Adipate 🌱 🐷 🐄
Mostly vegetable/synthetic, can also be partly animal. Salt of ► *adipic acid* and ► *cetyl alcohol*. Emollient, film forming agent, skin conditioner and plasticizer in cosmetics.

Dicetyl Ether 🌱 🐷 🐄
Mostly vegetable/synthetic, can also be animal. Compound of ► *cetyl alcohol*. Emollient and skin conditioner in cosmetics.

Dicetyl Phosphate 🌱 🐷 🐄
Mostly vegetable/synthetic, can also be animal. Salt of phosphoric acid and ► *cetyl alcohol*. Emulsifier in cosmetics.

Dicetyl Thiodipropionate 🌱 🐷 🐄
Mostly vegetable/synthetic, can also be partly animal. Salt of ► *propionic acid* and ► *cetyl alcohol*. Antioxidant in cosmetics.

Dicetyldimonium Chloride 🌱 🐷 🐄
Mostly vegetable/synthetic, can also be partly animal. Ammonium salt of ► *cetyl alcohol*. Antistatic, surfactant, emulsifier and hair conditioner in cosmetics.

Dicocoyl Pentaerythrityl Distearyl Citrate 🌱 🐷 🐄
Can be vegetable/synthetic or animal. Compound of citric acid, coconut derivatives and ► *stearyl alcohol*. Emollient in cosmetics.

Dierucic Acid ► *Erucic Acid*

Diethylene Tricaseinamide 🐄
From living and killed animals (► milk). Ammonia compound of ► *casein*. Antistatic and hair conditioner in cosmetics.

Digalloyl Trioleate 🌱 🐄
Can be vegetable or animal. Compound of ► *gallic acid* and ► *oleic acid*. Antioxidant in cosmetics.

Diglycerides ► *Glycerides*

Diglycerin 🌱 🐄 🐷
Mostly vegetable, can also be animal or synthetic. Chemical variant of ► *glycerol*. Humectant and solvent in cosmetics.

Diglyceryl Stearate Malate 🌱 🐄
Can be vegetable or animal. Compound of ► *glycerol*, ► *stearic acid* and malic acid. Viscosity controlling agent and emollient in cosmetics.

Dihexyldecyl Lauroyl Glutamate 🌱 🐷 🐄
Mostly vegetable/synthetic, can also be partly animal. Compound of ► *glutamic acid*, ► *decyl alcohol* and ► *lauric acid*. Emollient and skin conditioner in cosmetics.

Dihydrocholesterol 🐄 🐷
(Cholestanol)
Mostly animal, can also be synthetic. Variant of ► *cholesterol*. Emollient in cosmetics.

Dihydrocholesteryl Butyrate
Dihydrocholesteryl Isostearate
Dihydrocholesteryl Macadamiate
Dihydrocholesteryl Nonanoate
Dihydrocholesteryl Octyldecanoate
Dihydrocholesteryl Oleate

Mostly animal/vegetable, can also be vegetable/synthetic. Compounds of ► *dihydrocholesterol* and, respectively, ► *butyric acid*, ► *stearic acid*, macadamia nut fatty acids, nonanoic acid, ► *capric acid* and ► *oleic acid*. Skin conditioners and emollients in cosmetics.

Dihydrocholeth-n

Mostly animal, can also be synthetic. ► *PEG* compounds of ► *dihydrocholesterol*. Emulsifiers in cosmetics.

Dihydrogenated Tallow Benzylmonium Chloride

From killed animals. Chemically altered ► *tallow*. Antistatic, surfactant and hair conditioner in cosmetics.

Dihydrogenated Tallow Benzylmonium Hectorite

From killed animals. Chemically altered ► *tallow*. Antistatic, gelling agent and viscosity controlling agent in cosmetics.

Dihydrogenated Tallow Hydroxyethylmonium Methosulfate

From killed animals. Chemically altered ► *tallow*. Antistatic and hair conditioner in cosmetics.

Dihydrogenated Tallow Methylamine

From killed animals. Chemically altered ► *tallow*. Emulsifier, surfactant and hair conditioner in cosmetics.

Dihydrogenated Tallow Phthalate

From killed animals. Chemically altered ► *tallow*. Emollient and surfactant in cosmetics.

Dihydrogenated Tallow Phthalic Acid Amide

From killed animals. Chemically altered ► *tallow*. Emulsifier in cosmetics.

Dihydrogenated Tallowamidoethyl Hydroxyethylmonium Chloride
Dihydrogenated Tallowamidoethyl Hydroxyethylmonium Methosulfate
Dihydrogenated Tallowdimonium Chloride
Dihydrogenated Tallowethyl Hydroxyethylmonium Methosulfate
Dihydrogenated Tallowoylethyl Hydroxyethylmonium Methosulfate

Always partly from killed animals. Ammonium compounds of chemically altered ► *tallow*. Antistatics and hair conditioners in cosmetics.

Dihydrolanosterol

From living or killed animals. Compound of ► *lanosterol*. Emulsifier, skin conditioner and emulsion stabilizer in cosmetics.

Dihydrophytosteryl Octyldecanoate
Mostly vegetable, can also be partly animal. Compound of vegetable ► *steroids* and ► *capric acid.* Emollient in cosmetics.

Dihydroxyethyl Oleyl Glycinate
Can be vegetable or from killed animals. Compound of ► *oleyl alcohol* and ► *glycine.* Surfactant, antistatic and foam booster in cosmetics.

Dihydroxyethyl Stearamine Oxide
Can be vegetable/synthetic or animal. Ammonia compound of ► *stearic acid.* Antistatic, surfactant and foam booster in cosmetics.

Dihydroxyethyl Stearyl Glycinate
Can be vegetable or from killed animals. Compound of ► *stearyl alcohol* and ► *glycine.* Antistatic and hair conditioner in cosmetics.

Dihydroxyethyl Tallow Glycinate
From killed animals. Chemically altered ► *tallow.* Surfactant, foam booster and antistatic in cosmetics.

Dihydroxyethyl Tallowamine HCl
From killed animals. Chemically altered ► *tallow.* Surfactant, hair conditioner and antistatic in cosmetics.

Dihydroxyethyl Tallowamine Oleate
From killed animals. Chemically altered ► *tallow.* Surfactant and hair conditioner in cosmetics.

Dihydroxyethyl Tallowamine Oxide
From killed animals. Chemically altered ► *tallow.* Antistatic, emulsifiers, surfactant and foam booster in cosmetics.

Dihydroxyethyl Tallowamine/IPDI Copolymer
From killed animals. Chemically altered ► *tallow.* Film forming agent, hair and skin conditioner in cosmetics.

Dihydroxyethylamino Hydroxypropyl Oleate
Can be vegetable/synthetic or animal. Compound of ► *oleic acid.* Emollient and skin conditioner in cosmetics.

Diisocetyl Adipate
Mostly vegetable/synthetic, can theoretically also be partly animal. Compound of ► *adipic acid* and ► *cetyl alcohol.* Emollient in cosmetics.

Diisodecyl Adipate
Mostly vegetable/synthetic, can also be partly animal. Salt of ► *adipic acid* and ► *decyl alcohol.* Emollient in cosmetics.

Diisostearamidopropyl Epoxypropylmonium Chloride
Can be vegetable/synthetic or animal. Polymer compound of ► *stearic acid.* Antistatic and hair conditioner in cosmetics.

Diisostearoyl Trimethylolpropane Siloxy Silicate
Can be synthetic/mineral/vegetable or animal. Silicate compound of ► *stearic acid.* Skin conditioner in cosmetics.

Diisostearyl Adipate
Can be vegetable or animal. Compound of ► *adipic acid* and ► *stearyl alcohol.* Emollient in cosmetics.

Diisostearyl Dimer Dilinoleate
Can be vegetable or animal. Compound of ► *linoleic acid* and ► *stearyl alcohol.* Emollient in cosmetics.

Diisostearyl Fumarate
Can be vegetable/synthetic or animal. Compound of ► *fumaric acid* and ► *stearyl alcohol.* Emollient in cosmetics.

Diisostearyl Glutarate
Can be vegetable/synthetic or animal. Compound of glutaric acid (vegetable/synthetic) and ► *stearyl alcohol.* Emollient in cosmetics.

Diisostearyl Malate
Can be vegetable/synthetic or animal. Compound of ► *maleic acid* and ► *stearyl alcohol.* Emollient in cosmetics.

Dimethicone Copolyol Beeswax
From living animals. Chemically altered ► *beeswax.* Emollient in cosmetics.

Dimethicone Copolyol Cocoa Butterate
Synthetic/vegetable. Chemically altered ► *cocoa butter.* Emollient in cosmetics.

Dimethicone Copolyol Dhupa Butterate
Synthetic/vegetable. Chemically altered fat from seeds of the *Vateria indica* tree. Hair and skin conditioner, emollient in cosmetics.

Dimethicone Copolyol Hydroxystearate
Dimethicone Copolyol Isostearate
Can be vegetable/synthetic or animal. Silicone compounds of ► *stearic acid.* Humectants and emollients in cosmetics.

Dimethicone Copolyol Kokum Butterate
Synthetic/vegetable. Chemically altered ► *kokum butter.* Hair and skin conditioner, and emollient in cosmetics.

Dimethicone Copolyol Mango Butterate
Synthetic/vegetable. Chemically altered fat from mango fruit kernels. Hair and skin conditioner, and emollient in cosmetics.

Dimethicone Copolyol Mohwa Butterate
Synthetic/vegetable. Chemically altered fat from the seeds of the mahwa tree (*Madhuca longifolia*). Hair and skin conditioner, and emollient in cosmetics.

Dimethicone Copolyol Sal Butterate 🌿 🐄

Synthetic/vegetable. Chemically altered ► *Shorea robusta butter.* Hair and skin conditioner, emollient in cosmetics.

Dimethicone Copolyol Shea Butterate 🌿 🐄

Synthetic/vegetable. Chemically altered shea butter (► *Butyrospermum parkii butter*). Emollient and skin conditioner in cosmetics.

Dimethicone Copolyol Stearate 🌿 🐄 🐄

Can be vegetable/synthetic or animal. Silicone compound of ► *stearic acid.* Humectant, skin conditioner and emollient in cosmetics.

Dimethiconol Beeswax 🐄

From living animals. Chemically altered ► *beeswax.* Skin conditioner in cosmetics.

Dimethiconol Dhupa Butterate 🌿 🐄

Synthetic/vegetable. Chemically altered fat from seeds of the *Vateria indica* tree. Hair conditioner and emollient in cosmetics.

Dimethiconol Hydroxystearate 🌿 🐄 🐄

Can be vegetable/synthetic or animal. Silicone compound of ► *stearic acid.* Emollient in cosmetics.

Dimethiconol Illipe Butterate 🌿 🐄

Synthetic/vegetable. Chemically altered ► *illipé butter.* Skin conditioner and emollient in cosmetics.

Dimethiconol Isostearate 🌿 🐄 🐄

Can be vegetable/synthetic or animal. Silicone compound of ► *stearic acid.* Emollient in cosmetics.

Dimethiconol Kokum Butterate 🌿 🐄

Synthetic/vegetable. Chemically altered ► *kokum butter.* Skin conditioner and emollient in cosmetics.

Dimethiconol Lactate 🌿 🐄 🐄

Can be vegetable/synthetic or partly animal. Silicone compound of ► *lactic acid.* Hair and skin conditioner, and emollient in cosmetics.

Dimethiconol Mohwa Butterate 🌿 🐄

Synthetic/vegetable. Chemically altered fat from the seeds of the mahwa tree (*Madhuca longifolia*). Skin conditioner and emollient in cosmetics.

Dimethiconol Sal Butterate 🌿 🐄

Synthetic/vegetable. Chemically altered ► *Shorea robusta butter.* Skin conditioner and emollient in cosmetics.

Dimethiconol Stearate 🌿 🐄 🐄

Can be vegetable/synthetic or animal. Silicone compound of ► *stearic acid.* Emollient in cosmetics.

Dimethyl Cystinate
From living or killed animals, can also be microbiological or synthetic. Compound of ► *cystine*. Antistatic in cosmetics.

Dimethyl Diacetyl Cysteinate
From living or killed animals, can also be microbiological. Compound of ► *cysteine*. Hair conditioner in cosmetics.

Dimethyl Glutamic Acid
Mostly vegetable/synthetic, can theoretically also be partly animal. Compound of ► *glutamic acid*. Antistatic and hair conditioner in cosmetics.

Dimethyl Hydrogenated Tallowamine
From killed animals. Chemically altered ► *tallow*. Emulsifier, antistatic, emulsion stabilizer and hair conditioner in cosmetics.

Dimethyl Lauramine Isostearate
Can be vegetable/synthetic or animal. Compound of ► *stearic acid*. Emollient and emulsion stabilizer in cosmetics.

Dimethyl Lauramine Oleate
Can be vegetable/synthetic or animal. Compound of ► *oleic acid*. Antistatic and viscosity controlling agent in cosmetics.

Dimethyl Lauroyl Lysine
Synthetic/vegetable/microbiological, can theoretically also be partly animal. Compound of ► *lysine* and ► *lauric acid*. Skin conditioner in cosmetics.

Dimethyl PABA Ethyl Cetearyldimonium Tosylate
Can be vegetable/synthetic or animal. Ammonium compound of ► *cetostearyl alcohol*. UV absorber in cosmetics.

Dimethyl Palmitamine
Mostly vegetable/synthetic, can also be partly animal. Ammonia compound of ► *palmitic acid*. Antistatic, emulsifier and hair conditioner in cosmetics.

Dimethyl Stearamine
Can be vegetable/synthetic or animal. Ammonia compound of ► *stearic acid*. Antistatic, emulsifier and hair conditioner in cosmetics.

Dimethyl Tallowamine
From killed animals. Chemically altered ► *tallow*. Emollient, hair conditioner, emulsifier and antistatic in cosmetics.

Dimethylol Urea/Phenol/Sodium Phenolsulfonate Copolymer
Synthetic. Polymer compound of ► *urea*, among others. Viscosity controlling agent in cosmetics.

Dimethylsilanol Hyaluronate
Can be from killed animals or microbiological. Compound of ► *hyaluronic acid*. Humectant and moisturizer in cosmetics.

Dioctyldodeceth-2 Lauroyl Glutamate
Vegetable/synthetic, can theoretically also be partly animal. Compound of ► *lauric acid*, ► *lauryl alcohol* and ► *glutamic acid*. Surfactant and emollient in cosmetics.

Dioctyldodecyl Lauroyl Glutamate
Vegetable/synthetic, can theoretically also be partly animal. Compound of ► *lauric acid*, ► *lauryl alcohol* and ► *glutamic acid*. Surfactant and emollient in cosmetics.

Dioctyldodecyl Stearoyl Glutamate
Can be vegetable/synthetic or animal. Compound of ► *lauryl alcohol*, ► *stearic acid* and ► *glutamic acid*. Emulsifier and emollient in cosmetics.

Dioleoyl Edetolmonium Methosulfate
Can be vegetable/synthetic or animal. Compound of ► *oleic acid* with ammonia and salts of sulphur. Buffering agent, surfactant and emulsifier in cosmetics.

Dioleoyl EDTHP-Monium Methosulfate
Can be vegetable/synthetic or animal. Compound of ► *oleic acid* with ammonia and salts of sulphur. Antistatic and hair conditioner in cosmetics.

Dioleoylamidoethyl Hydroxyethylmonium Methosulfate
Can be vegetable/synthetic or animal. Compound of ► *oleic acid* with ammonia and salts of sulphur. Antistatic, surfactant and cleansing agent in cosmetics.

Dioleoylethyl Hydroxyethylmonium Methosulfate
Can be vegetable/synthetic or animal. Compound of ► *oleic acid* with ammonia and salts of sulphur. Antistatic and hair conditioner in cosmetics.

Dioleoylisopropyl Dimonium Methosulfate
Can be vegetable/synthetic or animal. Compound of ► *oleic acid* with ammonia and salts of sulphur. Antistatic and hair conditioner in cosmetics.

Dioleth-8 Phosphate
Can be vegetable or animal. Phosphoric acid salt of ► *oleyl alcohol*. Surfactant and emulsifier in cosmetics.

Dioleyl EDTHP-Monium Methosulfate
Can be vegetable/synthetic or animal. Compound of ► *oleic acid* with ammonia and salts of sulphur. Antistatic and hair conditioner in cosmetics.

Dioleyl Tocopheryl Methylsilanol
Can be vegetable or animal. Compound of ► *oleic acid* and ► *vitamin E*. Antioxidant, skin protecting substance and skin conditioner in cosmetics.

DIPA-Lanolate
From living or killed animals. Chemically altered ► *lanolin*. Emulsifier and surfactant in cosmetics.

Dipalmitoyl Cystine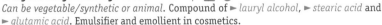
From living or killed animals, can also be microbiological or synthetic. Compound of ► *cetyl alcohol* and ► *cystine*. Antistatic in cosmetics.

Dipalmitoyl Glutathione
Can be vegetable or animal. Compound of ► *palmitic acid* and ► *glutathione.* Hair conditioner in cosmetics.

Dipentaerythrityl Hexacaprylate/Hexacaprate
Mostly vegetable, can also be animal. Compound of ► *caprylic acid* and ► *capric acid.* Emulsifier and smoothing agent in cosmetics.

Dipentaerythrityl Hexaheptanoate/Hexacaprylate/Hexacaprate
Mostly vegetable, can also be animal. Compound of heptanoic acid, ► *caprylic acid* and ► *capric acid.* Emollient and smoothing agent in cosmetics.

Dipentaerythrityl Hexahydroxystearate
Dipentaerythrityl Hexahydroxystearate/Isostearate
Dipentaerythrityl Hexahydroxystearate/Stearate/Rosinate
Can be vegetable or animal. Compounds of ► *stearic acid.* Emulsifiers and smoothing agents in cosmetics.

Dipentaerythrityl Pentaoctanoate/Behenate
Mostly vegetable, can also be partly animal. ► *Fatty acid* compound of ► *caprylic acid.* Emulsifier and smoothing agent in cosmetics.

Dipotassium Guanylate
(E 628. Potassium guanylate)
Microbiological/mineral. Potassium salt of ► *guanylic acid.* Flavour enhancer in foods.

Dipotassium Inosinate
(E 632. Potassium inosinate)
Microbiological/mineral. Potassium salt of ► *inosinic acid.* Flavour enhancer in foods.

Dipropylene Glycol Caprylate
Mostly vegetable/synthetic, can also be partly animal. ► *Glycol* compound of ► *caprylic acid.* Skin conditioner and emollient in cosmetics.

Disodium 5'-Ribonucleotides
(E 635. Sodium 5'-ribonucleotide)
Can be vegetable or animal. Sodium salts of ► *inosinic acid* and ► *guanylic acid.* Obtained from animal or plant cells. Flavour enhancer in foods.

Disodium Caproamphodiacetate
Mostly vegetable/synthetic/mineral, can also be partly animal. Acetic acid compound of ► *capric acid.* Antistatic, surfactant, hair conditioner, cleansing and foaming agent in cosmetics.

Disodium Caproamphodipropionate
Mostly vegetable/synthetic/mineral, can be partly animal. Compound of ► *propionic acid* and ► *capric acid.* Surfactant, hair conditioner, foaming and cleansing agent in cosmetics.

Disodium Capryloamphodiacetate
Mostly vegetable/synthetic/mineral, can also be partly animal. Compound of acetic acid

and ► *caprylic acid*. Antistatic, surfactant, hair conditioner, cleansing agent and foaming agent in cosmetics.

Disodium Capryloamphodipropionate
Mostly vegetable/synthetic/mineral, can also be partly animal. Compound of ► *propionic acid* and ► *caprylic acid*. Surfactant, foaming agent, hair conditioner and cleansing agent in cosmetics.

Disodium Cetearyl Sulfosuccinate
Can be vegetable/synthetic/mineral or animal. Sodium salt of ► *cetostearyl alcohol* and ► *succinic acid*. Surfactant, foaming agent, skin conditioner and cleansing agent in cosmetics.

Disodium Cetyl Phenyl Ether
Mostly vegetable/synthetic/mineral, can also be partly animal. Sodium salt of ► *cetyl alcohol*. Surfactant, cleansing agent, emulsifier and hydrotrope in cosmetics.

Disodium Deceth-n Sulfosuccinate
Mostly vegetable/synthetic/mineral, can also be partly animal. Sodium salt of ► *succinic acid* and ► *decyl alcohol*. Surfactant and cleansing agent in cosmetics.

Disodium Decyl Phenyl Ether Disulfonate
Mostly vegetable/synthetic/mineral, can also be partly animal. Sodium salt of ► *decyl alcohol*. Surfactant, cleansing agent, emulsifier and hydrotrope in cosmetics.

Disodium Diglyceryl Phosphate
Mostly vegetable/mineral, can also be partly animal. Compound of phosphoric acid and ► *glycerol* derivatives. Skin conditioner in cosmetics.

Disodium Guanylate
(E 627. Sodium guanylate)
Microbiological/mineral. Sodium salt of ► *guanylic acid*. Flavour enhancer in foods.

Disodium Hydrogenated Tallow Glutamate
From killed animals. Chemically altered ► *tallow*. Surfactant in cosmetics.

Disodium Inosinate
(E 631. Sodium inosinate)
Microbiological/mineral. Sodium salt of ► *inosinic acid*. Flavour enhancer in foods.

Disodium Isostearamido MEA-Sulfosuccinate
Can be vegetable/synthetic/mineral or animal. Compound of ► *succinic acid* and ► *stearic acid*. Surfactant, skin conditioner and foaming agent in cosmetics.

Disodium Isostearamido MIPA-Sulfosuccinate
Can be vegetable/synthetic/mineral or animal. Compound of ► *succinic acid* and ► *stearic acid*. Surfactant, skin conditioner and foaming agent in cosmetics.

Disodium Isostearoamphodiacetate
Can be vegetable/synthetic/mineral or animal. Acetic acid compound of ► *stearic acid*. Surfactant, foaming agent and cleansing agent in cosmetics.

Disodium Isostearoamphodipropionate

Can be vegetable/synthetic/mineral or animal. Compound of ► *stearic acid* and ► *propionic acid*. Surfactant, foaming agent and cleansing agent in cosmetics.

Disodium Isostearyl Sulfosuccinate

Can be vegetable/mineral or animal. Compound of ► *succinic acid* and ► *stearyl alcohol*. Used as a surfactant, cleansing agent, foaming agent and skin conditioner in cosmetics.

Disodium Laneth-5 Sulfosuccinate

From living or killed animals. Chemically altered ► *lanolin*. Surfactant in cosmetics.

Disodium Malyl Tyrosinate

Mostly from killed animals, can also be microbiological or synthetic. Sodium salt of ► *tyrosine*. Surfactant in cosmetics.

Disodium Oleamido MEA-Sulfosuccinate

Can be vegetable/synthetic/mineral or animal. Sodium salt of ► *succinic acid* and ► *oleic acid*. Surfactant in cosmetics.

Disodium Oleamido MIPA-Sulfosuccinate

Can be vegetable/synthetic/mineral or animal. Sodium salt of ► *succinic acid* and ► *oleic acid*. Surfactant in cosmetics.

Disodium Oleamido PEG-2 Sulfosuccinate

Can be vegetable/synthetic/mineral or animal. Sodium salt of ► *succinic acid* and ► *oleic acid*. Antistatic, surfactant, cleansing agent and foaming agent in cosmetics.

Disodium Oleoamphodipropionate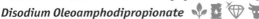

Can be vegetable/synthetic/mineral or animal. Sodium salt of ► *propionic acid* and ► *oleyl alcohol*. Surfactant, cleansing agent, antistatic and foaming agent in cosmetics.

Disodium Oleth-3 Sulfosuccinate

Can be vegetable/synthetic/mineral or animal. Sodium salt of ► *succinic acid* and ► *oleyl alcohol*. Surfactant in cosmetics.

Disodium Oleyl Phosphate

Can be vegetable/synthetic/mineral or animal. Sodium salt of phosphoric acid and ► *oleyl alcohol*. Emulsifier in cosmetics.

Disodium Oleyl Sulfosuccinate

Can be vegetable/synthetic/mineral or animal. Sodium salt of ► *succinic acid* and ► *oleyl alcohol*. Surfactant and cleansing agent in cosmetics.

Disodium PEG-8 Glyceryl Caprylate/Caprate

Mostly vegetable/synthetic/mineral, can also be partly animal. ► *PEG* compound of ► *glycerol*, ► *caprylic acid* and ► *capric acid*. Surfactant and emulsifier in cosmetics.

Disodium PPG-2-Isodeceth-7 Carboxyamphodiacetate

Mostly vegetable/synthetic/mineral, can also be partly animal. ► *PPG* and acetic acid compound of ► *decyl alcohol*. Surfactant in cosmetics.

D

Disodium Stearamido MEA-Sulfosuccinate
Can be vegetable/synthetic/mineral or animal. Compound of ► *succinic acid* and ► *stearic acid*. Surfactant, foam booster, cleansing agent and hydrotrope in cosmetics.

Disodium Steariminodipropionate
Can be vegetable/synthetic/mineral or animal. Compound of ► *stearic acid* and ► *propionic acid*. Antistatic, surfactant, hair conditioner and cleansing agent in cosmetics.

Disodium Stearoamphodiacetate
Can be vegetable/synthetic/mineral or animal. Acetic acid compound of ► *stearic acid*. Antistatic, surfactant, hydrotrope, hair conditioner, cleansing agent and foam booster in cosmetics.

Disodium Stearoyl Glutamate
Can be vegetable/synthetic/mineral or animal. Sodium salt of ► *glutamic acid* and ► *stearic acid*. Surfactant, hair conditioner, skin conditioner and cleansing agent in cosmetics.

Disodium Stearyl Sulfosuccinamate
Can be vegetable/synthetic/mineral or animal. Compound of ► *succinic acid* and ► *stearyl alcohol*. Surfactant in cosmetics.

Disodium Stearyl Sulfosuccinate
Can be vegetable/synthetic/mineral or animal. Compound of ► *succinic acid* and ► *stearyl alcohol*. Surfactant, foam booster, hydrotrope and cleansing agent in cosmetics.

Disodium Tallow Sulfosuccinamate
From killed animals. Chemically altered ► *tallow*. Surfactant, foam booster, hydrotrope and cleansing agent in cosmetics.

Disodium Tallowamphodiacetate
From killed animals. Chemically altered ► *tallow*. Surfactant, foam booster, hydrotrope, cleansing agent and hair conditioner in cosmetics.

Disodium Tallowiminodipropionate
From killed animals. Chemically altered ► *tallow*. Surfactant, antistatic, hair conditioner and cleansing agent in cosmetics.

Disodium Tridecylsulfosuccinate
Mostly vegetable/synthetic/mineral, can also be partly animal. Sodium salt of ► *succinic acid* and ► *decyl alcohol*. Surfactant, foam booster, hydrotrope and cleansing agent in cosmetics.

Distarch Glyceryl Ether
Mostly vegetable/synthetic, can also be partly animal. Compound of starch and ► *glycerol*. Binding agent, anticaking agent and absorbent in cosmetics.

Disteardimonium Hectorite
Can be vegetable/synthetic or animal. Ammonia compound of ► *stearic acid*. Stabilizer and viscosity controlling agent in cosmetics.

Disteareth-6 Dimonium Chloride

Can be vegetable/synthetic or animal. Ammonia compound of ▶ *stearyl alcohol*. Antistatic, emulsifier, surfactant and hair conditioner in cosmetics.

Disteareth-n Lauroyl Glutamate

Can be vegetable/synthetic or animal. Compounds of ▶ *stearyl alcohol*, ▶ *lauric acid* and ▶ *glutamic acid*. Surfactants, hair conditioners and soothing agents in cosmetics.

Distearoylethyl Dimonium Chloride
Distearoylethyl Hydroxyethylmonium Methosulfate
Distearoylpropyltrimonium Chloride
Distearyl Epoxypropylmonium Chloride

Can be vegetable/synthetic or animal. Ammonia compounds of ▶ *stearic acid*. Antistatics and hair conditioners in cosmetics.

Distearyl Ether

Can be vegetable/synthetic or animal. Compound of ▶ *stearyl alcohol*. Skin conditioner in cosmetics.

Distearyl Thiodipropionate

Can be vegetable/synthetic or animal. Compound of ▶ *stearyl alcohol* and ▶ *propionic acid*. Antioxidant in cosmetics.

Distearyldimethylamine Dilinoleate

Can be vegetable/synthetic or animal. Compound of ▶ *stearyl alcohol* and ▶ *linoleic acid*. Antistatic, emollient and hair conditioner in cosmetics.

Distearyldimonium Chloride

(Distearyl dimethyl ammonium chloride [DSDMAC])

Can be vegetable/synthetic or animal. A ▶ *cationic surfactant*, consisting of an ammonium compound of ▶ *stearic acid*. In fabric softeners (no longer in common usage). Antistatic and hair conditioner in cosmetics.

Ditallowamidoethyl Hydroxypropylamine
Ditallowamidoethyl Hydroxypropylmonium Methosulfate
Ditallowdimonium Cellulose Sulfate
Ditallowdimonium Chloride
Ditallowethyl Hydroxyethylmonium Methosulfate
Ditallowoylethyl Hydroxyethylmonium Methosulfate

From killed animals. Various forms of chemically altered ▶ *tallow*. Surfactants, hair conditioners and antistatics in cosmetics.

Ditridecyl Adipate

Mostly vegetable/synthetic, can also be partly animal. Compound of ▶ *decyl alcohol* and ▶ *adipic acid*. Emollient in cosmetics.

Ditridecyl Dimer Dilinoleate

Mostly vegetable/synthetic, can also be partly animal. Compound of ▶ *decyl alcohol* and

► *linoleic acid*. Soothing agent, skin conditioner, emollient, skin conditioner, moisturizer and smoothing agent in cosmetics.

Ditridecyl Sodium Sulfosuccinate

Mostly vegetable/synthetic/mineral, can also be partly animal. Compound of ► *decyl alcohol* and ► *propionic acid*. Antioxidant in cosmetics.

Ditridecyl Thiodipropionate

Mostly vegetable/synthetic, can also be partly animal. Compound of ► *decyl alcohol* and ► *propionic acid*. Antioxidant in cosmetics.

Ditridecyldimonium Chloride

Mostly vegetable/synthetic, can also be partly animal. Ammonium compound of ► *decyl alcohol*. Antistatic, surfactant and hair conditioner in cosmetics.

DNase ► Deoxyribonuclease

DNA

(Deoxyribonucleic acid)
Can be from living or killed animals, or vegetable. A biological molecule present in all living organisms and DNA viruses, and carrier of genetic information. Contains the genes responsible for coding ribonucleic acids and proteins necessary for an organism's biological development and cell metabolism. Skin conditioner in cosmetics.

Docosahexaenoic Acid

(DHA)
From killed animals or vegetable. An ► *omega-3 fatty acid*. Occurs naturally in the body oils of fishes such as salmon and herring as well as marine algae. Obtained from ► *fish oil* or algae. Antistatic and skin conditioner in cosmetics. In nutritional supplements.

Dodecanol ► Lauryl Alcohol

Dodecanedioic Acid/Cetearyl Alcohol/Glycol Copolymer

Mostly vegetable/synthetic, can also be partly animal. Polymer compound of ► *cetostearyl alcohol*. Film forming agent and viscosity controlling agent in cosmetics.

Dodecyl Alcohol ► Lauryl Alcohol

Dodecyl Gallate ► Gallates

Dog Fur. Dog Leather

From killed animals. The skin of dogs, with or without the hair. Used in many parts of the world for a long time, for instance in book printing or for clothing, shoes and accessories, sometimes under false designations. The trade and use of dog skins has been banned in the EU and the United States, but so far not in Canada.

Down (Feathers)

From living or killed animals. Soft, fluffy, warming feathers under the outer feathers, usually from geese or ducks. The feathers are "harvested" by "plucking" (tearing the feathers out manually or with machines). Plucking living animals is banned in North America and Europe, but up to the present day the ban is often circumvented. Tearing out the down and feathers from the animal's bodies inflicts intense pain and bloody injuries. Used as filling/insulation in pillows, quilts, duvets, cushions, jackets and sleeping bags.

Dripping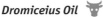

From killed animals. Animal ► *fat* melted out of roasted meats (usually pork, but also from beef). Traditionally used for frying or deep-frying foods, although vegetable fats, such as palm butter or coconut oil, are now more commonly used. Also see ► *frying fat*.

Dromiceius Oil

From killed animals. Oil from the fatty tissue of emus. Emollient in cosmetics.

Dry Milk ► *Milk Powder*

DSDMAC ► *Distearyldimonium Chloride*

Duodenum Suis ► *Organ Extracts*

E

Egg

From living and killed* animals. Developmental stage of birds and reptiles. The term is most commonly used to refer to chickens' eggs from factory farming. Ingredient for cooking and baking, raw material for influencing the properties of foods (baked goods, pasta, etc.) by means of flavour, yellow colour and physical properties (especially protein binding and emulsion). Used as a source of cosmetic ingredients (► *albumen*, ► *cephalins*, ► *ovum*, ► *ovum oil*, ► *ovum powder*, ► *ovum shell powder*, ► *luteum ovi extract*, ► *luteum ovi powder*) and food ingredients (e.g. ► *lecithin*, ► *lutein*, ► *lysozyme*). Used for manufacturing ► *vaccines*.

*Egg "production" inevitably involves killing the "useless" male chicks (hundreds of millions each year in North America alone). The laying hens themselves are killed after 1½ years at the most. (Hens' natural life expectancy can be up to 20 years!)

Egg Protein ► *Albumen*

Egg White ► *Albumen*

Egg Yolk

From living and killed animals (► egg). The yellow part of ► *eggs* that contains and sustains the developing embryo. Used as an ingredient in foods (for instance because of its colour and as an emulsifier) and as a pigment carrier in tempera painting.

Eicosapentaenoic Acid

(EPA)

From killed animals. An ► *omega-3 fatty acid*. Occurs naturally in living organisms, especially in fishes such as salmon and herring. Obtained from ► *fish oil*. Skin conditioner and emollient in cosmetics. In nutritional supplements.

Eiderdown

From living wild animals. ► *Down* feathers of the eider duck. The mother duck uses it to line the nest rather than as insulation for her own body. Eiderdown is collected by humans from the nests and cleaned mechanically. In Canada and Iceland it is collected from occupied nests (without destroying either the nests or their contents), whereas in Germany the down may only be collected from abandoned nests. Used as premium filling for bedcovers and pillows.

Elastin 🐂

From killed animals. An insoluble, elastic fibrous ► *protein*, naturally present in mammalian connective tissue. Obtained from elastic "slaughterhouse waste" rich in connective tissue, such as the nuchal (neck) ligaments and the aortae (largest arteries) of cattle. Smoothing agent and skin conditioner in cosmetics.

Elastin Amino Acids 🐂

(Animal elastin amino acids)
From killed animals. ► *Amino acids* from ► *elastin*. Hair conditioner and skin conditioner in cosmetics.

Elicina ► Snail Cream

Embryo Extract 🐂

From killed animals. Extract from unborn embryos of killed mammals. Moisturizer and skin conditioner in cosmetics.

Enalapril 🌿 ⚗ 🐂

Vegetable/microbiological, can theoretically be partly animal. An ACE inhibitor (pharmaceutical drug that lowers blood pressure). Produced biochemically from ► *proline*. In medication for treating high blood pressure.

E Numbers 🌿 🐂 ▦ ⬠ ⚗

European number codes for food additives. Includes vegetable, animal, synthetic, mineral and microbiological substances. Also see "Food additives" (introduction, page ix).

Enzymes 🌿 ⚗ 🐂

Can be vegetable, microbiological or from killed animals. ► *Proteins* that trigger or regulate biochemical reactions in all living cells, without themselves being altered by the reactions. Obtained from vegetable raw materials, yeast or bacterial cultures, or the organs of killed animals. Examples of enzymes used as ingredients: ► *amylase*, ► *batroxobin*, ► *deoxyribonuclease*, ► *invertase*, ► *lactase*, ► *lactoperoxidase*, ► *lipase*, ► *pancreatin*, ► *pepsin*, ► *proteases*, ► *rennin*, ► *urease*. Used as skin conditioners in cosmetics; in laundry and household detergents with the purpose of actively breaking down proteins, fat and carbohydrates; as food additives (e.g. in baked goods); as active agents in food supplements and medication.

EPA ► Eicosapentaenoic Acid

Epinephrin ► Adrenalin

Equae Lac ► Mare's Milk

Equus Extract 🐂

From killed animals. Extract from body tissue of horses. Skin conditioner in cosmetics.

Ergocalciferol 🌿

(Vitamin D_2)
Vegetable. Variant of ► *vitamin D*. Obtained by UV irradiation of ► *ergosterol*. In fortified foods and food supplements as an alternative to animal vitamin D_3.

Ergosterol 🌱
(Provitamin D$_2$)
Vegetable. Precursor of ► *ergocalciferol*. Occurs in cell membranes of fungi.

Erinoid ► *Galalith*

Estradiol. Estrone ► *Estrogen*

Estrogen 🐄 🐃
(Estrone. Estradiol)
Can be animal or synthetic. Collective term for female sexual hormones, produced especially in the ovaries of female animals, as well as in the adrenal glands and in lesser amounts in the testicles of male animals. The most important variant is estradiol. Obtained from mares' urine, ► *cholesterol* or synthetically from petroleum products. Active agents in oral hormonal contraceptives ("the pill"); for this purpose ethinylestradiol, a synthetic estradiol derivative, is normally used. In tablets/pills, creams, lotions and skin patches for treating hormonal disorders and as hormone substitution, for instance following surgical removal of ovaries or in menopause; in these cases, both synthetic and animal estrogens ("conjugated estrogens" or "extract from the urine of pregnant mares") are used.

Ethinylestradiol ► *Estrogen*

Ethyl Ester of Hydrolyzed Animal Protein 🐄
From killed animals. Chemically/enzymatically altered ► *protein* from various animal tissues. Antistatic, emollient, hair and skin conditioner in cosmetics.

Ethyl Ester of Hydrolyzed Keratin 🐄
From killed or living animals. Chemically altered ► *keratin*. Antistatic, hair and skin conditioner in cosmetics.

Ethyl Ester of Hydrolyzed Silk 🐄
From killed animals. Chemically altered ► *silk*. Antistatic, hair and skin conditioner in cosmetics.

Ethyl Glutamate 🌱 🐃 🐄
Mostly vegetable/synthetic, can theoretically also be partly animal. Compound of ► *glutamic acid*. Antistatic, hair and skin conditioner in cosmetics.

Ethyl Hydroxy Picolinium Lactate 🌱 🐃 🐄
Mostly vegetable/synthetic, can also be partly animal. Hydrocarbon compound of ► *lactic acid*. Skin conditioner in cosmetics.

Ethyl Isostearate 🌱 🐃 🐄
Can be vegetable/synthetic or animal. Ethyl ester of ► *stearic acid*. Used as a solvent in cosmetics.

Ethyl Lactate 🌱 🐃 🐄
Can be vegetable/synthetic or partly animal. Ethyl ester of ► *lactic acid*. Solvent in cosmetics.

Ethyl Minkate
From killed animals. Ethyl ester of ► *mink oil.* Emollient in cosmetics.

Ethyl Morrhuate
From killed animals. Ethyl ester of cod liver oil (► *fish liver oil*). Emollient in cosmetics.

Ethyl Oleate
Can be vegetable/synthetic or animal. Ethyl ester of ► *oleic acid.* Used as an emollient in cosmetics.

Ethyl Serinate
Can be animal or synthetic. Ethyl ester of ► *serine.* Antistatic, hair and skin conditioner in cosmetics.

Ethyl Stearate
Can be vegetable/synthetic or animal. Ethyl ester of ► *stearic acid.* Used as an emollient in cosmetics.

Ethylene Dihydrogenated Tallowamide
From killed animals. Chemically altered ► *tallow.* Emulsifier, viscosity controlling agent and skin conditioner in cosmetics.

Ethylene Distearamide
Can be vegetable/synthetic or animal. Compound of ► *stearic acid.* Viscosity controlling agent in cosmetics.

Ethylhexyl Acetoxystearate
Can be vegetable/synthetic or animal. Acetic acid compound of ► *stearic acid.* Emollient in cosmetics.

Ethylhexyl Caprylate/Caprate
Mostly vegetable/synthetic, can also be partly animal. Compound of ► *caprylic acid* and ► *capric acid.* Skin conditioner and emollient in cosmetics.

Ethylhexyl Gallate ► *Gallates*

Ethylhexyl Glyceryl Palmitate
Mostly vegetable/synthetic, can also be partly animal. Compound of ► *glycerol* and ► *palmitic acid.* Skin conditioner and emollient in cosmetics.

Ethylhexyl Hydroxystearate
Can be vegetable/synthetic or animal. Compound of ► *stearic acid.* Used as an emollient in cosmetics.

Ethylhexyl Hydroxystearate Benzoate
Can be vegetable/synthetic or animal. Compound of ► *stearic acid.* Skin conditioner and emollient in cosmetics.

Ethylhexyl Isopalmitate
Mostly vegetable/synthetic, can also be partly animal. Compound of ► *palmitic acid.* Emollient in cosmetics.

Ethylhexyl Isostearate

Can be vegetable/synthetic or animal. Compound of ► *stearic acid*. Used as an emollient in cosmetics.

Ethylhexyl Linoleoyl Stearate

Can be vegetable/synthetic or animal. Compound of ► *linoleic acid* and ► *stearic acid*. Emulsifier in cosmetics.

Ethylhexyl Oleate

Can be vegetable/synthetic or animal. Compound of ► *oleic acid*. Used as an emollient in cosmetics.

Ethylhexyl Palmitate

Mostly vegetable/synthetic, can also be partly animal. Compound of ► *palmitic acid*. Emollient in cosmetics.

Ethylhexyl Stearate

Can be vegetable/synthetic or animal. Compound of ► *stearic acid*. Used as an emollient in cosmetics.

Ethylhexylglycerin

Mostly vegetable/synthetic, can also be partly animal. Compound of ► *glycerol*. Skin conditioner in cosmetics.

Ethylhexylglyceryl Behenate

Mostly vegetable/synthetic, can also be partly animal. Compound of ► *glycerol* and behenic acid. Emulsifier in cosmetics.

Ethylhexylglyceryl Palmitate

Mostly synthetic/vegetable, can also be partly animal. Compound of ► *glycerol* and ► *palmitic acid*. Emollient in cosmetics.

Eucerit®

From living or killed animals. Trademark of the company Beiersdorf. Highly purified ► *lanolin alcohol*. Key ingredient (emulsifier) of Nivea® creme.

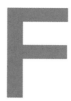

Fat

(Lipids)

Can be vegetable or from living or killed animals. Collective term for various compounds of ► *glycerol* and ► *fatty acids*. Fats are largely insoluble in water. They are also important energy carriers in foods and form important energy reservoirs in animal and plant tissues. Fats that are liquid at room temperature are referred to as "oil." Used in foods, pharmaceutical drugs, cosmetics, lubricants, polishes, paints, and much more. Also used as a source for a multitude of additional ingredients.

Examples of animal fats: ► *fish oil*, ► *lanolin oil*, ► *lard*, ► *marmot oil*, ► *mink oil*, ► *mustela oil*, ► *placental lipids*, ► *silk worm lipids*, ► *sphingolipids* ► *struthio oil*, ► *tallow*.

Examples of vegetable fats: coconut fat, linseed oil, corn oil, nut oils, olive oil, palm butter, rapeseed oil, safflower oil, sunflower oil.

Fat Mimetics

(Fat substitutes)

Can be vegetable or animal. Substances that imitate the sensory properties of ► *fat* without possessing its physical properties (such as the energy content). They are usually carbohydrates (e.g. maltodextrin or carrageenan) or proteins (e.g. Simplesse®, made from ► *whey protein*). Fat mimetics are sometimes also referred to as ► *fat substitutes*, however unlike such synthetic fats, fat mimetics are made using natural raw materials and are heat-unstable, making them unsuitable for frying or baking. Used especially in diet foods, in order to reduce the fat and calorie content.

Fat Substitutes

Can be vegetable/synthetic or animal. Artificial fats that possess the physical properties of fats, but chemically have nothing in common with natural fats. Usually they are compounds of ► *sucrose* with other carbohydrates and ► *fatty acids*, but also paraffins. Used in low-calorie foods, e.g. potato chips. The term "fat substitute" is also used to refer to ► *fat mimetics*.

Fatty Acids

(E 570)

Can be vegetable or from living or killed animals. Acids that are made up of hydrocarbon chains and are largely water-insoluble. Chemically they are subdivided into two groups:

► *saturated fatty acids* and ► *unsaturated fatty acids*. They are the main constituents of all vegetable and animal fats. As ingredients, they can as a matter of principle derive from vegetable fats or fats from living or killed animals. Fatty acids serve as raw materials for a multitude of chemical compounds in cosmetics, foods, household products, industrial processes and much more (also see ► *fatty acid esters*).

Examples of fatty acids that can be of animal origin: ► *arachidonic acid*, ► *butyric acid*, ► *capric acid*, ► *caproic acid*, ► *caprylic acid*, ► *linolenic acid*, ► *linoleic acid*, ► *oleic acid*, ► *palmitic acid*, ► *stearic acid*.

Fatty Acid Esters 🌱 🐮

Can be vegetable or from living or killed animals. Collective term for reaction products of various acids and glycerides of ► *fatty acids*.

Fatty acid esters used as ingredients in foods: ► *fatty acid esters of ascorbic acid*, ► *diacetyl tartaric acid esters of mono- and diglycerides of fatty acids*, ► *citric acid esters of mono- and diglycerides of fatty acids*, ► *acetic acid esters of mono- and diglycerides of fatty acids*, ► *mixed acetic and tartaric acid esters of mono- and diglycerides of fatty acids*, ► *polyglycerol esters of fatty acids*, ► *lactic acid esters of mono- and diglycerides of fatty acids*, ► *tartaric acid esters of mono- and diglycerides of fatty acids*, ► *sucrose esters of fatty acids*.

The fatty acid esters used in cosmetics are too numerous to name here, but these are a few examples: ► *cetearyl palmitate*, ► *cetearyl stearate*, ► *coco-caprylate/caprate*, ► *ethyl lactate*, ► *ethyl minkate*, ► *fish glycerides*, ► *glycereth-17 tallowate*, ► *glyceryl caprate*, ► *glyceryl caprylate*, ► *hexanediol beeswax*, ► *hexyldecyl ester of hydrolyzed collagen*, ► *lactoyl methylsilanol elastinate*.

Fatty Acid Esters of Ascorbic Acid 🌱 🐮

(Ascorbyl palmitate [E 304]. Ascorbyl stearate [E 304ii or E 305])
Can be vegetable or animal. Compounds of ascorbic acid (► *vitamin C*) and ► *palmitic acid* or ► *stearic acid*. Ascorbyl palmitate is obtained primarily from palm oil, but can also be from animal fats. Ascorbyl stearate is obtained from both vegetable and animal fats. Antioxidants and emulsifiers in foods, e.g. spreadable fats. Antioxidants in cosmetics.

Fatty Acid Esters of Glycerol 🌱 🐮

Can be vegetable or from living or killed animals. Term for diverse compounds of different ► *fatty acids* and ► *glycerol*. Are listed in this book alphabetically according to their standardized designations.

Some examples: ► *glyceryl adipate*, ► *glyceryl caprate*, ► *glyceryl caprylate*, ► *glyceryl lanolate*, ► *glyceryl oleate*, ► *glyceryl palmitate*, ► *glyceryl stearate*, ► *polyglyceryl-n caprate*, ► *polyglyceryl-n oleate*, ► *polyglyceryl-n palmitate*, ► *polyglyceryl-n stearate*.

Fatty Alcohols 🌱 🧪 🐮

Can be vegetable, synthetic or animal. Collective term for alcohols with long carbon chains. Primarily obtained from chemical reactions with ► *fatty acids*.

Examples of fatty alcohols: ► *capric alcohol*, ► *capryl alcohol*, ► *cetostearyl alcohol*, ► *cetyl alcohol*, ► *decyl alcohol*, ► *lauryl alcohol*, ► *oleyl alcohol*, ► *stearyl alcohol*.

Feathers

From living or killed animals. Epidermal structures consisting of ► *keratin* that form the outer covering of birds (plumage) and fulfil a number of functions, protecting against water or cold, providing colour (either as camouflage or a means of communication) and enabling flight. Obtained by plucking living or killed animals (also see ► *down*). Filling in pillows, duvets and mattresses, as well as in jackets and sleeping bags. Used as decoration and in ritual objects, as traditional writing implement (quills). Used in large quantities for the industrial production of ► *keratin*.

Felt

From living or killed animals. Fabric of matted fibres from unspun animal ► *hair* or ► *wool* that are mechanically subjected to friction in a soapy solution or in a dry condition using felting needles, creating a stable nonwoven fabric. In clothing and accessories (e.g. jackets, hats, shoes), musical instruments, furniture, insulation and sealings.

Ferrous Lactate

(E 585)

Partly mineral, partly vegetable or animal. Iron salt of ► *lactic acid*. Used for colouring green olives black, for fortifying foods with iron and in food supplements.

Fibrin

From killed animals. A ► *protein* that plays an important part in blood coagulation and hemostasis. Obtained from the ► *blood* of cattle. Used as an adhesive (fibrin glue) for surgical wound closure.

Fibroin ► Serica

Fibronectin

From killed animals. A sugar and ► *protein* compound that plays an important part in the body, in tissue repair and cellular processes. Obtained from the ► *blood* of cattle. Skin conditioner in cosmetics.

Fish

From killed animals. Aquatic poikilothermic (of varying body temperature) vertebrate animals. General term for the flesh of killed fishes of a variety of species. Used as food and food ingredients. Source of ► *fish glue*, ► *fish meal* and ► *fish oil*. Fish tissues are also used as a source of substances such as ► *alkylglycerols*, ► *fish silver*, ► *fish liver oil*, ► *scyllii pellis extract* and ► *thunnus extract*.

Fish Glue

From killed animals. Adhesive obtained by boiling and drying "waste" from industrial fishing. Used in conservation/restoration and plasterwork.

Fish Glycerides

From killed animals. ► *Fatty acid esters* from ► *fish oil*. From commercial fishing. Emollient in cosmetics.

Fish Liver Oil

From killed animals. Oil from the livers of ► *fishes* such as halibut, cod ("cod liver oil" or "gadi iecur oil") or sharks ("shark liver oil" or "squali iecur oil"). In refatting creams, lotions and ointments. In nutritional supplements. Also see ► *fish oil*, ► *hydrogenated shark liver oil*, ► *piscum iecur oil*, ► *salmo oil*, ► *squali iecur oil*.

Fish Meal

From killed animals. Dried, ground ► *fish* or parts thereof. Additive in animal feed, e.g. in aquaculture and for pigs and chickens.

Fish Oil

(Marine oil)

From killed animals. Body or liver oil of ► *fish* from commercial fishing. "Waste product" of ► *fish meal* production. Used as an ingredient in foods, e.g. margarine, in medication and in food supplements, for instance as a source of ► *omega-3 fatty acids*. Also see ► *brevoortia oil*, ► *dromiceius oil*, ► *fish liver oil*, ► *hoplostethus oil*, ► *hydrogenated fish oil*, ► *hydrogenated menhaden oil*, ► *hydrogenated orange roughy oil*, ► *hydrogenated shark liver oil*, ► *piscum iecur oil*, ► *salmon oil*, ► *squali iecur oil*. The term ► *"marine oil"* refers to both fish oil and oils from other marine animals, such as whales and seals.

Fish Silver

(Pearl essence)

From killed animals. Silver shimmering pigment rich in ► *guanine*. Obtained from the scales of killed whitefish. Used in painting and conservation/restoration. In imitation pearls. In cosmetics (e.g. eye shadow, lipstick).

Flavin Mononucleotide ► *Riboflavin-5′-Phosphate*

Flavour Enhancers

Can be animal, vegetable, synthetic or mineral. Collective term for different substances that intensify the flavour of foods and beverages. Canada does not have a definitive list of approved flavour enhancers, but these are some examples of commonly used substances: acesulfame, aspartame, calcium chloride, ► *calcium-5′-ribonucleotide*, ► *dinatrium-5′-ribonucleotide*, erythritol, ► *glutamic acid* and its salts (► *glutamates*), ► *glycine*, ► *guanylic acid* and its salts, ► *inosinic acid* and its salts, magnesium chloride, neohesperidin DC, potassium chloride, ► *succinic acid*, thaumatine, zinc acetate.

Flavouring

Can be vegetable, animal or synthetic. Collective term for substances that have the purpose of imparting a certain taste or smell to a product. Flavourings are obtained from living or killed animals, plants, microorganism (yeasts, bacteria) or synthetic substances. Ingredient in foods and cosmetics. Also see ► *natural flavouring* and the subsequent entries.

Foie Gras

From killed animals. The pathologically enlarged, fattened liver of geese or ducks, regarded as a delicacy and achieved by daily force-feeding large amounts of boiled feed (usually corn) using a metal tube inserted in the esophagus ("gavage"). This practice (but not the import or sale) is banned in several European countries, but not France, where foie gras is legally protected as part of the "cultural and gastronomical heritage."

Foie gras is also produced in the United States and Canada, although the State of California has banned both force-feeding and the sale of products that are the result of force-feeding effective July 1, 2012.

Folic Acid

(Folate. Vitamin B₉)

Synthetic/vegetable, can theoretically also be animal. A water-soluble ► *vitamin* that plays an important part in cell metabolism. Occurs naturally in leafy vegetables and whole grain products, as well as other vegetable and animal tissues. Industrial production from ► *glutamic acid*. Skin conditioner in cosmetics. In nutritional supplements and medications.

Freshwater Pearls ► *Pearls*

Frying Fat

Can be vegetable or from killed animals. ► *Fat* for frying/deep-frying foods. The composition can vary according to countries and regions. In Canada, vegetable fats are most commonly used, e.g. palm butter or coconut fat. Can also be a mixture of different vegetable and/or animal fats, or pure animal fat (e.g. ► *dripping* or ► *suet*).

Fumaric Acid

(E 297)

Vegetable or synthetic. An organic acid that occurs naturally in plants, fungi and lichens. Industrial production from petroleum products. Buffering agent in cosmetics. Source of additional cosmetic ingredients, e.g. compounds of ► *fatty acids*. Acidifier in foods.

Fungi ► *Mushrooms*

Fur

(Pelt)

From killed animals. The ► *hair* of mammals. Sometimes "fur" means only the hair, sometimes the entire coat of hair. In terms of usage as a product by humans, "fur" generally means the skin with the hair still attached, stripped off the animal and processed into ► *leather* (also called "pelt"). In clothing and fashion accessories, e.g. coats, hats, gloves, boots, trimmings, handbags, etc. Depending on the size of the animal and the article, a single item of clothing can be made of the fur of dozens of animals. Fur is obtained from many different animal species, whether rodents (such as muskrats, chinchillas and squirrels), hares and rabbits, members of the weasel family (e.g. minks, otters and sables), caniforms (such as foxes, dogs and wolves) and feliforms (such as cats, civets or leopards), bovines, sheep or marsupials. Dog and cat fur are banned in the European Union and the United States, but not in Canada. Also see ► *wool*.

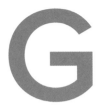

G

GABA ► *Aminobutyric Acid*

Gadi Iecur Oil ► *Fish Liver Oil*

Galalith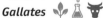
(Erinoid)
From living and killed animals (► milk). Synthetic plastic manufactured from ► *casein* in compound with formaldehyde. One of the first plastics ever made, it was used in large amounts during the first half of the twentieth century, for instance for buttons, combs, jewellery, handles, radio cases and insulation for electric cables, but has now been almost entirely replaced by synthetic oil-derived plastics. It is still used on a very small scale, for instance in some knitting needles.

Gallates
Mostly vegetable or microbiological, but can also be from killed animals. Compounds of ► *gallic acid* (propyl gallate, octyl gallate, dodecyl gallate). Antioxidant in foods and cosmetics.

Gall. Gall Soap ► *Ox Gall*

Gallic Acid
Mostly vegetable or microbiological, but can also be from killed animals. A component of vegetable tannins. Occurs naturally in oak bark and ► *oak apples*, as well as green tea. Usually obtained industrially from moulds, but also from oak apples. Antioxidant in foods and cosmetics. Used for making iron gall ink and tanning leather.

Gallus Extract
From killed animals. Extract obtained from the enzymatic decomposition of rooster (*Gallus*) cockscomb. Moisturizer and skin conditioner in cosmetics.

Gamma-Tocopherol ► *Vitamin E*

Gelatin
(Gelatine)
From killed animals. A gel-forming ► *protein*, obtained from ► *collagen* in connective tissue, e.g. skin and bone, especially from cattle and pigs. Used as a gelling agent, binding agent and thickener in foods (confectionery, desserts, cakes, etc. as well as meat

products, e.g. as ► *aspic*). Ingredient in many processed foods. Used for fining wine, fruit juice and other beverages. Viscosity controlling agent and film forming agent in cosmetics. Pharmaceutical excipient in hard and soft capsules, pills and tablets. Active agent in some infusion solutions. In hemostatic surgical sponges and some hydrocolloid wound dressings. Major constituent in the emulsion layer of photographic films (negatives, X-ray film, holograms, etc.) and papers (e.g. photographic prints and paper for inkjet printers). Auxiliary agent in painting and conservation/restoration, plaster work, etc. Modelling substance in make-up and special effects (film and theatre). Diverse uses as an auxiliary agent in many industrial processes, such as metalworking (e.g. in foundries and for electronics components such as circuits and batteries), in ammunition and explosives production. Used in cosmetic surgery in the form of anti-wrinkle injections.

Gelatin/Keratin Amino Acids/Lysine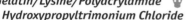
Hydroxypropyltrimonium Chloride
From killed animals. ► *Amino acids* from ► *gelatin* and ► *keratin*. Antistatic, hair and skin conditioner in cosmetics.

Gelatin/Lysine/Polyacrylamide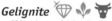
Hydroxypropyltrimonium Chloride
From killed animals. Chemically altered ► *gelatin*. Antistatic and hair conditioner in cosmetics.

Gelignite
(Blasting gelatin. Explosive jelly)
Can be mineral/vegetable or partly animal. An explosive consisting of ► *nitroglycerin* and cotton treated with nitric acid. Used in mining, for instance.

Gellan
(E 418)
Vegetable/microbiological. A polysaccharide produced by bacteria. ► *Gelling agent* in foods.

Gelling Agents
(Thickeners)
Can be vegetable or animal. Substances that absorb fluids (mostly water), swell and form viscous solutions or gels. Can be animal (especially ► *gelatin*) or vegetable (e.g. agar-agar, carrageenan and other algal extracts or ► *gellan*, pectin and other saccharides). Used for gelling or thickening foods, e.g. preserves, desserts and ► *aspic*. In many processed foods.

Ghee ► *Clarified Butter*

Glaze
(Icing)
Can be vegetable or animal. Coating applied to foods. Sweet glazes, e.g. chocolate glaze, often contain ► *fats* and emulsifiers, which can be of both animal or vegetable origin. Used for coating confectionery, cakes and pastries, and ice cream.

Glucocorticoids ► Corticosteriods

Glucosamine
From killed animals. An amino sugar compound. Obtained from ► *chitin* from ► *crustaceans*. Used as a dietary supplement for treating arthroses (benefit not scientifically verified). Hair and skin conditioner in cosmetics.

Glucose Glutamate
Vegetable, can theoretically also be partly animal. Sugar compound of ► *glutamic acid*. Humectant, hair and skin conditioner, and antistatic in cosmetics.

Glue
From killed animals, vegetable or synthetic. Liquid or semiliquid adhesive substances (can be animal, vegetable or synthetic). Animal glue consists of animal ► *proteins*, especially ► *gelatin* (obtained by boiling animal tissues: ► *bone glue*, ► *fish glue*, ► *isinglass*, ► *rabbit-skin glue*, ► *skin glue*) or ► *casein* (e.g. wood glue). Animal glues are traditionally used in paper and wood processing, bookbinding, painting, conservation/restoration, and for making musical instruments and furniture.

Glutamates
Vegetable, can theoretically also be partly animal. Salts and esters of ► *glutamic acid*: sodium glutamate (E 621), monosodium glutamate (MSG), potassium glutamate (E 622), calcium diglutamate (E 623), ammonium glutamate (E 624), magnesium glutamate (E 625). Occurs naturally in animal and vegetable tissues, also in fermented foods (e.g. soy sauce). Responsible for the basic taste "umami" (savoury, such as the flavour of meat or roasted foods). Can be obtained from animal tissues, however commercial production is based on the fermentation of starch products. Used as a flavour enhancer in seasonings. Hair and skin conditioners and surfactants in cosmetics. The glutamates named here and used as flavour enhancers are of vegetable origin, but the glutamates used in cosmetics can be chemically processed with the aid of animal substances. These glutamates are listed in this book according to their standardized INCI names.

Glutamic Acid
(E 620. L-glutamic acid. L-glutamate)
Vegetable, can theoretically also be animal. Nonessential ► *amino acid*. Occurs naturally in vegetable and animal tissues. Can be obtained from animal tissues, however commercial production is based on the fermentation of starch products. Flavour enhancer in foods. Antistatic, humectant and hair conditioner in cosmetics.

Glutamine
(L-glutamin[e], Levoglutamide)
Vegetable, can theoretically also be animal. An ► *amino acid* and salt of ► *glutamic acid*. Occurs naturally in vegetable and animal tissues. Produced via large-scale fermentation of glutamic acid. Hair and skin conditioner in cosmetics.

Glutamyl Histamine
Vegetable, can theoretically also be animal. Compound of ► *glutamine* and the natural messenger substance histamine. Hair conditioner in cosmetics.

Glutathione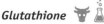
Can be from killed animals or microbiological. Compound of the amino acids ► *glutamic acid*, ► *cysteine* and ► *glycine*. Occurs naturally in almost all animal and vegetable cells. Can be obtained from liver and muscle, as well as from yeast cultures. Used as food supplement (antioxidant) and for the complementary treatment of cancer. Skin conditioner in cosmetics.

Glycereth-5 Lactate
Can be vegetable/synthetic or partly animal. Compound of ► *glycerol* and ► *lactic acid*. Emulsifier, solvent and emollient in cosmetics.

Glycereth-6 Laurate
Can be vegetable/synthetic or partly animal. Compound of ► *glycerol* and ► *lauric acid*. Surfactant and emulsifier in cosmetics.

Glycereth-7 Benzoate
Can be vegetable/synthetic or partly animal. Compound of ► *glycerol* and benzoic acid. Emulsifier, solvent, emulsion stabilizer and skin conditioner in cosmetics.

Glycereth-7 Diisononanoate
Can be vegetable/synthetic or partly animal. Compound of ► *glycerol* and vegetable nonanoic acid. Emulsifier, solvent, emulsion stabilizer and skin conditioner in cosmetics.

Glycereth-7 Hydroxystearate/IPDI Copolymer
Can be vegetable/synthetic or animal. Compound of ► *stearic acid* and ► *glycerol*. Film forming agent in cosmetics.

Glycereth-7 Triacetate
Can be vegetable/synthetic or partly animal. Compound of ► *glycerol* and acetic acid. Emollient in cosmetics.

Glycereth-7/IPDI Copolymer
Can be vegetable/synthetic or partly animal. Polymer compound of ► *glycerol*. Skin conditioner, viscosity controlling agent and film forming agent in cosmetics.

Glycereth-8 Hydroxystearate
Can be vegetable/synthetic or animal. Compound of ► *stearic acid* and ► *glycerol*. Emulsifier, emulsion stabilizer, surfactant and emollient in cosmetics.

Glycereth-17 Tallowate
From killed animals. Chemically altered ► *tallow*. Surfactant and emulsifier in cosmetics.

Glycereth-20 Stearate
Glycereth-25 PCA Isostearate
Can be vegetable/synthetic or animal. Compound of ► *glycerol* and ► *stearic acid*. Emulsifiers, emollients in cosmetics.

Glycereth-26 Phosphate
Can be synthetic/vegetable/mineral or partly animal. Phosphoric acid salt of ► *glycerol*. Emulsifier and chelating agent in cosmetics.

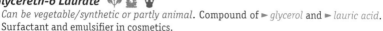

Glycereth-n

Can be synthetic/vegetable or partly animal. ► *PEG* compounds of the alcohol ► *glycerol.* Humectants, solvents and viscosity controlling agents in cosmetics.

Glycerides

(Acylglycerols)

Can be vegetable, synthetic or animal. Compounds of the alcohol ► *glycerol* with a maximum of three fatty acids (mono-, di- and triglycerides). Obtained from animal and vegetable fats, also partly from petroleum derivatives. In margarine, baking mixtures, confectionery and other foods (e.g. ► *mono- and diglycerides of fatty acids*), and cosmetics (e.g. ► *fish glycerides,* ► *glyceryl tallowate,* ► *lard glyceride,* ► *tall oil glycerides*), also further processed (e.g. ► *acetylated hydrogenated tallow glyceride,* ► *hydroxylated milk glycerides,* ► *lactic acid esters of mono- and diglycerides of fatty acids,* ► *PEG-8 hydrogenated fish glycerides,* ► *tartaric acid esters of mono- and diglycerides of fatty acids*).

Glycerin/Oxybutylene Copolymer Stearyl Ether

Can be vegetable/synthetic or animal. Compound of ► *glycerol* and ► *stearyl alcohol.* Emollient in cosmetics.

Glycerol

(Glycerin. Glycerine. E 422)

Mostly vegetable, can also be from killed animals. Viscous, sweet-tasting alcohol. By-product of the saponification/esterification of fats and oils, earlier in large quantities from animal fats, today obtained principally from vegetable oils, e.g. as a byproduct of biodiesel production. Humectant and solvent in cosmetics, foods, tobacco and pharmaceutical drugs. In lubricants, transmission oils, brake fluids, antifreeze and plastics. As nitroglycerin in medication and explosives.

Glycerol Diacetate ► *Diacetin*

Glycerol Monostearate ► *Glyceryl Stearate*

Glycerol Stearate ► *Glyceryl Stearate*

Glycerol Stearate, Self-emulsifying ► *Glyceryl Stearate SE*

Glycerol Trinitrate ► *Nitroglycerin*

Glycerol Tristearate ► *Tristearin*

Glyceryl Abietate

Can be vegetable/synthetic or partly animal. Compound of ► *glycerol* and vegetable abietic acid. Emollient in cosmetics.

Glyceryl Adipate

Can be vegetable/synthetic or partly animal. Compound of ► *glycerol* and ► *adipic acid.* Emollient in cosmetics.

Glyceryl Arachidate

Can be vegetable/synthetic or partly animal. Compound of ► *glycerol* and ► *arachidic acid.* Emollient and emulsifier in cosmetics.

Glyceryl Arachidonate
Can be vegetable/synthetic/microbiological or animal. Compound of ► *glycerol* and ► *arachidonic acid*. Emollient and emulsifier in cosmetics.

Glyceryl Behenate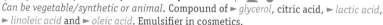
Can be vegetable/synthetic or partly animal. Compound of ► *glycerol* and vegetable behenic acid. Emollient and emulsifier in cosmetics.

Glyceryl Caprate
Can be vegetable/synthetic or partly animal. Compound of ► *glycerol* and ► *capric acid*. Emollient in cosmetics.

Glyceryl Caprylate
Can be vegetable/synthetic or partly animal. Compound of ► *glycerol* and ► *caprylic acid*. Emollient and emulsifier in cosmetics.

Glyceryl Caprylate/Caprate
Can be vegetable/synthetic or partly animal. Compound of ► *glycerol*, ► *capric acid* and ► *caprylic acid*. Emollient and emulsifier in cosmetics.

Glyceryl Citrate/Lactate/Linoleate/Oleate
Can be vegetable/synthetic or animal. Compound of ► *glycerol*, citric acid, ► *lactic acid*, ► *linoleic acid* and ► *oleic acid*. Emulsifier in cosmetics.

Glyceryl Collagenate
From killed animals. Chemically altered ► *collagen*. Hair and skin conditioner, and film forming agent in cosmetics.

Glyceryl Diacetate ► *Diacetin*

Glyceryl Diarachidate
Can be vegetable/synthetic or partly animal. Compound of ► *glycerol* and ► *arachidic acid*. Emollient in cosmetics.

Glyceryl Dibehenate
Glyceryl Dierucate
Can be vegetable/synthetic or partly animal. Compounds of ► *glycerol* and vegetable behenic acid or erucic acid. Emollients in cosmetics.

Glyceryl Dihydroxystearate
Can be vegetable/synthetic or animal. Compound of ► *glycerol* and ► *stearic acid*. Emollient in cosmetics.

Glyceryl Diisopalmitate
Can be vegetable/synthetic or partly animal. Compound of ► *glycerol* and ► *palmitic acid*. Emollient in cosmetics.

Glyceryl Diisostearate
Can be vegetable/synthetic or animal. Compound of ► *glycerol* and ► *stearic acid*. Emollient, emulsifier and opacifier in cosmetics.

G

Glyceryl Dilaurate

Can be vegetable/synthetic or partly animal. Compound of ► *glycerol* and ► *lauric acid.* Emollient and emulsifier in cosmetics.

Glyceryl Dilinoleate

Can be vegetable/synthetic or partly animal. Compound of ► *glycerol* and ► *linoleic acid.* Emollient in cosmetics.

Glyceryl Dimyristate

Can be vegetable/synthetic or partly animal. Compound of ► *glycerol* and ► *myristic acid.* Emollient in cosmetics.

Glyceryl Dioleate

Can be vegetable/synthetic or animal. Compound of ► *glycerol* and ► *oleic acid.* Emollient in cosmetics.

Glyceryl Dipalmitate

Can be vegetable/synthetic or partly animal. Compound of ► *glycerol* and ► *palmitic acid.* Emollient and emulsifier in cosmetics.

Glyceryl Dipalmitoleate

Can be vegetable/synthetic or partly animal. Compound of ► *glycerol* and ► *palmitoleic acid.* Emollient in cosmetics.

Glyceryl Diricinoleate

Can be vegetable/synthetic or partly animal. Compound of ► *glycerol* and vegetable ricinoleic acid. Emollient in cosmetics.

Glyceryl Distearate

Can be vegetable/synthetic or animal. Compound of ► *glycerol* and ► *stearic acid.* Antistatic and emollient in cosmetics.

Glyceryl Erucate

Can be vegetable/synthetic or partly animal. Compound of ► *glycerol* and vegetable erucic acid. Emollient and emulsifier in cosmetics.

Glyceryl Ethylhexanoate Dimethoxycinnamate

Can be vegetable/synthetic or partly animal. Compound of ► *glycerol,* ► *caproic acid* and vegetable cinnamic acid. UV absorber in cosmetics.

Glyceryl Ethylhexanoate/Stearate/Adipate

Can be vegetable/synthetic or partly animal. Compound of ► *glycerol,* ► *caproic acid,* ► *stearic acid* and ► *adipic acid.* Emollient in cosmetics.

Glyceryl Glycyrrhetinate

Can be vegetable/synthetic or partly animal. Compound of ► *glycerol* and ► *glycyrrhizin.* Emulsifier in cosmetics.

Glyceryl Hydrogenated Rosinate

Can be vegetable/synthetic or partly animal. Compound of ► *glycerol* and vegetable acids from tree resin. Film forming agent in cosmetics.

Glyceryl Lanolate

From living or killed animals. Compound of ► *glycerol* and ► *lanolin.* Antistatic, emollient and emulsifier in cosmetics.

Glyceryl Laurate

Can be vegetable or partly animal. Compound of ► *glycerol* and ► *lauric acid.* Emollient and emulsifier in cosmetics.

Glyceryl Laurate SE

Can be vegetable or partly animal. Variant of ► *glyceryl laurate.* Emulsifier in cosmetics.

Glyceryl Laurate/Oleate

Can be vegetable or animal. Compound of ► *glycerol,* ► *lauric acid* and ► *oleic acid.* Emollient in cosmetics.

Glyceryl Linoleate

Mostly vegetable, can also be partly animal. Compound of ► *glycerol* and ► *linoleic acid.* Emollient and emulsifier in cosmetics.

Glyceryl Linolenate

Mostly vegetable, can also be partly animal. Compound of ► *glycerol* and ► *linolenic acid.* Emollient in cosmetics.

Glyceryl Monostearate ► *Glyceryl Stearate*

Glyceryl Montanate

Mostly vegetable/mineral, can also be partly animal. Compound of ► *glycerol* and ► *montan wax.* Emulsifier in cosmetics.

Glyceryl Myristate

Mostly vegetable, can also be animal. Compound of ► *glycerol* and ► *myristic acid.* Emollient and emulsifier in cosmetics.

Glyceryl Oleate

Can be vegetable or animal. Compound of ► *glycerol* and ► *oleic acid.* Emollient and emulsifier cosmetics.

Glyceryl Oleate SE

Can be vegetable or animal. Variant of ► *glyceryl oleate.* Emulsifier in cosmetics.

Glyceryl Oleate/Elaidate

Can be vegetable or animal. Compound of ► *glycerol,* ► *oleic acid* and elaidic acid (fatty acid from hydrogenated fats). Skin conditioner, emollient, surfactant and emulsifier in cosmetics.

Glyceryl Palmitate

Mostly vegetable, can also be animal. Compound of ► *glycerol* and ► *palmitic acid.* Emollient in cosmetics.

Glyceryl Palmitate Lactate

Mostly vegetable, can also be animal. Compound of ► *glycerol,* ► *palmitic acid* and ► *lactic acid.* Emollient and emulsifier in cosmetics.

Glyceryl Palmitate/Stearate

Mostly vegetable, can also be animal. Compound of ► *glycerol,* ► *palmitic acid* and ► *stearic acid.* Emollient in cosmetics.

Glyceryl Palmitoleate

Can be vegetable or animal. Compound of ► *glycerol* and ► *palmitoleic acid.* Emulsifier in cosmetics.

Glyceryl Pentadecanoate

Mostly vegetable, can also be animal. Compound of ► *glycerol* and ► *capric acid.* Surfactant and emulsifier in cosmetics.

Glyceryl Polyacrylate

Mostly vegetable/synthetic, can also be partly animal. Compound of ► *glycerol* and acrylics. Film forming agent in cosmetics.

Glyceryl Polymethacrylate

Mostly vegetable/synthetic, can also be partly animal. Compound of ► *glycerol* and acrylics. Viscosity controlling agent in cosmetics.

Glyceryl Ricinoleate

Mostly vegetable, can also be partly animal. Compound of ► *glycerol* and ricinoleic acid (of vegetable origin). Emollient in cosmetics.

Glyceryl Ricinoleate SE

Mostly vegetable, can also be partly animal. Compound of ► *glycerol* and ricinoleic acid (of vegetable origin). Skin conditioner, emollient, surfactant and emulsifier in cosmetic products.

Glyceryl Rosinate

Mostly vegetable, can also be partly animal. Compound of ► *glycerol* and vegetable acids from tree resin. Film forming agent in cosmetics.

Glyceryl Sesquioleate

Can be vegetable or animal. Compound of ► *glycerol* and ► *oleic acid.* Emollient and emulsifier in cosmetics.

Glyceryl Starch

Mostly vegetable, can also be partly animal. Compound of ► *glycerol* and starch. Absorbing and binding agent in cosmetics.

Glyceryl Stearate

(Glyceryl monostearate. Glycerol monostearate)
Can be vegetable/synthetic or animal. Compound of ► *glycerol* and ► *stearic acid.* Emollient and emulsifier in cosmetics.

Glyceryl Stearate Citrate

Can be vegetable/synthetic or animal. Compound of ► *glycerol,* ► *stearic acid* and citric acid. Emollient, skin conditioner and emulsifier in cosmetics.

Glyceryl Stearate, Self-emulsifying ► Glyceryl Stearate SE

Glyceryl Stearate SE

(Glycerol stearate, self-emulsifying. Glyceryl stearate, self-emulsifying.)
Can be vegetable/synthetic or animal. Compound of ► *glycerol* and ► *stearic acid*. Emulsifier in cosmetics.

Glyceryl Triacetate ► *Triacetin*

Glyceryl Trinitrate ► *Nitroglycerin*

Glyceryl Tristearate ► *Tristearin*

Glycine

(E 640. Glycine and its sodium salt. Aminoacetic acid)
Mostly from killed animals, can also be synthetic or microbiological. A sweet-tasting nonessential ► *amino acid*. Important constituent of almost all ► *proteins*, with an important role in metabolism. Primarily found in ► *collagen*. Obtained for instance from cartilage or ► *gelatin*. Synthetically produced from chloroacetic acid and ammonia. Genetically produced using microorganisms. Antistatic, buffering agent, skin and hair conditioner in cosmetics. Flavour enhancer in sweet foods. Constituent of infusion solutions for parenteral nutrition.

Glycine Soja Extract

as well as
Glycine Soja Flour, Glycine Soja Germ Extract, Glycine Soja Oil, Glycine Soja Oil Unsaponifiables, Glycine Soja Protein, Glycine Soja Sprout Extract and Glycine Soja Sterol
Vegetable. Various products (flour, proteins, oils, etc.) of the soybean (*Glycine soja*). Not to be confused with the amino acid ► *glycine*. Used in cosmetics (e.g. skin and hair conditioners, and emollients) and foods (e.g. soy flour, soy oil and soy protein).

Glycogen

From killed animals. Polysaccharide that serves as energy storage in liver and muscle cells and is converted to blood sugar (glucose) as needed. Obtained from ► *oysters*, other ► *bivalves* or animal liver or muscle cells. Skin conditioner in cosmetics.

Glycol

(Ethandiol. [Mono]Ethylene glycol [MEG])
Synthetic. An alcohol. Obtained from petroleum products. Solvent, viscosity controlling agent and humectant in cosmetics. Is not itself animal, but part of many compounds of animal ► *fatty acids* (also see the following entries).

Glycol Cetearate

Can be vegetable/synthetic or animal. Compound of ► *glycol*, ► *stearic acid* and ► *palmitic acid*. Emulsion stabilizer, emollient, skin conditioner, stabilizer and emulsifier in cosmetics.

Glycol Diethylhexanoate

Can be vegetable/synthetic or partly animal. Compound of ► *glycol* and ► *caproic acid*. Emollient, skin conditioner and viscosity controlling agent in cosmetics.

Glycol Dioleate 🌱 ⬛ 🐃
Can be vegetable/synthetic or animal. Compound of ► *glycol* and ► *oleic acid*. Emollient, skin conditioner and viscosity controlling agent in cosmetics.

Glycol Distearate 🌱 ⬛ 🐃
Can be vegetable/synthetic or animal. Compound of ► *glycol* and ► *stearic acid*. Emollient, skin conditioner, emulsifier, opacifier and viscosity controlling agent in cosmetics, also used as a pearlescent.

Glycol Ditallowate 🐃
From killed animals. Chemically altered ► *tallow*. Emollient, viscosity controlling agent, opacifier and skin conditioner in cosmetics.

Glycol Ethylhexanoate 🌱 ⬛ 🐃
Mostly vegetable/synthetic, can also be partly animal. Compound of ► *glycol* and ► *caproic acid*. Emulsifier and skin conditioner in cosmetics.

Glycol Hydroxystearate 🌱 ⬛ 🐃
Can be vegetable/synthetic or animal. Compound of ► *glycol* and ► *stearic acid*. Emollient, skin conditioner, emulsifier and opacifier in cosmetics.

Glycol Oleate 🌱 ⬛ 🐃
Can be vegetable/synthetic or animal. Compound of ► *glycol* and ► *oleic acid*. Antistatic, emulsifier, emollient and skin conditioner in cosmetics.

Glycol Palmitate 🌱 ⬛ 🐃
Can be vegetable/synthetic or partly animal. Compound of ► *glycol* and ► *palmitic acid*. Emulsifier, opacifier and skin conditioner in cosmetics.

Glycol Stearate 🌱 ⬛ 🐃
Can be vegetable/synthetic or animal. Compound of ► *glycol* and ► *stearic acid*. Emollient, emulsifier, opacifier and surfactant in cosmetics.

Glycol Stearate SE 🌱 ⬛ 🐃
Can be vegetable/synthetic or animal. Compound of ► *glycol* and ► *stearic acid*. Emulsifier and surfactant in cosmetics.

Glycolamide Stearate 🌱 ⬛ 🐃
Can be vegetable/synthetic or animal. Compound of ► *glycol* and ► *stearic acid*. Skin conditioner in cosmetics.

Glycoproteins 🐃
From living and killed animals (► milk). ► *Protein* and saccharide compounds from ► *whey*. Skin and hair conditioner in cosmetics.

Glycosaminoglycans 🐃
(Mucopolysaccharides)
From killed animals. Polysaccharide compounds, including ► *heparin*, ► *hyaluronic acid* and ► *chondroitin sulfate*. Obtained from the skin, connective tissue or internal organs of mammals, or from ► *bivalves*). Emollient, skin conditioner and film forming agent in

cosmetics. In nutritional supplements and the complemetary treatment of rheumatic complaints and arthritis.

Glycosphingolipids
From killed animals. Carbohydrate and fat compounds belonging to the group of the ► *sphingolipids*. Emollient and skin conditioner in cosmetics.

Glycyl Glycine
Mostly from killed animals, can also be synthetic or microbiological. Variant of ► *glycine*. Hair and skin conditioner in cosmetics.

Glycyrrhetinic Acid
Vegetable. Degradation product of ► *glycyrrhizin*. Skin conditioner in cosmetics.

Glycyrrhetinyl Stearate
Can be vegetable/synthetic or animal. Compound of ► *glycyrrhetinic acid* and ► *stearic acid*. Humectant and skin conditioner in cosmetics.

Glycyrrhizin
(Glycyrrhizinic acid. Glycyrrhizic acid)
Vegetable. Saccharide, naturally occurs for instance in licorice root. Humectant and skin conditioner in cosmetics.

Goat Butter
(Caprae butyrum)
From living animals. Semi-firm fat from ► *goat milk* (also see ► *butter*). Skin conditioner and emollient in cosmetics.

Goat Cheese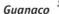
From living animals. ► *Cheese* from ► *goat milk*. Food and food ingredient.

Goat Milk
(Caprae lac)
From living animals. ► *Milk* from goats. Skin conditioner in cosmetics. Food and food ingredient.

Grège ► Silk

Guanaco
From living or killed animals. ► *Wool* or pelt (► *fur*) of a South American camelid. In textiles, clothing, etc.

Guanidine
Synthetic. An organic base, derivative of ► *guanine*. Occurs naturally in ► *arginine*, ► *creatine* and ► *creatinine*. Industrial production from ► *urea*. Used for manufacturing plastics and explosives. Source for cosmetic ingredients.

Guanidine Carbonate
Synthetic. Compound of ► *guanidine*. Industrially produced from ► *guanidine*. Buffering agent and skin conditioner in cosmetics. Used for manufacturing antibiotics, in flame retardants and in explosives.

Guanidine HCl
Synthetic. Compound of ► *guanidine*. Buffering agent in cosmetics.

Guanidine Phosphate
Synthetic. Compound of ► *guanidine*. Skin conditioner in cosmetics.

Guanine
(CI 75170)
Can be from killed animals or synthetic. One of the bases of ► *RNA* and ► *DNA*. In all animal and vegetable tissues. Pearlescent constituent of fish scales (► *fish silver*). Industrially manufactured from the scales and skin of ► *fish*. Can also be produced from ► *uric acid*. Opacifier and colourant (pearlescent pigment) in cosmetics, e.g. shampoos, nail polish, eye shadow. Pearlescent in paints, lacquers and plastics.

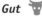

Guanosin Monophosphate ► *Guanylic Acid*

Guanosine
From killed animals, microbiological or vegetable. Compound of ► *guanine* and a saccharide, constituent of ► *RNA* and ► *DNA*. Skin conditioner and opacifier in cosmetics.

Guanylic Acid
(E 626. Guanylate. Guanosine monophosphate [GMP])
Can be from killed animals, microbiological or vegetable. Phosphoric acid ester of ► *guanosine*. Occurs naturally in all living cells. Can be produced from dried ► *fish*. Can also be produced from dried seaweed or with the aid of microorganisms. Guanylic acid and its salts disodium guanylate, dipotassium guanylate and calcium guanylate are used as flavour enhancers in foods, often in combination with ► *glutamates*.

Gum Lac ► *Shellac*

Gut
(Natural gut)
From killed animals. The intestine, the tube-shaped part of the digestive tract between the stomach and anus of animals (in this context, mammals). Is responsible for digesting food, regulating the body's fluid balance and excreting metabolic end products. Is obtained especially from industrial animal slughtering. Used as ► *gut strings*, and as skin for meat sausages.

Gut Strings
From killed animals. Strong, ► *collagen*-rich strings made from the ► *gut* of mammals. Used in surgical sutures (► *catgut*) and as strings for musical instruments and tennis rackets.

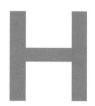

Hair

From living or killed animals. Filaments comprising ► *horn* that grow from and cover the skin of mammals, forming the ► *fur* or ► *wool*. Hair fulfills a variety of important biological functions, especially thermal insulation, protection against external influences and sensory perception (touch). Also plays an important part in the appearance of animals (e.g. camouflage), sometimes also as part of visual signals. Hair from a multitude of domesticated and feral species is used, e.g. badgers, beavers, camelids, cattle, goats, horses, pigs, rabbits, squirrels and weasels. Obtained by shearing or plucking the fur of living or killed animals. Used in knitted and woven textiles for clothing, in blankets, carpets, mattresses, furniture, etc. Also in wigs, brushes and brooms. Also see: ► *badger hair*, ► *bristles*, ► *brushes*, ► *camel hair*, ► *felt*, ► *horsehair*, ► *wool*.

Hard Fat

(Adeps solidus)

Vegetable, can be partly animal. Solid mixed ► *glycerides* with a high proportion of ► *saturated fatty acids* (especially ► *lauric acid*) and a defined melting point. Obtained from palm kernel oil and coconut oil, hydrogenated and esterified with ► *glycerol*. Used as the base (carrier substance) for medicinal suppositories.

Hartshorn. Hartshorn Salt ► *Ammonium Carbonate*

Heart Extract

From killed animals. Extract from animals' hearts. Skin conditioner in cosmetics.

Heart Hydrolysate

From killed animals. Chemically altered heart tissue from killed mammals. Anticaking agent and hair conditioner in cosmetics.

Hematin

From killed animals. Iron compound from the red blood cells in the ► *blood* of killed animals. Hair conditioner in cosmetics.

Hemoglobin

From killed animals. An iron-containing ► *protein* in red blood cells in the ► *blood* of vertebrate animals. Is responsible for transporting oxygen and for the red colour of blood. Obtained from the blood of killed mammals (especially cattle and pigs). Can be contained in cigarette filters (in order to bind toxins). Additive in some meat products or pet foods (as a colour or a source of protein).

Hepar (Lysat.) Bovis ▸ *Organ Extracts*

Hepar Suis ▸ *Organ Extracts*

Hepar Sulfuris
(Liver of sulphur)
Mineral/vegetable. Mixed salts of sulphur. Obtained from sulphur and potash. "Liver of sulphur" merely refers to the red-brown colour. Traditionally used in medicinal baths for skin disorders. Used in copper work. Can be confused with ▸ *hepar sulfuris calcareum*.

Hepar Sulfuris Calcareum
(Liver of sulphur)
From killed animals. Preparation of ▸ *hepar sulfuris* using the ground shells of ▸ *oysters.* In ▸ *homeopathic medicines*.

Heparin
From killed animals. A polysaccharide compound (▸ *glycosaminoglycans*) that inhibits blood clotting. Is usually obtained from the intestinal mucous membranes of pigs, but also from the lung tissue of cattle. Is used routinely as a medicinal active agent for preventing and treating blood clots following severe injuries, after surgery or in the case of bedridden patients, either as subcutaneous injections or continual infusions. In ointments for the topical treatment of swelling and inflammation. Skin conditioner in cosmetics.

Hexacosyl Glycol Isostearate
Can be vegetable/synthetic or animal. Hydrocarbon compound of ▸ *stearic acid*. Emulsifier and skin conditioner in cosmetics.

Hexadecanol ▸ *Cetyl Alcohol*

Hexadecenoic Acid ▸ *Palmitoleic Acid*

Hexadecyltrimethylammonium Bromide ▸ *Cetrimonium Bromide*

Hexanediol Beeswax
From living animals. Chemically altered ▸ *beeswax*. Humectant and skin conditioner in cosmetics.

Hexanetriol Beeswax
From living animals. Chemically altered ▸ *beeswax*. Humectant and viscosity controlling agent in cosmetics.

Hexanoic Acid ▸ *Caproic acid*

Hexyl Isostearate
Can be vegetable/synthetic or animal. Hydrocarbon compound of ▸ *stearic acid*. Emollient and skin conditioner in cosmetics.

Hexyldecanol ▸ *Decyl Alcohol*

Hexyldeceth-2

Mostly vegetable/synthetic, can also be partly animal. Polymer compound of ► *decyl alcohol.* Emulsifier, solvent, antifoaming agent, viscosity controlling agent and skin conditioner in cosmetics.

Hexyldeceth-20

Mostly vegetable/synthetic, can also be partly animal. Polymer compound of► *decyl alcohol.* Emulsifier, humectant and solvent in cosmetics.

Hexyldecyl Ester of Hydrolyzed Collagen

From killed animals. Chemically/enzymatically altered ► *collagen.* Hair and skin conditioner in cosmetics.

Hexyldecyl Ethylhexanoate

Mostly vegetable/synthetic, can also be partly animal. Compound of ► *caproic acid* and ► *decyl alcohol.* Skin conditioner and emollient in cosmetics.

Hexyldecyl Isostearate

Can be vegetable/synthetic or animal. Compound of ► *stearic acid* and ► *decyl alcohol.* Skin conditioner in cosmetics.

Hexyldecyl Oleate

Can be vegetable/synthetic or animal. Compound of ► *oleic acid* and ► *decyl alcohol.* Emollient, skin conditioner, surfactant and emulsifier in cosmetics.

Hexyldecyl Stearate

Can be vegetable/synthetic or animal. Compound of ► *stearic acid* and ► *decyl alcohol.* Skin conditioner and emollient in cosmetics.

Hirudin

From living or killed animals or microbiological. A ► *protein* from leeches (*Hirudo medicinalis*) that inhibits blood clotting, obtained either by directly attaching living leeches to patients (for treating hematomas and improving wound healing) or as an extract of killed leeches. Is also produced using genetically modified microorganisms. Used for preventing and treating blood clots (thromboses), also as an alternative to ► *heparin.*

Hirudo Extract

From killed animals. Extract of whole leeches. Skin conditioner and masking agent in cosmetics.

Histidine

Can be animal, vegetable or microbiological. A semiessential ► *amino acid.* Occurs naturally in young plant tissue, soy, seeds, ► *blood*, muscle tissue and ► *milk* products. Can be obtained from animal or vegetable sources, as well as microorganisms. Antistatic, humectant and skin conditioner in cosmetics. In nutritional supplements.

Histidine Hydrochloride

Can be animal, vegetable or microbiological. Salt of ► *histidine.* Antioxidant and reducing agent in cosmetics.

Hog Bristles ► China Bristles

Homeopathic Medicine

From living or killed animals, vegetable or mineral. Preparations (tablets, globuli, drops, tinctures, ointments and injectible solutions) of substances that are in several steps repeatedly diluted in carrier fluids and "succussed" (rhythmically shaken) until the substances themselves are barely or no longer detectable. Solid and unsoluble substances are first ground with ► *lactose*. Source materials can be whole animals or parts thereof, whole plants or parts thereof, or minerals. Used for treating diverse acute and chronic ailments. For this purpose, preparations are used of which the source materials would in healthy persons trigger the ailment to be healed, or similar symptoms. The described succussion is intended to induce a "potentization" that, despite the dilution, is supposed to alleviate or heal exactly those ailments in the afflicted persons. The efficacy of homoeopathy is subject to debate. Several substances are listed in this book according to their respective homeopathic denominations, as well as under ► *organ extracts*.

Honey
(Mel)

From living animals. Food made by ► *bees* from nectar from flowers or ► *honeydew* and stored in wax honeycombs as food for the hive. Beekeepers obtain the honey by removing the honeycomb from the hive. The honey is then usually extracted (centrifuged) from the honeycomb and sometimes additionally treated or processed as needed, but is also sometimes left untreated in the honeycomb. Used as food, and as soothing agent, moisturizer and humectant in cosmetics. Special kinds of honey are used medicinally in topical wound treatment.

Honeydew

From living animals. Sugary excretion of insects (mostly scale insects or aphids) that feed on tree sap. Is either collected directly by humans from trees or used by ► *bees* for producing ► *honey*. Used as a sweetener in foods.

Hoplostethus Oil

From killed animals. Oil from the subcutaneous fat tissue of the orange roughy (*Hoplostethus atlanticus*), a deep sea fish. Emollient in cosmetics.

Horn

From living or killed animals. Hard, tough, fibrous ► *protein* substance mostly comprising ► *keratin*. Horn makes up the outer layer of skin, as well as hair, nails, feathers, scales, hoofs and horns. Most horn is from killed animals. Used in buttons, combs, eyeglass frames, knife handles, imitation ► *tortoisehell*, etc.

Horn Meal. Horn Shavings

From living or killed animals. Ground or chipped ► *horn*. Used as a biological fertilizer.

Horsehair

From living or killed animals. The ► *hair* of horses, especially the long mane or tail hair. Used as stuffing in upholstered furniture and for stringing the bows of string instruments (violin, cello, etc.). In traditional wigs.

Horse Leather
(Cordovan. Shell cordovan)
From killed animals. The skin of killed horses. The skin of adult horses is referred to in general as "horse leather," whereas the skin of the hindquarters is known as "(shell) cordovan." The skin of young horses may be referred to as "foalskin." In clothing (e.g. coats and jackets). Cordovan leather is used in shoes and in gloves and finger tabs for archers.

Huanaco ► *Guanaco*
Hyaluronic Acid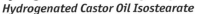
(Hyaluronate. Hyaluronan)
Can be from killed animals or microbiological. ► *Protein* and saccharide compound. Important constituent of the connective tissue and joint fluid of vertebrates. Also plays an important part in wound healing. Obtained from animal tissue (e.g. cockscomb) or from bacterial cultures. Used in eye surgery, for treating joint complaints and skin disorders, and in aesthetic surgery and cosmetics for targeted skin smoothing (injections and creams). Antistatic, humectant, moisturizer and skin conditioner in cosmetics.

Hydrogenated Castor Oil Hydroxystearate
Hydrogenated Castor Oil Isostearate
Hydrogenated Castor Oil Stearate
Hydrogenated Castor Oil Triisostearate
Hydrogenated Castor Oil Triisostearin Esters
Can be vegetable or animal. Compounds of vegetable ricinoleic acid and ► *stearic acid*. Viscosity controlling agents and skin conditioners in cosmetics.

Hydrogenated Fish Oil
From killed animals. Hydrogenated ► *fish oil*. Emollient and skin conditioner in cosmetics. Ingredient in foods.

Hydrogenated Honey
From living animals. Hydrogenated ► *honey*. Used as a humectant and skin conditioner in cosmetics.

Hydrogenated Laneth-n
From living or killed animals. Compounds of hydrogenated ► *lanolin alcohol*. Emulsifiers in cosmetics (hydrogenated laneth-5 is also used as a bulking agent and skin conditioner in cosmetics, hydrogenated laneth-20 and hydrogenated laneth-25 are also used as stabilizers).

Hydrogenated Lanolin
From living or killed animals. Hydrogenated ► *lanolin*. Antistatic, emollient, hair and skin conditioner in cosmetics.

Hydrogenated Lanolin Alcohol
From living or killed animals. Hydrogenated ► *lanolin alcohol*. Emulsion stabilizer and skin conditioner in cosmetics.

Hydrogenated Lard
From killed animals. Hydrogenated ► *lard*. Emollient and skin conditioner in cosmetics.

Hydrogenated Lard Glyceride
Hydrogenated Lard Glycerides
From killed animals. Hydrogenated ► *glycerides* from ► *lard*. Emulsifiers and skin conditioners in cosmetics.

Hydrogenated Lecithin
Mostly vegetable, can also be animal. Hydrogenated ► *lecithin*. Emulsifier and skin conditioner in cosmetics.

Hydrogenated Menhaden Acid
From killed animals. Hydrogenated ► *fatty acids* from menhaden oil (► *Brevoortia oil*). Emulsifier, surfactant and cleansing agent in cosmetics.

Hydrogenated Menhaden Oil
From killed animals. Hydrogenated menhaden oil (► *Brevoortia oil*). Emollient, skin conditioner and solvent in cosmetics.

Hydrogenated Milk Lipids
From living and killed animals (► *milk*). Hydrogenated ► *butterfat*. Skin conditioner in cosmetics.

Hydrogenated Mink Oil
From killed animals. Hydrogenated ► *mink oil*. Used as an emollient and skin conditioner in cosmetics.

Hydrogenated Orange Roughy Oil
From killed animals. Hydrogenated orange roughy oil (► *Hoplostethus oil*). Emollient and skin conditioner in cosmetics.

Hydrogenated Shark Liver Oil
From killed animals. Hydrogenated oil from the livers of killed sharks. Emollient and skin conditioner in cosmetics.

Hydrogenated Tallow
From killed animals. Hydrogenated ► *tallow*. Emollient, skin conditioner, emulsifier and viscosity controlling agent in cosmetics.

Hydrogenated Tallow Acid
From killed animals. Hydrogenated ► *fatty acids* from ► *tallow*. Emollient, emulsifier, opacifier, cleansing agent and surfactant in cosmetics.

Hydrogenated Tallow Alcohol
From killed animals. Alcohol from ► *tallow*. Emollient, skin conditioner, stabilizer, foam booster, surfactant, emulsifier and viscosity controlling agent in cosmetics.

Hydrogenated Tallow Amide
From killed animals. Chemically altered ► *tallow*. Emulsifier, emulsion stabilizer, surfactant, viscosity controlling agent, opacifier and hair conditioner in cosmetics.

Hydrogenated Tallow Betaine
From killed animals. Chemically altered ► *tallow*. Surfactant, hair conditioner, antistatic, cleansing agent, foam booster and viscosity controlling agent in cosmetics.

Hydrogenated Tallow Glyceride
Hydrogenated Tallow Glycerides
Hydrogenated Tallow Glyceride Citrate
Hydrogenated Tallow Glycerides Citrate
Hydrogenated Tallow Glyceride Lactate
From killed animals. Various forms of hydrogenated ► *glycerides* from ► *tallow*. Emollients, skin conditioners and emulsifiers in cosmetics.

Hydrogenated Tallowalkonium Chloride
From killed animals. Chemically altered ► *tallow*. Preservative, antistatic and hair conditioner in cosmetics.

Hydrogenated Tallowamide DEA
From killed animals. Chemically altered ► *tallow*. Surfactant, foam booster, viscosity controlling agent and stabilizer in cosmetics.

Hydrogenated Tallowamine
From killed animals. Chemically altered ► *tallow*. Emulsifier, surfactant, antistatic, viscosity controlling agent and stabilizer in cosmetics.

Hydrogenated Tallowamine Oxide
From killed animals. Chemically altered ► *tallow*. Antistatic, surfactant, foam booster, hydrotrope, cleansing agent and viscosity controlling agent in cosmetics.

Hydrogenated Talloweth-n
From killed animals. Chemically altered ► *tallow*. Emulsifiers and surfactants in cosmetics. hydrogenated talloweth-12 also used as a stabilizer and viscosity controlling agent, hydrogenated talloweth-25 also as a cleansing agent.

Hydrogenated Talloweth-60 Myristyl Glycol
From killed animals. Chemically altered ► *tallow*. Emulsifier, stabilizer and surfactant in cosmetics.

Hydrogenated Tallowoyl Glutamic Acid
From killed animals. Chemically altered ► *tallow*. Cleansing agent, hair and skin conditioner, and surfactant in cosmetics.

Hydrogenated Tallowtrimonium Chloride
From killed animals. Chemically altered ► *tallow*. Antistatic, surfactant, hair conditioner and preservative in cosmetics.

Hydrolyzed Actin
From killed animals. Chemically/enzymatically altered actin, a ► *protein* found in all vegetable and animal cells, especially in muscle cells. Obtained from mammal muscle tissue. Skin and hair conditioner in cosmetics.

Hydrolyzed Albumen
From living animals. Chemically/enzymatically altered ► *albumen*. Antistatic, skin and hair conditioner, and viscosity controlling agent in cosmetics.

Hydrolyzed Animal Elastin ► Hydrolyzed Elastin

Hydrolyzed Animal Protein
(Protein hydrolysate)
From killed animals. Collective term for chemically/enzymatically altered ► *proteins* from different animal tissues (e.g. connective tissue, hair, horn, bone, muscle tissue) or fluids (blood, milk, egg constituents) and mixtures thereof. The individual substances are described in the entries from ► *hydrolyzed albumen* to ► *hydrolyzed spinal protein*.

Hydrolyzed Beeswax
From living animals. Chemically/enzymatically altered ► *beeswax*. Surfactant, emulsifier, emulsion stabilizer and stabilizer in cosmetics.

Hydrolyzed Casein
(Casein hydrolysate)
From living and killed animals (► milk). Chemically/enzymatically altered ► *casein*. Antistatic, skin and hair conditioner in cosmetics.

Hydrolyzed Collagen
(Collagen hydrolysate)
From killed animals. Chemically/enzymatically altered ► *collagen*. Obtained primarily from the horns and hoofs of cattle. Antistatic, emollient, skin and hair conditioner, film forming agent and humectant in cosmetics. Excipient in pharmaceutical drugs (pills, capsules, tablets). Ingredient in nutritional supplements.

Hydrolyzed Conchiorin Protein
From killed animals. Chemically/enzymatically altered ► *proteins* from ► *oysters*. Skin and hair conditioner in cosmetics.

Hydrolyzed DNA
Can be vegetable, animal or microbiological. Chemically/enzymatically altered ► *DNA*. Skin and hair conditioner in cosmetics.

Hydrolyzed Egg Protein
From living and killed animals (► egg). Chemically/enzymatically altered ► *proteins* from ► *eggs*. Hair conditioner in cosmetics.

Hydrolyzed Egg Shell Membrane
From living and killed animals (► egg). Chemically/enzymatically altered ► *proteins* from the shell membranes of ► *eggs*. Skin conditioner in cosmetics.

Hydrolyzed Elastin
(Hydrolyzed animal elastin. Elastin hydrolysate)
From killed animals. Chemically/enzymatically altered ► *elastin*. Film forming agent in cosmetics, e.g. hair care, masks.

Hydrolyzed Fibroin ► Hydrolyzed Silk

Hydrolyzed Fibronectin
From killed animals. Chemically/enzymatically altered ► *fibronectin*. Hair and skin conditioner in cosmetics.

Hydrolyzed Gadidae Protein
From killed animals. Chemically/enzymatically altered ► *protein* from cod. From industrial fishing. Skin conditioner in cosmetics.

Hydrolyzed Gelatin
From killed animals. Chemically/enzymatically altered ► *gelatin*. Skin conditioner in cosmetics.

Hydrolyzed Glycosaminoglycans
From killed animals. Chemically/enzymatically altered ► *glycosaminoglycans*. Humectant, hair and skin conditioner in cosmetics.

Hydrolyzed Hair Keratin
From killed or living animals. Chemically/enzymatically altered ► *keratin* from ► *hair*. Antistatic, skin and hair conditioner in cosmetics.

Hydrolyzed Hemoglobin
From killed animals. Chemically/enzymatically altered ► *hemoglobin*. Skin and hair conditioner in cosmetics.

Hydrolyzed Human Placental Protein
From humans. Chemically/enzymatically altered ► *proteins* from human ► *placenta* tissue. Antistatic, skin and hair conditioner in cosmetics.

Hydrolyzed Keratin
From killed or living animals. Chemically/enzymatically altered ► *keratin*. Antistatic, film forming agent, humectant, skin and hair conditioner in cosmetics.

Hydrolyzed Milk Protein
From living and killed animals (► *milk).* Chemically/enzymatically altered ► *milk protein*. Antistatic, skin and hair conditioner in cosmetics.

Hydrolyzed Pearl
From killed animals. Chemically/enzymatically altered ► *pearls*. Skin conditioner in cosmetics.

Hydrolyzed Placental Protein
From living or killed animals. Chemically/enzymatically altered ► *protein* from mammal ► *placenta* tissue. Antistatic, skin and hair conditioner in cosmetics.

Hydrolyzed Protein
(Protein hydrolysate)
Can be vegetable, animal or microbiological. Collective term for chemically/enzymatically altered ► *protein* from plants (e.g. maize, cereals and legumes), yeasts and animals (► *hydrolyzed animal protein*). Used especially as cosmetic hair and skin conditioners.

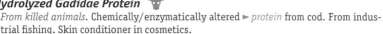

Hydrolyzed Red Blood Cells
From killed animals. Chemically/enzymatically altered red blood cells from the ► *blood* of killed mammals. Skin conditioner in cosmetics.

Hydrolyzed Reticulin
From killed animals. Chemically/enzymatically altered fibres from the connective tissue of killed mammals. Skin and hair conditioner in cosmetics.

Hydrolyzed RNA
Can be vegetable, animal or microbiological. Chemically/enzymatically altered ► *RNA*. Skin and hair conditioner in cosmetics.

Hydrolyzed Roe
From killed animals. Chemically/enzymatically altered fish eggs. The eggs are cut out of killed female ► *fish*. Skin conditioner in cosmetics.

Hydrolyzed Serum Protein
From killed animals. Chemically/enzymatically altered ► *proteins* from the ► *blood* of mammals (► *serum protein*). Antistatic, skin and hair conditioner in cosmetics.

Hydrolyzed Silk
From killed animals. Chemically/enzymatically altered ► *proteins* from ► *silk*. Antistatic, humectant, hair and skin conditioner in cosmetics.

Hydrolyzed Spinal Protein
From killed animals. Chemically/enzymatically altered ► *proteins* from the spinal cords of killed mammals. Antistatic, hair and skin conditioner in cosmetics.

Hydroxycapric Acid
Mostly vegetable, can also be animal. Compound of ► *capric acid*. Skin conditioner in cosmetics.

Hydroxycaproyl Phytosphingosine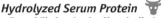
Mostly vegetable/microbiological, can also be partly animal. Compound of ► *caproic acid* and ► *phytosphingosine*. Skin and hair conditioner in cosmetics.

Hydroxycaprylic Acid
Mostly vegetable, can also be animal. Compound of ► *caprylic acid*. Skin conditioner in cosmetics.

Hydroxycapryloyl Phytosphingosine
Mostly vegetable/microbiological, can also be partly animal. Compound of ► *caprylic acid* and ► *phytosphingosine*. Skin and hair conditioner in cosmetics.

Hydroxyceteth-60
Mostly vegetable/synthetic, can theoretically also be animal. Polymer compound of ► *cetyl alcohol*. Surfactant and cleansing agent in cosmetics.

Hydroxycetyl Isostearate
Can be vegetable or animal. Compound of ► *cetyl alcohol* and ► *stearic acid*. Emulsifier, emollient and skin conditioner in cosmetics.

Hydroxyethyl Chitosan
From killed animals. Chemically altered ▶ *chitosan*. Film forming agent and viscosity controlling agent in cosmetics.

Hydroxyethyl Palmityl Oxyhydroxypropyl Palmitamide
Mostly vegetable/synthetic, can also be partly animal. Chemically altered ▶ *palmitic acid*. Emollient and humectant in cosmetics.

Hydroxyethyl Stearamide-MIPA
Can be vegetable/synthetic or animal. Chemically altered ▶ *stearic acid*. Antistatic, viscosity controlling agent and opacifier in cosmetics.

Hydroxyethyl Tallowdimonium Chloride
From killed animals. Chemically altered ▶ *tallow*. Antistatic and hair conditioner in cosmetics.

Hydroxylated Lanolin
From living or killed animals. Chemically altered ▶ *lanolin*. Antistatic, emollient, skin conditioner, emulsifier, film forming agent and binding agent in cosmetics.

Hydroxylated Milk Glycerides
From living and killed animals (▶ *milk*). Chemically altered ▶ *glycerides* from ▶ *milk*. Emollient and skin conditioner in cosmetics.

Hydroxylauroyl Phytosphingosine
Can be animal, vegetable or microbiological. Compound of ▶ *lauric acid* and ▶ *phytosphingosine*. Skin and hair conditioner in cosmetics.

Hydroxyoctacosanyl Hydroxystearate
Can be vegetable/synthetic or animal. Chemically altered ▶ *stearic acid*. Emollient and skin conditioner in cosmetics.

Hydroxypropyl Biscetearyldimonium Chloride
Can be vegetable/synthetic or animal. Ammonium compound of ▶ *cetyl alcohol* and ▶ *stearyl alcohol*. Antistatic and hair conditioner in cosmetics.

Hydroxypropyl Bisisostearamidopropyldimonium Chloride
Can be vegetable/synthetic or animal. Ammonium compound of ▶ *stearic acid*. Antistatic and hair conditioner in cosmetics.

Hydroxypropyl Bisstearyldimonium Chloride
Can be vegetable/synthetic or animal. Ammonium compound of ▶ *stearyl alcohol*. Antistatic and hair conditioner in cosmetics.

Hydroxypropyl Chitosan
From killed animals. Reaction product of ▶ *chitosan* and petroleum products. Film forming agent in cosmetics.

Hydroxypropyltrimonium Amylopectin/Glycerin Crosspolymer
Can be vegetable/synthetic or partly animal. Polymer compound of ammonium and ▶ *glycerol*. Antistatic, hair and skin conditioner in cosmetics.

Hydroxypropyltrimonium Gelatin
From killed animals. Chemically altered ► *gelatin.* Antistatic, hair and skin conditioner in cosmetics.

Hydroxypropyltrimonium Honey
From living animals. Chemically altered ► *honey.* Antistatic and hair conditioner in cosmetics.

Hydroxypropyltrimonium Hydrolyzed Casein
From living and killed animals (► milk). Chemically altered ► *casein.* Antistatic, hair and skin conditioner in cosmetics.

Hydroxypropyltrimonium Hydrolyzed Collagen
From killed animals. Chemically/enzymatically altered ► *collagen.* Antistatic, hair and skin conditioner in cosmetics.

Hydroxypropyltrimonium Hydrolyzed Keratin
From killed or living animals. Chemically/enzymatically altered ► *keratin.* Antistatic, hair and skin conditioner in cosmetics.

Hydroxypropyltrimonium Hydrolyzed Silk
From killed animals. Chemically/enzymatically altered ► *silk.* Antistatic, hair and skin conditioner in cosmetics.

Hydroxystearamide MEA
Can be vegetable/synthetic or animal. Chemically altered ► *stearic acid.* Antistatic, viscosity controlling agent and hair dye in cosmetics.

Hydroxystearamidopropyl Trimonium Chloride
Can be vegetable/synthetic or animal. Ammonium compound of ► *stearic acid.* Antistatic and hair conditioner in cosmetics.

Hydroxystearamidopropyl Trimonium Methosulfate
Can be vegetable/synthetic or animal. Ammonium compound of ► *stearic acid.* Antistatic and hair conditioner in cosmetics.

Hydroxystearic Acid
Can be vegetable or animal. Chemically altered ► *stearic acid.* Emulsifier, cleansing agent and surfactant in cosmetics.

Hydroxystearyl Methylglucamine
Can be vegetable/synthetic or animal. Compound of ► *stearyl alcohol* and the sugar alcohol sorbitol. Antistatic in cosmetics.

Icing ► *Glaze*

Icosanoic acid ► *Arachidic Acid*

Illipé Butter

(Bassia latifolia butter. Shorea stenoptera butter)
Vegetable. Denomination for fat from two different tree species: 1. from the seeds of *Bassia latifolia*; 2. from the fruits and seeds of *Shorea stenoptera*. Not to be confused with animal ► *butter*. Emollients in cosmetics. Used as edible fat, e.g. partial substitute for ► *cocoa butter* in chocolate products.

Imidazolidinyl Urea

Synthetic. Compound of ► *urea*. Preservative in cosmetics.

Inosine

Microbiological, can also be animal. Constituent of ► *RNA*. In all living cells. Industrial production from yeasts. In pharmaceutical drugs and food supplements.

Inosinic Acid

(E 630. Inosinate. Inosine monophosphate [IMP])
Microbiological, can theoretically alao be animal. Derivative of ► *inosine* that plays an important part in metabolism. Present in greater quantities in ► *blood* and muscle tissue. Industrial production with the aid of microorganisms. Used as a flavour enhancer in foods, often together with ► *glutamates*.

Insulin

Microbiological, can sometimes be from killed animals. A ► *hormone* that regulates blood sugar level and energy balance in the body. Obtained earlier from the pancreases of pigs and cattle. "Human insulins" from genetically engineered yeasts are now standard. Animal insulins are only used in exceptional cases and are unmistakeably labelled as such. Used as injections for treating diabetes mellitus. Insulin products contain not only the active agent but also excipients that may be animal, e.g. ► *glycerol*.

Invertase

(E 1103)
Microbiological. An ► *enzyme* that breaks down sucrose (► *sugar*) to fructose and glucose. The resulting mixture of sucrose, fructose and glucose is called ► *inverted sugar*.

Occurs naturally in bacteria, yeasts and plants. Is also produced by ► *bees*, in order to convert nectar to ► *honey*. Industrially produced from yeast cultures. Used for producing ► *inverted sugar* and as a humectant in confectionery.

Inverted Sugar

Vegetable, can also have been partly treated with animal substances. Mixture of sucrose, fructose and glucose. Produced by breaking down ► *sugar* with the enzyme ► *invertase* or using acids. Can also be obtained from starch. Sweetening ingredient in foods and source material for sugar substitutes.

Inverted Sugar Cream

(Artificial honey. Invertzuckercreme [German])

Vegetable, can also be partly animal. A sugar cream with properties similar to those of ► *honey*. Consists mainly of ► *inverted sugar* enriched with starch or glucose syrup, can also contain ► *honey* (for instance, according to German regulations the honey must only be labelled when the proportion of honey exceeds 10%). Used as a substitute for honey in gingerbread, chocolates, etc.

Inverted Sugar Syrup

(Invert sugar syrup. Glucose-fructose syrup)

Vegetable, can also have been partly treated with animal substances. Solution with more than 50% ► *inverted sugar*. Sweetening ingredient in foods.

Isinglass

From killed animals. Expensive ► *fish glue* from the dried air bladders of sturgeons. Used for fining ► *wine*, ► *beer* (but not beer brewed according to the German *Reinheitsgebot* ["Purity Law"]) and other beverages. Adhesive in conservation/restoration and for building musical instruments. In certain photochemical print methods. Sturgeons are now protected species and genuine isinglass is seldom available, so that the swim bladders of other fishes are also sold under the same name. The name "isinglass" also refers to sheets of mica, a glittering silicate mineral. However, the two substances have nothing in common apart from the name, and mica is entirely mineral and therefore vegan.

Isobutyl Palmitate

Synthetic/vegetable, can also be partly animal. Chemically altered ► *palmitic acid*. Emollient and skin conditioner in cosmetics.

Isobutyl Stearate

Can be synthetic/vegetable or animal. Chemically altered ► *stearic acid*. Emollient and skin conditioner in cosmetics.

Isobutyl Tallowate

From killed animals. Chemically altered ► *tallow*. Emollient and skin conditioner in cosmetics.

Isobutylated Lanolin Oil

From living or killed animals. Chemically altered ► *lanolin oil*. Antistatic, emollient, skin and hair conditioner in cosmetics.

Isobutyric Acid
Mostly synthetic, can also be animal or vegetable. Variant of ► *butyric acid.* Cosmetic buffering agent. For treating rubber and plastics, and producing aromatic substances.

Isoceteareth-8 Stearate
Can be vegetable/synthetic or animal. Compound of chemically altered ► *cetostearyl alcohol* and ► *stearic acid.* Emulsifier and surfactant in cosmetics.

Isoceteth-10 Stearate
Can be vegetable/synthetic or animal. Compound of chemically altered ► *cetyl alcohol* and ► *stearic acid.* Emulsifier in cosmetics.

Isoceteth-n
Vegetable/synthetic, can theoretically also be partly animal. Chemically altered ► *cetyl alcohol.* Emulsifiers and surfactants in cosmetics.

Isocetyl Alcohol
Mostly vegetable/synthetic, can also be animal. Chemically altered ► *cetyl alcohol.* Emollient, skin conditioner and viscosity controlling agent in cosmetics.

Isocetyl Behenate
Mostly vegetable/synthetic, can also be partly animal. Compound of vegetable behenic acid and ► *cetyl alcohol.* Emollient and skin conditioner in cosmetics.

Isocetyl Ethylhexanoate
Mostly vegetable/synthetic, can also be partly animal. Compound of ► *caproic acid* and ► *cetyl alcohol.* Skin conditioner and emollient in cosmetics.

Isocetyl Isodecanoate
Mostly vegetable/synthetic, can also be partly animal. Compound of ► *capric acid* and ► *cetyl alcohol.* Emollient and skin conditioner in cosmetics.

Isocetyl Isostearate
Can be vegetable/synthetic or animal. Compound of ► *stearic acid* and ► *cetyl alcohol.* Skin conditioner and emollient in cosmetics.

Isocetyl Laurate
Mostly vegetable/synthetic, can also be partly animal. Compound of ► *lauric acid* and ► *cetyl alcohol.* Skin conditioner and emollient in cosmetics.

Isocetyl Linoleoyl Stearate
Can be vegetable/synthetic or animal. Compound of ► *stearic acid,* ► *cetyl alcohol* and ► *linoleic acid.* Emollient and skin conditioner in cosmetics.

Isocetyl Myristate
Mostly vegetable/synthetic, can also be partly animal. Compound of ► *myristic acid* and ► *cetyl alcohol.* Emollient and skin conditioner in cosmetics.

Isocetyl Palmitate
Mostly vegetable/synthetic, can also be partly animal. Compound of ► *palmitic acid* and ► *cetyl alcohol.* Emollient and skin conditioner in cosmetics.

Isocetyl Salicylate
Mostly synthetic/vegetable, can also be partly animal. Compound of salicylic acid and ► *cetyl alcohol.* Solvent, emollient and skin conditioner in cosmetics.

Isocetyl Stearate
Can be vegetable/synthetic or animal. Compound of ► *stearic acid* and ► *cetyl alcohol.* Emollient and skin conditioner in cosmetics.

Isocetyl Stearoyl Stearate
Vegetable/synthetic or animal. Compound of ► *stearic acid,* ► *stearyl alcohol* and ► *cetyl alcohol.* Emollient, skin conditioner and viscosity controlling agent in cosmetics.

Isodeceth-2 Cocoate
Mostly vegetable/synthetic, can also be partly animal. ► *PEG* compound of ► *decyl alcohol* and coconut fatty acids. Emollient, emulsifier and surfactant in cosmetics.

Isodeceth-n
Mostly vegetable/synthetic, can also be partly animal. ► *PEG* compound of ► *decyl alcohol.* Emulsifier and surfactant in cosmetics.

Isodecyl Citrate
Mostly vegetable/synthetic, can also be partly animal. Compound of ► *decyl alcohol* and citric acid. Emollient and skin conditioner, plasticizer in cosmetics.

Isodecyl Cocoate
Mostly vegetable/synthetic, can also be partly animal. Compound of ► *decyl alcohol* and coconut fatty acids. Emollient and skin conditioner in cosmetics.

Isodecyl Ethylhexanoate
Mostly vegetable/synthetic, can also be partly animal. Compound of ► *decyl alcohol* and ► *caproic acid.* Emollient, skin conditioner in cosmetics.

Isodecyl Hydroxystearate
Can be vegetable/synthetic or animal. Compound of ► *decyl alcohol* and ► *stearic acid.* Emollient and skin conditioner in cosmetics.

Isodecyl Isononanoate
Mostly vegetable/synthetic, can also be partly animal. Compound of ► *decyl alcohol* and vegetable nonanoic acid. Antistatic and emollient, skin conditioner in cosmetics.

Isodecyl Laurate
Mostly vegetable/synthetic, can also be partly animal. Compound of ► *decyl alcohol* and ► *lauric acid.* Emollient, skin conditioner in cosmetics.

Isodecyl Myristate
Mostly vegetable/synthetic, can also be partly animal. Compound of ► *decyl alcohol* and ► *myristic acid.* Emollient and skin conditioner in cosmetics.

Isodecyl Neopentanoate
Mostly vegetable, can also be partly animal. Compound of ► *decyl alcohol* and vegetable valeric acid. Emollient and skin conditioner in cosmetics.

Isodecyl Oleate 🌿 ⬛ 🐄
Can be vegetable/synthetic or animal. Compound of ► *decyl alcohol* and ► *oleic acid*. Emollient and skin conditioner in cosmetics.

Isodecyl Palmitate 🌿 ⬛ 🐄
Mostly vegetable/synthetic, can also be partly animal. Compound of ► *decyl alcohol* and ► *palmitic acid*. Emollient and skin conditioner in cosmetics.

Isodecyl Salicylate 🌿 ⬛ 🐄
Mostly vegetable/synthetic, can also be partly animal. Compound of ► *decyl alcohol* and salicylic acid. Antistatic and skin conditioner in cosmetics.

Isodecyl Stearate 🌿 ⬛ 🐄
Can be vegetable/synthetic or animal. Compound of ► *decyl alcohol* and ► *stearic acid*. Emollient and skin conditioner in cosmetics.

Isodecylparaben 🌿 ⬛ 🐄
Mostly vegetable/synthetic, can also be partly animal. Compound of ► *decyl alcohol* and benzoic acid. Antimicrobial agent in cosmetics.

Isohexyl Palmitate 🌿 ⬛ 🐄
Mostly vegetable/synthetic, can also be partly animal. Compound of ► *palmitic acid*. Emollient and skin conditioner in cosmetics.

Isoleucine 🧪 ⬛ 🌿 🐄
Can be microbiological, synthetic, vegetable or animal. An essential ► *amino acid*. Constituent of animal and vegetable ► *proteins*. Obtained principally by microbiological fermentation of glucose solutions, but also from hydrocarbons or ► *hydrolyzed protein*, which can be either vegetable or animal. Antistatic, skin conditioner and hair dye in cosmetics. Also used in microbiology, in solutions for parenteral nutrition and special diets.

Isopropyl Hydroxycetyl Ether 🌿 ⬛ 🐄
Mostly vegetable/synthetic, can also be partly animal. Alcohol compound of ► *cetyl alcohol*. Surfactant and skin conditioner in cosmetics.

Isopropyl Hydroxystearate 🌿 ⬛ 🐄
Can be vegetable/synthetic or animal. Alcohol compound of ► *stearic acid*. Emollient and skin conditioner in cosmetics.

Isopropyl Isostearate 🌿 ⬛ 🐄
Can be vegetable/synthetic or animal. Alcohol compound of ► *stearic acid*. Emollient, skin conditioner and binding agent in cosmetics.

Isopropyl Lanolate 🐄
From living or killed animals. Chemically altered ► *fatty acids* from ► *lanolin*. Antistatic, emollient, skin conditioner, emulsifier and binding agent in cosmetics.

Isopropyl Linoleate ⬛ 🌿
Synthetic/vegetable. Alcohol compound of ► *linoleic acid*. Emollient, skin conditioner and binding agent in cosmetics.

Isopropyl Oleate 🌱 🧪 🐄
Can be vegetable/synthetic or animal. Alcohol compound of ► *oleic acid*. Emollient, skin conditioner and binding agent in cosmetics.

Isopropyl Palmitate 🌱 🧪 🐄
Mostly vegetable/synthetic, can also be partly animal. Alcohol compound of ► *palmitic acid*. Used as antistatic, binding agent, emollient, skin conditioner and solvent in cosmetics.

Isopropyl PPG-2-Isodeceth-7 Carboxylate 🌱 🧪 🐄
Mostly vegetable/synthetic, can also be partly animal. Polymer compound of ► *decyl alcohol*. Emollient, skin conditioner and solvent in cosmetics.

Isopropyl Stearate 🌱 🧪 🐄
Can be vegetable/synthetic or animal. Alcohol compound of ► *stearic acid*. Binding agent and emollient, skin conditioner in cosmetics.

Isopropyl Tallowate 🐄
From killed animals. Chemically altered ► *tallow*. Emollient, skin conditioner and binding agent in cosmetics.

Isopropyl Titanium Triisostearate 🧪 🌱 💎 🐄
Synthetic/vegetable/mineral or animal. Alcohol compound of ► *stearic acid*. Emollient and emulsifier in cosmetics.

Isostearamide DEA 🌱 🧪 🐄
Isostearamide MEA
Isostearamide MIPA
Can be vegetable/synthetic or animal. Alcohol compounds of ► *stearic acid*. Antistatics, viscosity controlling agents, foam boosters and surfactants in cosmetics.

Isostearamidomorpholine Stearate 🌱 🧪 🐄
Can be vegetable/synthetic or animal. Hydrocarbon compound of ► *stearic acid*. Surfactant and emulsifier in cosmetics.

Isostearamidopropyl Betaine 🌱 🧪 🐄
Can be vegetable/synthetic or animal. Ammonium compound of ► *stearic acid*. Used as antistatic, surfactant, skin and hair conditioner, foam booster and cleansing agent in cosmetics.

Isostearamidopropyl Dimethylamine 🌱 🧪 🐄
Isostearamidopropyl Dimethylamine Gluconate
Isostearamidopropyl Dimethylamine Glycolate
Can be vegetable/synthetic or animal. Ammonium compounds of ► *stearic acid*. Used as antistatics in cosmetics.

Isostearamidopropyl Dimethylamine Lactate 🌱 🧪 🐄
Can be vegetable/synthetic or animal. Ammonium compound of ► *stearic acid* and ► *lactic acid*. Antistatic in cosmetics.

Isostearamidopropyl Epoxypropyldimonium Chloride
Can be vegetable/synthetic or animal. Ammonium and resin compound of ► *stearic acid.*
Antistatic in cosmetics.

Isostearamidopropyl Epoxypropylmorpholinium Chloride
Can be vegetable/synthetic or animal. Ammonium and resin compound of ► *stearic acid.*
Hair conditioner in cosmetics.

Isostearamidopropyl Ethyldimonium Ethosulfate
Isostearamidopropyl Ethylmorpholinium Ethosulfate
Can be vegetable/synthetic or animal. Ammonium and sulphur compounds of ► *stearic acid.* Antistatics and hair conditioners in cosmetics.

Isostearamidopropyl Laurylacetodimonium Chloride
Can be vegetable/synthetic or animal. Ammonium compound of ► *stearic acid.* Antistatic and hair conditioner in cosmetics.

Isostearamidopropyl Morpholine
Can be vegetable/synthetic or animal. Ammonium compound of ► *stearic acid.* Antistatic in cosmetics.

Isostearamidopropyl Morpholine Lactate
Can be vegetable/synthetic or animal. Ammonium compound of ► *stearic acid* and ► *lactic acid.* Antistatic in cosmetics.

Isostearamidopropyl Morpholine Oxide
Can be vegetable/synthetic or animal. Ammonium compound of ► *stearic acid.* Used as a surfactant, foam booster, hydrotrope, hair conditioner and cleansing agent in cosmetics.

Isostearamidopropyl PG-Dimonium Chloride
Can be vegetable/synthetic or animal. Ammonium compound of ► *stearic acid.* Antistatic and hair conditioner in cosmetics.

Isostearamidopropylamine Oxide
Can be vegetable/synthetic or animal. Nitrogen compound of ► *stearic acid.* Surfactant, foam booster, hydrotrope, hair conditioner and cleansing agent in cosmetics.

Isostearaminopropalkonium Chloride
Can be vegetable/synthetic or animal. Ammonium compound of ► *stearic acid.* Antistatic and hair conditioner in cosmetics.

Isosteareth-10 Stearate
Can be vegetable/synthetic or animal. ► *PEG* compound of ► *stearyl alcohol* and ► *stearic acid.* Emulsifier, skin conditioner and emollient in cosmetics.

Isosteareth-n
Isosteareth-n Carboxylic Acid
Can be vegetable/synthetic or animal. ► *PEG* compounds of ► *stearic acid.* Emulsifiers and surfactants in cosmetics.

Isostearic Acid
Can be vegetable or animal. Variant of ► *stearic acid*. Binding agent, emulsifier, surfactant and cleansing agent in cosmetics.

Isostearic/Myristic Glycerides
Can be vegetable or animal. ► *Glycerides* of ► *stearic acid* and ► *myristic acid*. Emulsifier and skin conditioner in cosmetics.

Isostearoyl Hydrolyzed Collagen
From killed animals. Chemically/enzymatically altered ► *collagen*. Antistatic, surfactant, skin and hair conditioner, and cleansing agent in cosmetics.

Isostearoyl Isostearyl Stearate
Can be vegetable or animal. Compound of ► *stearyl alcohol* and ► *stearic acid*. Emulsifier and skin conditioner in cosmetics.

Isostearoyl PG-Trimonium Chloride
Can be vegetable/synthetic or animal. Ammonium compound of ► *stearyl alcohol*. Antistatic and hair conditioner in cosmetics.

Isostearyl Alcohol
Can be vegetable or animal. Compound of ► *stearyl alcohol*. Emollient, skin conditioner and viscosity controlling agent in cosmetics.

Isostearyl Avocadate
Can be vegetable or animal. Compound of ► *stearyl alcohol* and fatty acids from avocado oil. Emollient and skin conditioner in cosmetics.

Isostearyl Behenate
Can be vegetable or animal. Compound of ► *stearyl alcohol* and vegetable behenic acid. Emollient and skin conditioner in cosmetics.

Isostearyl Benzoate
Can be vegetable/synthetic or animal. Compound of ► *stearyl alcohol* and benzoic acid (vegetable/synthetic). Emollient, skin conditioner in cosmetics.

Isostearyl Benzylimidonium Chloride
Can be vegetable/synthetic or animal. Ammonium compound of ► *stearyl alcohol*. Antistatic and binding agent in cosmetics.

Isostearyl Diglyceryl Succinate
Can be vegetable/synthetic or animal. Compound of ► *stearyl alcohol*, ► *glycerol* and ► *succinic acid*. Antistatic and skin conditioner in cosmetics.

Isostearyl Erucate
Can be vegetable or animal. Compound of ► *stearyl alcohol* and vegetable erucic acid. Emollient and skin conditioner in cosmetics.

Isostearyl Ethyldimonium Chloride
Can be vegetable/synthetic or animal. Ammonium compound of ► *stearyl alcohol*. Antistatic and hair conditioner in cosmetics.

Isostearyl Ethylhexanoate
Can be vegetable or animal. Compound of ► *stearyl alcohol* and ► *caproic acid.* Emollient and skin conditioner in cosmetics.

Isostearyl Ethylimidonium Ethosulfate
Can be vegetable/synthetic or animal. Ammonium and sulphur compound of ► *stearyl alcohol.* Antistatic and hair conditioner in cosmetics.

Isostearyl Glyceryl Pentaerythrityl Ether
Can be vegetable/synthetic or animal. Carbon compound of ► *stearyl alcohol* and ► *glycerol.* Emollient and skin conditioner in cosmetics.

Isostearyl Hydroxyethyl Imidazoline
Can be vegetable/synthetic or animal. Nitrogen carbon compound of ► *stearyl alcohol.* Antistatic and hair conditioner in cosmetics.

Isostearyl Isononanoate
Can be vegetable or animal. Compound of ► *stearyl alcohol* and vegetable nonanoic acid. Emollient, skin conditioner in cosmetics.

Isostearyl Isostearate
Can be vegetable or animal. Compound of ► *stearyl alcohol* and ► *stearic acid.* Binding agent, emollient and skin conditioner in cosmetics.

Isostearyl Lactate
Can be vegetable/synthetic or animal. Compound of ► *stearyl alcohol* and ► *lactic acid.* Emollient and skin conditioner in cosmetics.

Isostearyl Laurate
Can be vegetable/synthetic or animal. Compound of ► *stearyl alcohol* and ► *lauric acid.* Emollient and skin conditioner in cosmetics.

Isostearyl Laurdimonium Chloride
Can be vegetable/synthetic or animal. Ammonium compound of ► *stearyl alcohol.* Antistatic in cosmetics.

Isostearyl Myristate
Can be vegetable/synthetic or animal. Compound of ► *stearyl alcohol* and ► *myristic acid.* Emollient, skin conditioner and binding agent in cosmetics.

Isostearyl Neopentanoate
Can be vegetable or animal. Compound of ► *stearyl alcohol* and vegetable valeric acid. Emollient, skin conditioner and binding agent in cosmetics.

Isostearyl Palmitate
Can be vegetable or animal. Compound of ► *stearyl alcohol* and ► *palmitic acid.* Emollient, skin conditioner and binding agent in cosmetics.

Isostearyl Stearoyl Stearate
Can be vegetable or animal. Compound of ► *stearyl alcohol* and ► *stearic acid.* Emollient, skin conditioner and viscosity controlling agent in cosmetics.

Isotridecyl Isononanoate

Mostly vegetable/synthetic, can also be partly animal. Compound of ► *decyl alcohol* and vegetable nonanoic acid. Emollient, skin conditioner in cosmetics.

Isotridecyl Myristate

Mostly vegetable/synthetic, can also be partly animal. Compound of ► *decyl alcohol* and ► *myristic acid*. Emollient, skin and hair conditioner.

Ivory

From killed animals. Material of certain animal teeth, usually elephant tusks, sometimes also "fossil ivory" of extinct mammoths. More broadly also the canines or incisors of walruses, narwals and hippopotami. Earlier, whole elephant herds were slaughtered for ivory, and poaching still poses an acute threat to the animals. Trade in ivory—except fossil ivory—is subject to worldwide restrictions, but not entirely banned. Most recently, in 2008, over 100 metric tons of ivory were legally auctioned. Used for jewellery, piano keys, ivory carving, chess pieces, billiard balls, etc.

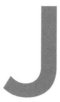

Japan Wax
(Rhus succedanea cera. Rhus verniciflua cera)
Vegetable. A waxy mixture of fats from the berries of certain Asian trees, especially the Japanese wax tree *(Rhus succedanea)*. Emollient in cosmetics. In candles and soaps, and used in general as a substitute for ► *beeswax*.

Japanese Gelatin
(Japanese isinglass)
Vegetable. Alternative name for agar-agar, a gelling agent obtained from marine algae. The name is misleading in that it is not actually ► *gelatin* from animal tissue, but rather a substitute.

Jelly
Can be vegetable or animal. Umbrella term for a gelled food, e.g. fruit jelly or ► *aspic*. Made using ► *gelling agents*.

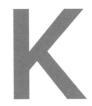

K

Karakul
(Astrakhan. Qaraqul)
From killed animals. The pelt (► *fur*) of unborn, stillborn, premature or newborn lambs of karakul sheep, with mostly black wool forming small, tight curls. The lambs are killed shortly after birth. They can also be aborted or cut out of their mothers. In clothing, e.g. coats, caps.

Karité Butter ► *Butyrospermum Parkii Butter*

Katsuobushi ► *Bonito Flakes*

Keratin
From killed or living animals. Water-insoluble fibrous ► *proteins*. Main constituent of ► *horn* in the hair, horns, feathers, claws, nails and scales of animals. Obtained from ground horns, hooves, claws, nails, hair, scales and feathers of diverse vertebrates. Hair and skin conditioner in cosmetics. In fertilizers. Source for the industrial production of ► *cystine*, ► *cysteine*, ► *tyrosine* and other ► *amino acids*.

Keratin Amino Acids
From killed or living animals. ► *Amino acids* obtained from ► *keratin*. Antistatic, hair and skin conditioner in cosmetics.

Keratin Hydrolysate ► *Hydrolyzed Keratin*

Kokum Butter
Vegetable. Fat from the seeds of the kokum tree *Garcinia indica*. Not to be confused with animal ► *butter*. Used as a partial substitute for ► *cocoa butter* in chocolate products. Source of cosmetic ingredients.

Kolinsky ► *Brushes*

Kopi Luwak
(Café alamid. Coffee alamid. Civet coffee)
From living animals. Rare and very expensive coffee variety. The coffee berries are eaten by civets and the coffee beans are excreted—fermented, but undigested. The beans are collected from the animals' feces, washed and lightly roasted.

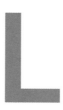

L-DOPA ► *Levodopa*

L-Thyroxine ► *Thyroxine*

Labilin® ► *Hydrolyzed Milk Protein*

Lac 1. ► *Shellac*
     2. ► *Milk*

Lac Caninum
From living animals. ► *Milk* from dogs. In ► *homeopathic medicines.*

Lac Powder
From living and killed animals (► milk*).* Powdered dried cow's ► *milk*. Skin conditioner in cosmetics.

Laccaic Acid
(C.I. natural red 25. Lac dye)
From killed animals. Red powder from ground lac scale insects (similar to ► *carmine*). In hair dyes, paints and textile dyes.

Lachesis
(Lachesis lanceolatus. L. muta. L. mutus. Bothrops lanceolatus. Trigonocephalus lachesis)
From living or killed animals. Snake venom from American lanceheads or pitvipers. In ► *homeopathic medicines.*

Lactamide MEA
Can be vegetable/synthetic or partly animal. Derivative of ► *lactic acid*. Skin and hair conditioner in cosmetics.

Lactamidopropyl Trimonium Chloride
Can be vegetable/synthetic or partly animal. Ammonium compound of ► *lactic acid*. Antistatic in cosmetics.

Lactase
Microbiological. An ► *enzyme* that breaks down ► *lactose*. Occurs naturally in animals and some plants; is produced by many moulds, yeasts and bacteria. Required by animals to digest ► *milk*; a deficiency causes lactose intolerance. Obtained commercially from

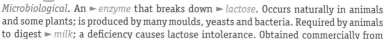

yeasts. Active agent in tablets/capsules for lactose intolerance. Used for making lactose-free dairy products for people with lactose intolerance, and in the production of dairy ice cream, to make it sweeter and prevent the formation of ice crystals.

Lactic Acid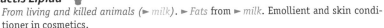

(L-lactic acid. E 270. Sodium lactate. Acidum lacticum)
Mostly vegetable/microbiological, can also be animal. An acid that is the result of fermenting various sugars with ► *lactic acid bacteria*. Its salts are called lactates. Found in soured milk and ► *yogurt*, as well as pickled vegetables. Also present in blood and muscle tissue as the result of biochemical processes. Commercially produced lactic acid is usually—but not always—obtained by fermenting vegetable sugars (starch, vegetable bio-mass). Some lactic acid is still obtained from ► *milk*/► *whey*. Skin protecting substance, humectant and skin conditioner in cosmetics. In adhesives and plasticizers. Excipient in pharmaceutical drugs. Acidifier and preservative in foods. Is permitted as an additive in ► *beer*. Used as ► *polylactic acid* in new, biologically degradable plastics.

Lactic Acid Bacteria

Microbiological, can be grown on vegetable or animal nutrient media. Bacteria that convert sugars to ► *lactic acid*. Occur naturally on plants, in the gut and on mucous membranes of animals, including humans. Play an important part in biological degradation processes and the fermentation of foods. The bacterial cultures can be grown on vegetable nutrient media (e.g. starch) or animal media (e.g. ► *whey*).

Lactic Acid Esters of Mono- and Diglycerides of Fatty Acids

(E 472b. Lactoglycerides)
Can be vegetable or animal. Compound of ► *lactic acid* and ► *glycerides* of ► *fatty acids*. Emulsifier, flour treating agent, stabilizer and carrier in foods.

Lactide

Mostly microbiological/vegetable, can also be animal. Compound of ► *lactic acid*. Can be produced from lactic acid, but is normally obtained biotechnologically from glucose and molasses (e.g. from biomass). Used for producing ► *polylactic acid*.

Lactis Faex

From living and killed animals (► milk). Yeast obtained from ► *milk*. Skin conditioner in cosmetics.

Lactis Lipida

From living and killed animals (► milk). ► *Fats* from ► *milk*. Emollient and skin conditioner in cosmetics.

Lactis Proteinum

From living and killed animals (► milk). ► *Proteins* from ► *milk*. Hair and skin conditioner in cosmetics.

Lactis Proteinum Extract

From living and killed animals (► milk). Extract of milk proteins (► *lactis proteinum*). Skin conditioner in cosmetics.

Lactis Serum Proteinum
From living and killed animals (► milk). ► *Protein* from the hydrous fraction of milk (► *whey*). Hair and skin conditioner in cosmetics.

Lactitol
(E 966. Lacty®. Importal®)
From living and killed animals (► milk). A sugar alcohol that does not occur naturally, but is chemically produced from ► *lactose*. Used as a sugar substitute or sweetener in (reduced-calorie) foods. Also active agent in laxatives. Humectant and skin conditioner in cosmetics.

Lactobacillus Acidophilus (L. Acidophilus) ► *Yogurt Cultures*

Lactobacillus/Algae Ferment
Microbiological/vegetable. Product obtained by the fermentation of algae extract by ► *lactic acid bacteria*. Skin protecting substance in cosmetics.

Lactobacillus Bulgaricus (L. Bulgaricus) ► *Yogurt Cultures*

Lactobacillus/Eichornia Crassipes Ferment
Microbiological/vegetable. Product obtained by the fermentation of water hyacinth by ► *lactic acid bacteria*. Skin protecting substance in cosmetics.

Lactobacillus Ferment
Microbiological, can be of animal origin. Product obtained from the fermentation of ► *lactic acid bacteria*. The denomination does not provide any information as to whether vegetable or animal raw materials were fermented. Skin conditioner in cosmetics.

Lactobacillus/Glycerin/Hydrolyzed Casein/Lactose/ Catharantus Roseus Seed/Faex Extract Ferment
Microbiological/animal/vegetable. Product obtained from the fermentation of ► *glycerol*, ► *hydrolyzed casein*, ► *lactose*, plant matter and yeast extract by ► *lactic acid bacteria*. Skin conditioner in cosmetics.

Lactobacillus Lac/Calcium/Phosphorous/Magnesium/Zinc Ferment
Microbiological/animal. Extract of a fermentation product of ► *milk* by ► *lactic acid bacteria* in the presence of calcium, phosphorous, magnesium and zinc. Skin protecting substance in cosmetics.

Lactobacillus/Lac Ferment
Microbiological/animal. Product obtained by the fermentation of ► *whey* by ► *lactic acid bacteria*. Skin conditioner in cosmetics.

Lactobacillus/Malpighia Glabra Ferment
Microbiological/vegetable. Product obtained by the fermentation of acerola cherry by ► *lactic acid bacteria*. Skin protecting substance in cosmetics.

Lactobacillus/Porphyridium Ferment
Microbiological/vegetable. Product obtained by the fermentation of red algae by ► *lactic acid bacteria*. Skin protecting substance in cosmetics.

Lactobacillus/Skeletonema Ferment

Microbiological/vegetable. Product obtained by the fermentation of phytoplankton by ► *lactic acid bacteria.* Skin protecting substance in cosmetics.

Lactococcus Ferment

Can be microbiological or animal. Product obtained from or extract of the bacterial culture derived from ► *lactic acid bacteria.* The denomination does not provide any information as to whether vegetable or animal raw materials were fermented. Humectant, skin conditioner and skin protecting substance in cosmetics.

Lactococcus/Lac Ferment Lysate

From living and killed animals (► milk). Product obtained by fermenting ► *milk* using ► *lactic acid bacteria,* thus breaking down the microorganism cells. Skin conditioner in cosmetics.

Lactococcus Lysate

Can be microbiological or animal. Broken down ► *lactic acid bacteria.* The nutrient medium can have been animal (e.g. ► *milk*). Skin protecting substance in cosmetics.

Lactoferrin

From living and killed animals (► milk). Iron-binding ► *protein* from ► *milk.* Skin and hair conditioner in cosmetics.

Lactoflavin ► Riboflavin

Lactoglobulin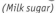

From living and killed animals (► milk). ► *Protein* from ► *whey.* Antistatic, skin and hair conditioner in cosmetics.

Lactoperoxidase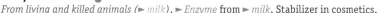

From living and killed animals (► milk). ► *Enzyme* from ► *milk.* Stabilizer in cosmetics.

Lactose

(Milk sugar)

From living and killed animals (► milk). A sugar in ► *milk.* Obtained from the ► *whey* of cow's milk. Carrier substance for flavour enhancers and flavouring substances in many processed foods, e.g. soups, sauces, potato chips, confectionery. In infant formulas and dietetic foods. Bulking agent and binding agent in medication (tablets/pills). Source material for producing ► *lactic acid,* ► *lactitol* and ► *lactulose.* Humectant and skin conditioner in cosmetics.

Lactose Syrup

(Glucose-galactose syrup)

From living and killed animals (► milk). Mixture of the sugars glucose, galactose and ► *lactose* obtained by enzymatic breakdown of ► *lactose* or ► *whey.* Sweetener in foods.

Lactoyl Methylsilanol Elastinate

From killed animals. Chemically altered ► *elastin.* Antistatic, skin and hair conditioner in cosmetics.

Lactoyl Phytosphingosine
Can be vegetable/synthetic or animal. Compound of ► *lactic acid* and ► *phytosphingosine*. Skin conditioner in cosmetics.

Lactulose
From living and killed animals. A synthetic disaccharide derived from ► *lactose*. Used as a laxative. In medication for treating brain damage resulting from liver diseases.

Lacty® ► Lactitol

Lambskin
From killed animals. The pelt (see ► *fur*) of young sheep. On paint rollers, as car seat covers, in carpets, shoe linings, warm clothing, baby blankets, etc.

Lambswool
From living animals. The ► *wool* from the first shearing of young sheep. In textiles for clothing, accessories, blankets, etc.

Laneth-n
From living or killed animals. Compounds of chemically altered ► *lanolin alcohol*. Emulsifiers, surfactants, cleansing agents and viscosity controlling agent in cosmetics.

Laneth-n-Acetate
From living or killed animals. Compounds of chemically altered ► *lanolin alcohol*. Emulsifiers, surfactants, cleansing agents and viscosity controlling agents in cosmetics.

Lanolate
From living or killed animals. Compound of ► *fatty acids* from ► *lanolin*. Emulsifier and surfactant in cosmetics.

Lanolic Acid ► Lanolin Acid

Lanolin
(Adeps lanae. Wool wax. Wool grease)
From living or killed animals. Secretion of the sebaceous glands of sheep. Is washed out of the ► *wool* of shorn or slaughtered sheep and purified. Antistatic, emollient, hair and skin conditioner, surfactant and carrier in many cosmetics. In medications (ointments) as a skin care substance, healing aid or carrier. In wood care products. Source material for many other substances, e.g. ► *vitamin D*, ► *acetylated lanolin alcohol*, ► *laneth-n* compounds, ► *Eucerit®*, ► *lanolin oil*, etc.

Lanolin Acid
From living or killed animals. ► *Fatty acids* from ► *lanolin*. Antistatic, emollient, skin conditioner, emulsifier, viscosity controlling agent and binding agent in cosmetics.

Lanolin Alcohol
(Alcoholes adipis lanae. Wool wax alcohol. Eucerit®)
From living or killed animals. Mixed alcohols from ► *lanolin* treated with lye. Antistatic, emollient, hair conditioner, emulsifier, viscosity controlling agent and binding agent in cosmetics. The purest lanolin alcohol is Eucerit®, the emulsifier in Nivea® creme.

Lanolin, Anhydrous

From living or killed animals. Pure, water-free ► *lanolin.*

Lanolin Cera

(Cera lanae. Lanolin wax)

From living or killed animals. Fraction of ► *lanolin* that remains after separating the ► *lanolin oil.* Antistatic, emollient, hair and skin conditioner, emulsifier, film forming agent, binding agent and foam booster in cosmetics.

Lanolin Linoleate

From living or killed animals. Chemically altered ► *lanolin.* Antistatic, emollient, hair and skin conditioner in cosmetics.

Lanolin Oil

(Wool wax oil)

From living or killed animals. Liquid fraction of ► *lanolin.* Antistatic, emollient, hair conditioner, solvent, emulsifier and binding agent in cosmetics.

Lanolin Ricinoleate

From living or killed animals. Chemically altered ► *lanolin.* Antistatic, emollient, hair conditioner, solvent, emulsifier and binding agent in cosmetics.

Lanolin Wax ► Lanolin Cera

Lanolin, Ethoxylated ► PEG-n Lanolate

Lanolinamide DEA

From living or killed animals. Alcohol compound of ► *fatty acids* from ► *lanolin.* Emulsifier, emulsion stabilizer, surfactant and viscosity controlling agent in cosmetics.

Lanosterol

From living or killed animals. A ► *steroid* compound, related to ► *cholesterol.* Obtained from ► *lanolin.* Antistatic, emollient, skin and hair conditioner in cosmetics.

Lard

From killed animals. ► *Fat* melted out of the fat tissues of pigs and geese. Used for frying, cooking and baking, also as an ingredient in processed foods. Raw material for cosmetic ingredients, e.g. ► *acetylated hydrogenated lard glyceride,* ► *acetylated lard glyceride,* ► *hydrogenated lard,* ► *lard glyceride.* Used as a source of ► *fatty acids.*

Lard Glyceride(s)

From killed animals. ► *Glycerides* from ► *lard.* Emulsifiers, skin conditioners and viscosity controlling agents in cosmetics.

Lauric Acid

(Dodecanoic acid)

Vegetable, can theoretically also be animal. A ► *saturated fatty acid.* Occurs naturally in copious amounts in coconut oil, palm kernel oil, laurel berries and ► *milk.* Obtained industrially from the aforementioned plants. Lauric acid and its derivatives (laurates) are used as emulsifiers, surfactants and cleansing substances in cosmetics.

Lauric/Palmitic/Oleic Triglyceride
Can be vegetable or animal. ► *Glycerides* of ► *lauric acid*, ► *palmitic acid* and ► *oleic acid*. Emollient, skin conditioner in cosmetics.

Lauroyl Collagen Amino Acids
From killed animals. Chemically altered ► *amino acids* from ► *collagen*. Antistatic, cleansing agent and hair conditioner in cosmetics.

Lauroyl Glutamic Acid
Mostly vegetable, can theoretically also be animal. Compound of ► *lauryl alcohol* and ► *glutamic acid*. Skin conditioner in cosmetics.

Lauroyl Hydrolyzed Collagen
From killed animals. Chemically/enzymatically altered ► *collagen*. Antistatic, surfactant, hair and skin conditioner in cosmetics.

Lauroyl Hydrolyzed Elastin
From killed animals. Chemically/enzymatically altered ► *elastin*. Skin and hair conditioner in cosmetics.

Lauroyl Lactylic Acid
Can be vegetable/microbiological or partly animal. Compound of ► *lauryl alcohol* and ► *lactic acid*. Surfactant in cosmetics.

Lauroyl Lysine
Vegetable/microbiological, can theoretically also be partly animal. Compound of ► *lauryl alcohol* and ► *lysine*. Used as viscosity controlling agent, hair and skin conditioner in cosmetics.

Lauroyl Sarcosine
Can be vegetable/synthetic or animal. Compound of ► *lauryl alcohol* and ► *sarcosine*. Antistatic, surfactant, cleansing agent and hair conditioner in cosmetics.

Lauryl Alcohol
(Dodecanol. Dodecyl alcohol)
Vegetable, can theoretically also be animal. A ► *fatty alcohol*, obtained from ► *fatty acids*, e.g. ► *lauric acid*. Emollient, emulsifier, emulsion stabilizer and viscosity controlling agent in cosmetics.

Lauryl Aminopropylglycine
Mostly vegetable/animal, can also be vegetable/synthetic/microbiological. Compound of ► *lauryl alcohol* and ► *glycine*. Antistatic, hair and skin conditioner in cosmetics.

Lauryl Diethylenediaminoglycine
Mostly vegetable/animal, can also be vegetable/synthetic/microbiological. Compound of ► *lauryl alcohol* and ► *glycine*. Antistatic, hair and skin conditioner in cosmetics.

Lauryl Glycol
Vegetable/synthetic, can theoretically also be partly animal. Compound of ► *lauryl alcohol* and ► *glycol*. Antistatic, emollient, hair and skin conditioner in cosmetics.

Lauryl Isostearate

Can be vegetable or animal. Compound of ► *lauryl alcohol* and ► *stearic acid.* Skin conditioner and emollient in cosmetics.

Lauryl Lactate

Can be vegetable/microbiological or partly animal. Compound of ► *lauryl alcohol* and ► *lactic acid.* Emollient, skin conditioner in cosmetics.

Lauryl Oleate

Can be vegetable or animal. Compound of ► *lauryl alcohol* and ► *oleic acid.* Emollient, skin conditioner in cosmetics.

Lauryl Palmitate

Mostly vegetable, can also be partly animal. Compound of ► *lauryl alcohol* and ► *palmitic acid.* Antistatic and emollient, skin conditioner in cosmetics.

Lauryl Polyglyceryl-6 Cetearyl Glycol Ether

Can be vegetable/synthetic or partly animal. ► *Glycol* compound of ► *lauryl alcohol,* ► *glycerol* and ► *cetostearyl alcohol.* Emulsifier and skin conditioner in cosmetics.

Lauryl Stearate

Can be vegetable or animal. Compound of ► *lauryl alcohol* and ► *stearic acid.* Emollient, skin conditioner in cosmetics.

Lauryldimonium Hydroxypropyl Hydrolyzed Casein

From living and killed animals (► milk). Chemically/enzymatically altered ► *casein.* Antistatic, hair and skin conditioner in cosmetics.

Lauryldimonium Hydroxypropyl Hydrolyzed Collagen

From killed animals. Chemically/enzymatically altered ► *collagen.* Antistatic, emollient, hair and skin conditioner in cosmetics.

Lauryldimonium Hydroxypropyl Hydrolyzed Keratin

From killed or living animals. Chemically/enzymatically altered ► *keratin.* Antistatic, skin and hair conditioner in cosmetics.

Lauryldimonium Hydroxypropyl Hydrolyzed Silk

From killed animals. Chemically/enzymatically altered ► *silk.* Antistatic, skin and hair conditioner in cosmetics.

Leather

From killed animals. The skin of dead animals, stripped off and made durable by means of chemical treatment (tanning). Primarily from cattle/calves, but also from other animals, such as sheep, goats, horses, pigs, dogs, cats, kangaroos, ostriches, snakes, crocodiles and fishes. In footwear, jackets, belts, hats, purses, bags and handbags, jewellery, upholstery, car interiors, etc.

Lecithin

(Choline bitartrate. E 322)
Mostly vegetable, can also be animal. Complex compound of ► *fatty acids,* ► *glycerol,*

phosphoric acid and ► *choline*. Occurs naturally in animal and vegetable tissues. Can be obtained from animal cells, e.g. ► *egg yolk*. Industrially produced lecithin is usually from soybeans, also from sunflower and other oilseeds, and often so labelled. Widely used as an emulsifier in foods. Antistatic, emollient, emulsifier, skin conditioner in cosmetics. Excipient in medicines. Diverse industrial applications as emulsifier or surfactant.

Lecithinamide DEA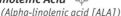
Mostly vegetable/synthetic, can also be partly animal. Chemically altered ► *lecithin*. Antistatic, viscosity controlling agent, foam booster and hair conditioner in cosmetics.

Leucine
Can be vegetable, microbiological or animal. An essential ► *amino acid* important for muscle growth and protein metabolism. Occurs in animal ► *proteins* (e.g. muscle tissue, ► *albumen* and ► *casein*), as well as in plants (cereals and pulses). Obtained by isolation from either vegetable or animal proteins, or using bacterial cultures. Antistatic, hair and skin conditioner in cosmetics. In nutritional supplements and infusion solutions.

Leukocyte Extract
From killed animals. Extract of white blood cells from the ► *blood* of killed mammals. Skin conditioner in cosmetics.

Levodopa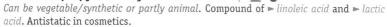
(L-DOPA. Madopar. L-3,4-dihydroxyphenylalanine)
Can be animal or microbiological/vegetable. An ► *amino acid* produced in mammals' bodies from ► *tyrosine* and phenylalanine. Precursor of the neurotransmitters ► *adrenalin*, noradrenalin and dopamine, and the pigment ► *melanin*. Industrially produced from tyrosine. In medication for treating Parkinson's disease and neurological disorders.

Levothyroxine ► *Thyroxine*

Linoleamidopropyl Dimethylamine Lactate
Can be vegetable/synthetic or partly animal. Compound of ► *linoleic acid* and ► *lactic acid*. Antistatic in cosmetics.

Linoleic Acid
Vegetable. An ► *omega-6 fatty acid*. Occurs naturally in vegetable oils such as safflower, sunflower, soy and corn germ oil. Antistatic, emollient, skin and hair conditioner, surfactant and cleansing agent in cosmetics.

Linolenic Acid
(Alpha-linolenic acid [ALA])
Vegetable. An essential ► *omega-3 fatty acid*. Occurs naturally in many vegetable oils, e.g. linseed, chia and perilla oils. Natural constituent of vegetable foods. Antistatic, emollient, skin and hair conditioner, surfactant and cleansing agent in cosmetics. Products of linolenic acid are also used as additives in varnishes and lacquers.

Linoleyl Lactate
Can be vegetable/microbiological or partly animal. Compound of linoleyl alcohol (► *fatty alcohol* of ► *linoleic acid*) and ► *lactic acid*. Emollient and skin conditioner in cosmetics.

Lipase

Can be from killed animals or microbiological. ► *Enzymes* produced in the pancreas that break down ► *lipids* in the intestine as part of the digestion process. Obtained from the pancreases of animals (usually pigs) or from microorganisms (e.g. moulds or bacteria). Added to many laundry detergents in order to improve the cleansing affect and in soap production. Used for processing ► *fatty acids* and flavourings in the food industry (not subject to mandatory labelling). Ingredient in medication for substituting enzymes in the case of pancreas diseases.

Lipids

Can be vegetable or from living or killed animals. Collective term for ► *fats* and fat-like substances. Occur naturally in all animal and vegetable tissues. Most lipids are water insoluble. The term "lipids" is often applied to fats and oils only, however it also includes the fat-like substances, such as hydrocarbons (e.g. ► *alkylglycerols,* ► *squalane* and ► *squalene*), ► *fatty alcohols,* ► *fatty acids,* ► *glycerides,* ► *waxes* and ► *ceramides.*

Liquid Crystals

Can be animal or synthetic. Substances that are liquid, but possess similar physical (especially optical) characteristics to solid crystals. Many liquid crystals are based on the chemical structure of ► *cholesterol* (see ► *cholesteryl benzoate* and the subsequent entries). Used as cosmetic ingredients. In technical appliances, e.g. LCD screens in computers, televisions, digital cameras, etc., and thermosensitive pigments in liquid crystal thermometers.

Lisinopril

Vegetable/microbiological, can theoretically be partly animal. An important ACE inhibitor (pharmaceutical drug that lowers blood pressure). Originally synthesized on the basis of proteins found in snake venom. Is now biochemically produced from ► *proline,* which is derived from ► *glutamic acid.* Active agent in medication for treating high blood pressure.

Lithium Stearate

Can be mineral/vegetable or animal. Compound of ► *stearic acid.* Opacifier, viscosity controlling agent, anticaking agent and binding agent in cosmetics.

Liver Extract

From killed animals. Extract from the livers of mammals. Skin conditioner in cosmetics.

Liver Hydrolysate

From killed animals. Chemically/enzymatically altered ► *proteins* from the livers of killed mammals. Skin conditioner in cosmetics.

Liver of Sulphur ► *Hepar Sulfuris*

Lobster

Killed animals. Marine ► *crustaceans.* Are caught in lobster traps, and often transported and stored alive for as long as several months in tiered tanks or crates with circulating cold salt water. Finally they are cooked alive in boiling water. Lobsters are regarded by some as a delicacy and also as an ► *aphrodisiac*. The exoskeletons can be used for obtaining ► *chitin*.

Lutein
(E 161b)
Can be vegetable or animal. Natural orange pigment that belongs to the carotenoids. Occurs naturally in dark vegetable leaves, marigold petals and ► *egg yolk*. Can be industrially obtained from both plants, e.g. marigold or lucerne, and egg yolks. Colour in foods and animal feed.

Luteum Ovi Extract
From living and killed animals (► egg). Extract of ► *egg yolk*. Skin and hair conditioner in cosmetics.

Luteum Ovi Powder
From living and killed animals (► egg). Dried, powdered ► *egg yolk*. Abrasive in cosmetics.

Lysine
Microbiological, can theoretically be animal. An essential ► *amino acid*. Occurs naturally in ► *milk* and animal muscle protein. Obtained industrially via fermentation. Antistatic, hair and skin conditioner in cosmetics. In nutritional supplements. Excipient in pharmaceutical drugs.

Lysine Aspartate
Microbiological/vegetable, can theoretically also be partly animal. Compound of ► *lysine* and ► *aspartic acid*. Skin and hair conditioner in cosmetics.

Lysine Carboxymethyl Cysteinate
From living or killed animals, can also be microbiological or synthetic. Compound of ► *lysine* and ► *cysteine*. Skin conditioner in cosmetics.

Lysine Cocoate
Microbiological/vegetable, can theoretically also be partly animal. Compound of ► *lysine* and coconut ► *fatty acids*. Surfactant in cosmetics.

Lysine Glutamate
Microbiological/vegetable, can theoretically also be partly animal. Compound of ► *lysine* and ► *glutamic acid*. Skin conditioner in cosmetics.

Lysine Hydrochloride
Microbiological/mineral, can theoretically also be partly animal. Salt of ► *lysine*. Antioxidant, reducing agent and skin conditioner in cosmetics.

Lysine Lauroyl Methionate
Vegetable/microbiological/synthetic, can theoretically also be animal. Compound of ► *lysine*, ► *lauric acid* and ► *methionine*. Skin conditioner in cosmetics.

Lysine PCA
Vegetable/microbiological, can also be partly animal. Compound of ► *lysine* and ► *glutamic acid*. Antistatic, humectant and skin conditioner in cosmetics.

Lysine Thiazolidine Carboxylate

Synthetic/microbiological, can theoretically also be partly animal. Carbon compound of ► *lysine.* Surfactant and skin conditioner in cosmetics.

Lysolecithin

Can be from living or killed animals or vegetable/microbiological. ► *Lecithin,* chemically altered using ► *phospholipase A₂.* Emulsifier in cosmetics.

Lysozyme

(E 1105)

Mostly animal, can also be microbiological. Antibacterial ► *enzyme,* for instance in saliva, tears, eggs and some microorganisms. Obtained primarily from egg white (► *albumen*), but also from genetically altered microorganisms. Preservative in mature cheese. Used as an additive in ► *wine,* in order to prevent the growth of certain bacteria.

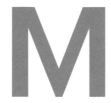

Macrogol ► *PEG*

Macrogolglycerol Oleate ► *PEG-n Glyceryl Oleate*

Macrogolglycerol Ricinoleate ► *PEG-n Glyceryl Ricinoleate*

Macrogolglycerol Stearate ► *PEG-n Glyceryl Stearate*

Magnesium Diglutamate ► *Glutamates*

Magnesium Distearate ► *Magnesium Stearate*

Magnesium Glutamate ► *Glutamates*

Magnesium Lanolate
From living or killed animals. Chemically altered ► *fatty acids* from ► *lanolin*. Emulsifier, surfactant, anticaking agent and viscosity controlling agent in cosmetics.

Magnesium Oleth Sulfate
Can be vegetable or animal. Magnesium and sulphur compound of ► *oleyl alcohol*. Surfactant and cleansing agent in cosmetics.

Magnesium Orotate ► *Orotic Acid*

Magnesium Palmitate
Mostly vegetable, can also be animal. Magnesium salt of ► *palmitic acid*. opacifier, viscosity controlling agent and anticaking agent in cosmetics.

Magnesium Salts of Fatty Acids ► *Magnesium Stearate*

Magnesium Stearate
(E 470 b. Magnesium salts of fatty acids. Magnesium distearate)
Can be vegetable or from killed animals. Magnesium salt of ► *stearic acid*. Colourant, moisturizer, bulking agent and anticaking agent in cosmetics. Carrier, anticaking agent and glazing agent in processed foods, e.g. baking powder, decorating sugar, seasonings. Ingredient in infant formulas. Bulking agent in medicinal tablets/pills).

Magnesium Tallowate
From killed animals. Chemically altered ► *tallow*. Emulsifier, surfactant, anticaking agent and bulking agent in cosmetics.

Mammarian Hydrolysate

From killed animals. Chemically/enzymatically altered ► *proteins* from the mammary gland tissue of female mammals. Skin protecting substance in cosmetics.

Mammary Extract

From killed animals. Extract from the mammary glands of female mammals. Skin protecting substance in cosmetics.

Mango Butter

Vegetable. Fat from mango seeds. Not to be confused with similarly named animal ► *butter.* Souce of cosmetic ingredients. Partial substitute for ► *cocoa butter* in chocolate products.

Mare's Milk

(Equae lac)
From living animals. ► *Milk* of horses. Hair conditioner in cosmetics.

Margarita Powder

From killed animals. Powder from ground ► *pearls.* Abrasive in cosmetics.

Marine Oils

From killed animals. Oils from the body fat or livers of marine animals, especially ► *fish oil,* but also from whales and seals (► *train oil*).

Marmota Oil ► *Marmot Oil*

Marmot Oil

(Marmota oil)
From killed animals. Oil from the fat tissue of marmots. Hair conditioner in cosmetics.

Marrow Extract

From killed animals. Extract from the bone marrow of mammals. Skin conditioner in cosmetics.

MEA-Hydrolyzed Collagen

From killed animals. Chemically/enzymatically altered ► *collagen.* Skin and hair conditioner in cosmetics.

MEA-Hydrolyzed Silk

From killed animals. Chemically/enzymatically altered ► *silk.* Skin and hair conditioner in cosmetics.

MEA-PPG-8-Steareth-7 Carboxylate

Can be vegetable/synthetic or animal. Polymer compound of ► *stearyl alcohol.* Emulsifier and cleansing agent in cosmetics.

Meat. Meat Products

From killed animals. Collective term for the soft tissue or flesh (especially muscle tissue) of all kinds of animals, most commonly used in reference to the flesh of birds, mammals and reptiles. Used as food/food ingredient. Several cosmetic ingredients are obtained from meat or meat constituents, e.g. from connective tissue (► *connective tissue extract,*

► *collagen,* ► *sarcosine*), muscle tissue (► *carnitine*, ► *carnosine*, ► *cytochrome C*, ► *glu-tathione*, ► *glycogen*, ► *heart extract*, ► *heart hydrolysate* ► *histidine*, ► *muscle extract*) and fat tissue (► *fats*).

Meat and Bone Meal

From killed animals. Ground animal tissue of all kinds, "slaughterhouse waste." Used as animal feed for "livestock" (now banned EU-wide as a possible transmission path for BSE). Is still used as a fertilizer and especially as fuel for energy production.

Meat Broth ► Broth

Medium-Chain Triglycerides

(MCT)

Mostly vegetable, can theoretically also be animal. ► *Triglycerides* of ► *capric acid*, ► *caproic acid*, ► *caprylic acid* and ► *lauric acid*. Occur naturally in certain ► *fats*, especially in coconut oil, also palm oil and ► *milk*. Industrially produced primarily from coconut oil, isolating above all ► *tricaprin* and ► *tricaprylin*. Medium-chain triglycerides have a special status compared with other fats, having an especially low melting point and being water-soluble; they are especially easy to metabolize, as they need not be broken down first. This makes them suitable as a readily available, low-stress source of energy. In certain dietetic foods, food supplements (e.g. for gaining weight or high performance athletics), special diets and infusion therapies (e.g. in the case of digestive disorders). Carrier substance in medicinal creams.

Mel ► Honey

Mel Extract

From living animals. Extract from ► *honey*. Moisturizer in cosmetics.

Melamine

Synthetic. A compound of carbon and nitrogen. Obtained industrially from ► *urea*. In flame retardants. Additive in concrete mixtures. Used for making ► *melamine resin*; the term "melamine" is also often used as a synonym for ► *melamine resin*.

Melamine/Formaldehyde Resin ► Melamine Resin

Melamine Resin

(Melamine/formaldehyde resin. Melamine [casual usage])

Synthetic. A hard plastic. Reaction product of ► *melamine* and formaldehyde, commonly referred to (incorrectly) as "melamine." Film forming agent in cosmetics. In resins for treating textiles and paper, in wood glues and laminate coatings. In unbreakable tableware, kitchen utensils, etc. In acoustic and thermal insulation. In "dirt erasers."

Melanin

Can be animal or synthetic. A natural pigment, either brown-black or reddish. Occurs naturally in numerous animals and plants. Main constituent of squid ink (► *sepia*). Is responsible in varying combinations and concentrations for the skin and hair colour of humans. Can be chemically produced from ► *tyrosin* or ► *levodopa* or derived from ► *sepia*. Skin protecting substance in cosmetics. In some UV-blocking sunglasses.

Melatonin

Can be from killed animals or synthetic. A hormone with an important role in regulating the circadian rhythms of animals and plants. Can be obtained from animal tissue, but also from petroleum products. Antioxidant in cosmetics. Approved as medication for treating sleep disorders. Available over the counter in Canada and the United States as a dietary supplement (it is supposed to combat the effects of shift work and jetlag; the efficacy is disputed). Melatonin is a prescription drug in many other countries.

Melissic Acid

(Triacontanoic acid)
Can be animal or synthetic. A ► *saturated fatty acid*, important constituent of ► *beeswax*. Can be obtained from ► *beeswax*, ► *shellac* or ► *montan wax*. Viscosity controlling agent in cosmetics. In "metallic" effect coatings.

Menadione ► *Vitamin K*

Metatartaric Acid

(E 353)
Vegetable, source materials may have been treated with animal substances. ► *Tartaric acid*, chemically altered by means of heat treatment. Acidifier in wine.

Methionine

Synthetic. An essential ► *amino acid*. Occurs naturally in various animal and vegetable ► *proteins*. Industrially produced from petroleum products. Hair and skin conditioner in cosmetics. Used for treating liver diseases and heavy metal poisoning, also in infusions for parenteral nutrition. Additive in animal feed.

Methyl Caproate

Mostly vegetable/synthetic, can also be partly animal. Compound of methanol and ► *caproic acid*. Emollient and skin conditioner in cosmetics.

Methyl Caprylate

Mostly vegetable/synthetic, can also be partly animal. Compound of methanol and ► *caprylic acid*. Emollient, skin conditioner in cosmetics.

Methyl Caprylate/Caprate

Mostly vegetable/synthetic, can also be partly animal. Compound of methanol, ► *caproic acid* and ► *capric acid*. Emollient and skin conditioner in cosmetics.

Methyl Glucose Dioleate

Can be vegetable/synthetic or animal. Compound of ► *oleic acid*. Emollient, humectant and skin conditioner incosmetics.

Methyl Glucose Isostearate

Can be vegetable/synthetic or animal. Compound of methanol and ► *stearic acid*. Emulsifier and skin conditioner in cosmetics.

Methyl Glucose Sesquicaprylate/Sesquicaprate

Mostly vegetable/synthetic, can also be partly animal. Compound of methanol, ► *caproic acid* and ► *capric acid*. Emollient, skin conditioner and emulsifier in cosmetics.

M

Methyl Glucose Sesquiisostearate
Can be vegetable/synthetic or animal. Compound of methanol with glucose and ► *stearic acid*. Emollient, skin conditioner and emulsifier in cosmetics.

Methyl Glucose Sesquioleate
Can be vegetable/synthetic or animal. Compound of methanol with glucose and ► *oleic acid*. Emollient, skin conditioner and emulsifier in cosmetics.

Methyl Glucose Sesquistearate
Can be vegetable/synthetic or animal. Compound of ► *stearic acid*. Emollient, skin conditioner and emulsifier in cosmetics.

Methyl Glutamic Acid
Vegetable/synthetic, can theoretically also be partly animal. Compound of ► *glutamic acid*. Antistatic, skin and hair conditioner in cosmetics.

Methyl Hydroxycetyl Glucaminium Lactate
Mostly vegetable/synthetic, can also be partly animal. Compound of methanol, ► *cetyl alcohol*, the sugar alcohol sorbitol and ► *lactic acid*. Antistatic, skin and hair conditioner in cosmetics.

Methyl Hydroxystearate
Can be vegetable/synthetic or animal. Compound of methanol and ► *stearic acid*. Emollient and skin conditioner in cosmetics.

Methyl Isostearate
Can be vegetable/synthetic or animal. Compound of methanol and ► *stearic acid*. Emulsifier and skin conditioner in cosmetics.

Methyl Linoleate
Synthetic/vegetable. Compound of methanol and ► *linoleic acid*. Emulsifier and skin conditioner in cosmetics.

Methyl Oleate
Can be vegetable/synthetic or animal. Compound of methanol and ► *oleic acid*. Emollient and skin conditioner in cosmetics.

Methyl Palmitate
Mostly vegetable/synthetic, can also be partly animal. Compound of methanol and ► *palmitic acid*. Emollient and skin conditioner in cosmetics.

Methyl Stearate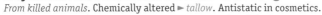
Can be vegetable/synthetic or animal. Compound of methanol and ► *stearic acid*. Emollient and skin conditioner in cosmetics.

Methylenebis Tallow Acetamidodimonium Chloride
From killed animals. Chemically altered ► *tallow*. Antistatic in cosmetics.

Methylglucose Dioleate/Hydroxystearate
Can be vegetable/synthetic or animal. Sugar compound of ► *oleic acid* and ► *stearic acid*. Surfactant and emulsifier in cosmetics.

M

Methylsilanol Elastinate
From killed animals. Chemically altered ► *elastin*. Antistatic and skin conditioner in cosmetics.

Microcrystalline Wax
(Cera microcristallina. E 905)
Synthetic. Mixture of various hydrocarbons, ► *wax* with a particularly fine crystalline structure, one of the natural constituents of petroleum. Obtained with the aid of chemical and physical methods from the residues of petroleum distillation, or from peat, slate, lignite or natural asphalt/bitumen deposits. Binding agent, emulsion stabilizer, opacifier and viscosity controlling agent in cosmetics. Base for ► *chewable mass* in chewing gum. Food additive for surface treatment of confectionery (except chocolate), chewing gum, melons, mango, papaya and avocado.

Milk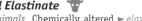
(Lac)
From living and killed* animals. White, opaque, energy-rich fluid, produced in the mammary glands of female mammals for feeding their own offspring. Quantity and composition are suited to the requirements of the young of the respective species. Traditionally obtained by humans by manual extraction (squeezing and pulling) from the teats of the mother animals (mainly cows, but also sheep, goats and horses). Milk is now usually extracted with suction pumps. Used as food (beverages, cooking and baking ingredients, in desserts). Skin conditioner in cosmetics. Constituents or derivatives of milk are also used in a multitude of industrially produced foods, food supplements, cosmetics and pharmaceutical drugs. Some examples: amino acids (► *milk amino acids*) and proteins (► *casein*, ► *lactoglobulin*, ► *hydrolyzed milk protein*), fats (► *butter*, ► *butterfat*, ► *hydrogenated milk lipids*) and ► *cream*, carbohydrates (► *lactose*), liquids (► *buttermilk*, ► *whey*), ► *cheese* and fermented products (► *lactic acid*, ► *yogurt*). Legally, only cows' mik may be labelled simply as "milk." Milk from other animals must be labelled specifically according to the origin, e.g. "buffalo milk," "sheep milk," "mare's milk" or "goat milk." Vegetable milks (e.g. from soy, rice, almonds, hemp or oats) may not, with the exception of coconut milk, be sold as "milk" at all, but only under alternative names (such as "soy drink").

*Milk production inevitably involves killing animals. Cows must give birth once a year in order to be able to produce milk. This is generally achieved by artificial insemination. The "useless" male calves are separated from their mothers after birth, fattened, killed and processed to meat, leather, gelatin, bone meal, etc. A few are spared and used as breeding bulls. Dairy cows, who would otherwise have a natural life expectancy of at least 20 years, are generally slaughtered within 4 years (i.e. at an age of about 6 years) due to sinking milk production or increasing health problems caused by the constant stress of milking. Their bodies are processed just as those of the calves are. Therefore, milk is by no means only from living, but also from killed animals, as their death and economic exploitation are immediately interconnected.

Milk Acid ► *Lactic Acid*

Milk Amino Acids

From living and killed animals (► milk*).* ► *Amino acids* obtained from ► milk by hydrolysis. Antistatic, hair and skin conditioner in cosmetics.

Milk Products ► *Dairy Products*

Milk Protein

From living and killed animals (► milk*).* Collective term for the ► *proteins* in ► milk. The term usually refers to ► *casein*, but also includes ► *whey protein*. Bodybuilding protein formulas and food supplements can often contain milk protein.

Milk Powder

(Lac powder. Dried milk. Powdered milk. Whole milk powder. Skim milk powder)

From living and killed animals (► milk*).* Dried, powdered cow's ► milk. Food ingredient, e.g. in baked goods, ► *yogurt*, ice cream, chocolates, desserts, soups and sauces. Ingredient in some infant formulas. In nutritional supplements. Skin conditioner in cosmetics. Used in the production of animal feed.

Milk Serum

From living and killed animals (► milk*).* Deproteinized ► *whey*. Refreshment beverage. Cosmetic ingredient, usually under the name "Lac" (► milk).

Milk Sugar ► *Lactose*

Milkamidopropyl Amine Oxide

From living and killed animals (► milk*).* Chemical compound of ► *butterfat*. Hair conditioner in cosmetics.

Milkamidopropyl Betaine

From living and killed animals (► milk*).* Chemical compound of ► *butterfat*. Surfactant, cleansing agent and skin conditioner in cosmetics.

Milkfat ► *Butterfat*

Mink

From killed animals. Name for two species of the weasel family, the European mink (*Mustela lutreola*) and the American mink (*Neovison vison*), as well as for the ► *fur* of those animals. It usually refers to the American mink, bred and kept in cages in mink farms for its fur. In clothing and fashion accessories, either as fur trimming or used for making complete clothing items (e.g. coats), a single item of clothing requiring the skin of several animals.

Mink Oil

(Mustela oil)

From killed animals. Oil from the body fat of killed ► *minks*. Emollient, skin and hair conditioner in cosmetics. In some leather care products.

Mink Oil PEG-13 Esters

From killed animals. Chemically altered ► *mink oil*. Emollient, hair and skin conditioner in cosmetics.

M

Minkamide DEA

From killed animals. Ammonia compound of ► *mink oil.* Surfactant and foam booster in cosmetics.

Minkamidopropalkonium Chloride

From killed animals. Ammonia compound of ► *mink oil.* Antistatic and hair conditioner in cosmetics.

Minkamidopropyl Amine Oxide

From killed animals. Ammonia compound of ► *mink oil.* Surfactant, hydrotrope, cleansing agent, hair conditioner and foam booster in cosmetics.

Minkamidopropyl Betaine

From killed animals. Ammonia compound of ► *mink oil.* Surfactant, skin and hair conditioner, foam booster and cleansing agent in cosmetics.

Minkamidopropyl Dimethylamine

From killed animals. Ammonia compound of ► *mink oil.* Antistatic, emulsifier and surfactant in cosmetics.

Minkamidopropyl Ethyldimonium Ethosulfate

From killed animals. Ammonia compound of ► *mink oil.* Antistatic and hair conditioner in cosmetics.

Mixed Acetic and Tartaric Acid Esters of Mono- and Diglycerides of Fatty Acids
(E 472f)

Can be vegetable or animal. Reaction product of acetic acid and ► *tartaric acid* with ► *glycerides* of ► *fatty acids* (chemical composition and activity identical to those of ► *mono- and diacetyl tartaric acid esters of mono- and diglycerides of fatty acids*). Emulsifiers and flour treatment agents in baked foods.

Mixed Isopropanolamines Lanolate

From living or killed animals. Chemically altered ► *lanolin.* Emulsifier and surfactant in cosmetics.

Mohair

Mostly from living, also from killed animals. ► *Hair* of angora goats, obtained by shearing living animals, but also from killed animals. Used as knitting yarn, in clothing, blankets, doll hair, etc.

Mono- and Diacetyl Tartaric Acid Esters of Mono- and Diglycerides of Fatty Acids
(E 472e. Diacetyl tartaric acid ester of mono- and diglycerides. DATEM)

Mostly vegetable, can also be from killed or living animals. Reaction product of acetic acid, ► *tartaric acid* and ► *fatty acids.* Obtained primarily from vegetable ► *fats* (e.g. from soy oil), however can also be derived from animal fats. Emulsifier in foods, especially baked goods. Emollient, hair and skin conditioner, surfactant and emulsifier in cosmetics.

Mono- and Diglycerides of Fatty Acids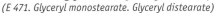
(E 471. Glyceryl monostearate. Glyceryl distearate)
Can be vegetable or animal. Collective term for degradation products of ► *fatty acids.*
Mostly from vegetable ► *fats* (e.g. soy oil), but can also be derived from animal fats.
Widespread use as emulsifier and flour treatment agent in foods.

Monoammonium Glutamate ► *Glutamate*

Monopotassium Glutamate ► *Glutamates*

Monopotassium Tartrate ► *Potassium Bitartrate*

Monosaccharide Lactate Condensate
Mostly vegetable/microbiological, can also be partly animal. Reaction product of ► *lactic acid* with various sugars. Antistatic and skin conditioner in cosmetics.

Monosodium Glutamate ► *Glutamates*

Monostearin ► *Glyceryl Stearate*

Montan Acid Wax
Synthetic. ► *Fatty acids* from ► *montan wax.* Antistatic, binding agent and viscosity controlling agent in cosmetics.

Montan Cera ► *Montan Wax*

Montan Wax
(Montan cera)
Mineral. ► *Wax* derived from lignite. Antistatic, binding agent, opacifier and viscosity controlling agent in cosmetics.

Mother of Pearl
(Nacre)
From killed animals. A solid composite material of calcium carbonate and organic substances produced by molluscs such as ► *bivalves* as a protective inner layer of their shells. Used for its optical qualities (► *pearlescence*) in jewellery, arts and crafts, buttons for shirts and blouses, and inlays in furniture and musical instruments.

MSG ► *Glutamates*

Mucopolysaccharides ► *Glycosaminoglycans*

Mucosa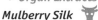
(Mucosa coli suis. Mucosa ductus choledochi. Mucosa ilei suis. Mucosa jejuni suis. Mucosa nasalis suis. Mucosa oculi suis. Mucosa oesophagi suis. Mucosa oris suis. Mucosa pulmonis suis. Mucosa pylori suis. Mucosa recti suis. Mucosa vesicae felleae suis)
► *Organ Extracts*

Mulberry Silk
From killed animals. ► *Silk* from unhatched silkworm cocoons. The silkworms are killed with hot water or steam before they can hatch. After that the silk filament is unwound from the cocoon in one piece. Used in fine, smooth textiles (clothing, décor, covers).

M

Muscle Extract

From killed animals. Extract from the muscle tissue of killed mammals. Skin protective substance in cosmetics.

Muscone

Mostly synthetic, can also be from killed animals. The main substance responsible for the odour of ► *musk.* Can be isolated from musk, is now primarily synthesized from petroleum derivatives. Used in perfumes, air fresheners, etc.

Muscopyridin

Mostly synthetic, can also be from killed animals. Fragrant substance in ► *musk.* Is now primarily synthesized from petroleum derivatives. Used in perfumes, air fresheners, etc.

Mushrooms

Vegetable within the context of this book, but also grown using animal substances. Mushrooms are fungi, organisms that possess cell nuclei and make up a distinct biological kingdom alongside plants and animals. Fungi also include unicellular yeasts and moulds. Mushrooms as referred to in daily usage (both edible and inedible/poisonous) are the fruiting bodies of multicellular fungi. In terms of appearance, mushrooms are closer to plants than animals; however, genetically and metabolically they are more closely related to animals. In this book, we have for simplicity's sake categorized yeasts, moulds and bacteria as "microbiological," multicellular fungi as "vegetable." In this context, edible mushrooms are thus "vegetable." They are, however, often grown on a substrate of animal excrement (e.g. chicken and horse manure), so that, strictly speaking, they are not vegan as long as the manure comes from animal husbandry, and its "disposal" and the animal husbandry itself are economically related.

Musk

From killed or living animals. Substance with a strong smell, secreted from glands of male musk deer, native to the mountains of southern Asia. Can be obtained by capturing the animals and pressing out the glands, however wild animals are often killed and the entire glands cut out and dried (for this reason, musk deer are now classified as an endangered species). Musk is used as a fragrance in perfumes. Also used in traditional traditional Chinese medicine and as an ► *aphrodisiac.* Synthetic ► *muscone* or ► *musk ketone* are now used in modern perfumes.

Musk Ketone

Synthetic. A fragrance derived from petroleum and used as a substitute for genuine ► *musk.* In perfumes, air fresheners, etc. Masking agent in cosmetics.

Mussels ► *Bivalves*

Mustela Cera

From killed animals. Solid constituents of ► *mink oil.* Emollient, skin and hair conditioner, and film forming agent in cosmetics.

Mustela Oil ► *Mink Oil*

Mycoprotein

Microbiological, can be partly animal. ► *Protein* from moulds. Is sold in some countries by the name of "Quorn" as a meat substitute (can contain ► *albumen* as a binding agent)

Myristic Acid

Mostly vegetable, can also be animal. A ► *saturated fatty acid.* Occurs naturally in vegetable fats, but also in animal fats, e.g. ► *butterfat* or ► *fish oil.* Industrially obtained primarily from coconut or palm oil. Emulsifier and cleansing agent in cosmetics. In flavourings/aromas and essential oils. Used in soap production. Constituent of many other cosmetic ingredients.

Myristoyl Glutamic Acid

Mostly vegetable, can also be partly animal. Compound of ► *myristic acid* and ► *glutamic acid.* Skin and hair conditioner in cosmetics.

Myristoyl Glycine/Histidine/Lysine Polypeptide

Mostly animal, can also be synthetic/vegetable/microbiological. ► *Protein* compound of ► *myristic acid,* ► *glycine,* ► *histidine* and ► *lysine.* Skin and hair conditioner in cosmetics.

Myristoyl Hydrolyzed Collagen

From killed animals. Chemically/enzymatically altered ► *collagen.* Antistatic, emollient, skin and hair conditioner, cleansing agent and surfactant in cosmetics.

Myristoyl Lactylic Acid

Mostly vegetable, can also be animal. Compound of ► *myristic acid and* ► *lactic acid.* Surfactant and emulsifier in cosmetics.

Myristoyl Sarcosine

Can be animal or vegetable/microbiological. Compound of ► *myristic acid* and ► *sarcosine.* Antistatic, surfactant, hair conditioner and cleansing agent in cosmetics.

Myristyl Lactate

Mostly vegetable, can also be animal. Compound of myristyl alcohol (from ► *myristic acid*) and ► *lactic acid.* Emollient and skin conditioner in cosmetics.

Myristyl Stearate

Can be vegetable or animal. Compound of myristyl alcohol (from ► *myristic acid*) and ► *stearic acid.* Emollient and skin conditioner in cosmetics.

Mytilus Extract

From killed animals. Extract from mussels. Skin conditioner in cosmetics.

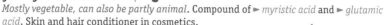

N

Naja Tripudians
From living animals. Venom of the Indian cobra. In ▶ *homeopathic medicines*.

Natural Flavouring
Can be vegetable, animal or microbiological. Flavouring substance or mixture of flavouring substances obtained by appropriate physical, enzymatic or microbiological processes from material of vegetable, animal or microbiological origin and chemically identical to naturally occurring substances. Used for flavouring foods and aromatizing natural cosmetics. If processing leads to any (albeit temporary) alteration of the molecular structure, it is no longer a natural flavouring but a ▶ *nature-identical flavouring*.

Nature-Identical Flavouring
Mostly synthetic or microbiological, can also be of vegetable or animal origin. Chemically defined synthesized flavouring substance, or composition of flavouring substances, chemically identical to a ▶ *natural flavouring*. It is a copy of a natural flavouring, can also be derived from natural substances, but is usually of synthetic or microbiological origin (e.g. mould). The best known example is vanillin (byproduct of cellulose manufacturing or from petroleum derivatives). The term "nature-identical" is not universally used within the European Union, and in Canada such flavours are classed as "artificial."

Neatsfoot Oil
(Bubulum oil)
From killed animals. Purified oil from the shinbones and feet of cattle. Used as a leather care product. Emollient and solvent in cosmetics.

Neopentyl Glycol Dicaprylate/Dicaprate
Mostly vegetable/synthetic, can also be partly animal. ▶ *Glycol* compound of ▶ *caprylic acid* and ▶ *capric acid*. Emollient, skin conditioner in cosmetics.

Neopentyl Glycol Dicaprylate/Dipelargonate/Dicaprate
Mostly vegetable/synthetic, can also be partly animal. ▶ *Glycol* compound of ▶ *caprylic acid*, ▶ *capric acid* and nonanoic acid. Emollient and skin conditioner in cosmetics.

Neopentyl Glycol Diisostearate
Can be vegetable/synthetic or animal. ▶ *Glycol* compound of ▶ *stearic acid*. Emulsifier and skin conditioner in cosmetics.

Neural Extract
From killed animals. Extract from mammal nerve tissue. Skin conditioner in cosmetics.

Niacin
(Nicotinic acid. Nicotinamide. Vitamin B₃ [outdated])
Synthetic/vegetable. A water-soluble ► *vitamin* that plays an important part in cell metabolism. Occurs mainly as nicotinamide in animal body tissues, but also as nicotinic acid in whole grain products and legumes. Industrial manufacture from vegetable raw materials and petroleum derivatives. Antistatic and smoothing agent in cosmetics. Active ingredient in medication for treating niacin deficiency or lowering blood lipids. Auxiliary agent in the metalworking industry.

Nicotinamide ► *Niacin*

Nicotinic Acid ► *Niacin*

Nisin
(E 234)
Microbiological/animal. Antibacterial ► *protein* compound that occurs naturally in raw ► *milk.* Obtained from milk modified by ► *lactic acid bacteria.* Preservative in foods (desserts, cheese, processed cheese). Antimicrobial substance in cosmetics. Also used as medical antibiotic.

Nitroglycerin
(Glyceroltrinitrat. Glyceryl trinitrate)
Mostly vegetable, can also be from killed animals. Nitrate compound of ► *glycerol.* Used as an explosive, is a constituent of dynamite. Active ingredient in medication for treating high blood pressure, e.g. in emergency medicine (inhalers).

Noil 🐄
From killed animals. ► *Silk* with short fibres and a matte surface. In textiles.

Nonfat Dry Milk ► *Sine Adipe Lac*

Nonionic Surfactants 🌱🐄
Can be vegetable or animal. ► *Surfactants* with neither positively nor negatively charged hydrophilic groups. Also include ► *sugar surfactants.* In cosmetics, laundry detergents, household cleaners, dish soap, etc. Some potentially animal examples: ► *cetyl alcohol*, ► *stearyl alcohol*, ► *cetostearyl alcohol*, ► *oleyl alcohol*, ► *glyceryl laurate*.

Nubuck 🐄
From killed animals. ► *Leather* with a velvet-like surface that has been buffed or sanded on the upper side. Made from calf hides. In upholstered furniture, handbags, clothing, footwear and gloves, etc.

Nutritional Supplement ► *Food Supplement*

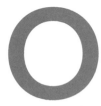

Oak Apple

Both vegetable and animal. Round outgrowths on oak leaves and branches caused by wasp eggs and the larvae that hatch from them, but also by infections (bacteria, viruses). One possible source of ► *gallic acid.*

Octacosanyl Glycol Isostearate

Can be vegetable/synthetic or animal. ► *Glycol* compound of ► *stearic acid* and lignite derivatives. Emollient in cosmetics.

Octadecanol ► *Stearyl Alcohol*

Octadecylamin ► *Stearamine*

Octanoic Acid ► *Caprylic Acid*

Octyl Gallate ► *Gallates*

Octyldecanol

Mostly vegetable/synthetic, can also be animal. Compound of ► *decyl alcohol.* Emollient in cosmetics.

Octyldodecanol

Mostly vegetable/synthetic, can also be animal. Compound of ► *decyl alcohol.* Emollient and solvent in cosmetics.

Octyldodecyl Hydroxystearate
Octyldodecyl Isostearate

Can be vegetable/synthetic or animal. Compounds of ► *decyl alcohol* and ► *stearic acid.* Skin conditioner in cosmetics.

Octyldodecyl Lactate

Mostly vegetable/microbiological/synthetic, can also be animal. Compound of ► *decyl alcohol* and ► *lactic acid.* Emollient in cosmetics.

Octyldodecyl Lanolate

From living or killed animals. Chemically altered acids from ► *lanolin.* Hair and skin conditioner in cosmetics.

Oil ► *Fat*

Oleamidopropyl Dimethylamine Hydrolyzed Collagen
From killed animals. Chemically/enzymatically altered ► *collagen*. Antistatic, hair and skin conditioner in cosmetics.

Oleamidopropyl Dimethylamine Lactate
Can be vegetable/microbiological/synthetic or animal. Compound of ► *oleic acid* and ► *lactic acid*. Antistatic and hair conditioner in cosmetics.

Oleamidopropyldimonium Hydroxypropyl Hydrolyzed Collagen
From killed animals. Chemically/enzymatically altered ► *collagen*. Antistatic, hair and skin conditioner in cosmetics.

Oleamine Bishydroxypropyltrimonium Chloride
Can be vegetable/synthetic or animal. Ammonium compound of ► *oleic acid*. Antistatic and hair conditioner in cosmetics.

Oleamine Oxide
Can be vegetable or animal. Compound of ► *oleic acid*. Antistatic, surfactant, foam booster, hair conditioner, cleansing agent and hydrotrope in cosmetics.

Oleic Acid
Can be vegetable or from killed animals. Most important ► *unsaturated fatty acid*. Occurs naturally in large amounts in animal and vegetable fats. Obtained from ► *tallow* or vegetable oils (e.g. sunflower oil). In foods and animal feed. Emollient and emulsifier in cosmetics. In soaps, detergents and lubricants. Many oleic acid compounds are used as cosmetic ingredients (hair and skin conditioners, ointments, creams, make-up, etc.).

Oleic/Linoleic Triglyceride
Can be vegetable or animal. Mixed ► *glycerides* of ► *oleic acid* and ► *linoleic acid*. Emollient in cosmetics.

Oleic/Palmitic/Lauric/Myristic/Linoleic Triglyceride
Can be vegetable or animal. Mixed ► *glycerides* of ► *oleic acid*, ► *palmitic acid*, ► *lauric acid*, ► *myristic acid* and ► *linoleic acid*. Emollient in cosmetics.

Oleoyl Ethyl Glucoside
Can be vegetable or animal. Sugar compound of ► *oleic acid*. Emulsifier in cosmetics.

Oleoyl Hydrolyzed Collagen
From killed animals. Chemically/enzymatically altered ► *collagen*. Antistatic, emollient, hair and skin conditioner, cleansing agent, film forming agent and surfactant in cosmetics.

Oleoyl PG-Trimonium Chloride
Can be vegetable/synthetic or animal. Ammonium compound of ► *oleic acid*. Antistatic and hair conditioner in cosmetics.

Oleoyl Sarcosine
Can be from killed animals or vegetable/synthetic. Compound of ► *oleic acid* and ► *sarcosine*. Antistatic, surfactant, cleansing agent and hair conditioner in cosmetics.

Oleoyl Tyrosine

Can be animal, microbiological or vegetable. Compound of ▶ *oleic acid* and ▶ *tyrosine*. Skin protecting substance and skin conditioner in cosmetics.

Oleth-2 Benzoate

Can be vegetable/synthetic or animal. ▶ *PEG* compound of ▶ *oleic acid*. Skin conditioner and emollient in cosmetics.

Oleth-n

Can be vegetable/synthetic or animal. ▶ *PEG* compounds of ▶ *oleyl alcohol*. Emulsifiers, surfactants and cleansing substances in cosmetics.

Oleth-n Carboxylic Acid

Can be vegetable/synthetic or animal. ▶ *PEG* compounds of ▶ *oleyl alcohol*. Surfactants and cleansing substances in cosmetics.

Oleth-n Phosphate

Can be vegetable/synthetic or animal. ▶ *PEG* and phosphoric acid compounds of ▶ *oleyl alcohol*. Surfactants in cosmetics. Some also used as emulsifiers.

Oleyl Acetate

Can be vegetable/synthetic or animal. Compound of ▶ *oleyl alcohol* and acetic acid. Emollient in cosmetics.

Oleyl Alcohol

(Octadecenol)

Can be vegetable or animal. A ▶ *fatty alcohol*, derived from ▶ *oleic acid*. Occurs naturally in ▶ *tallow* and ▶ *fish oil*. Emollient, emulsifier, opacifier and viscosity controlling agent in cosmetics.

Oleyl Arachidate

Can be vegetable or animal. Compound of ▶ *oleyl alcohol* and ▶ *arachidic acid*. Emollient in cosmetics.

Oleyl Betaine

Can be vegetable/synthetic or animal. Ammonium compound of ▶ *oleyl alcohol*. Antistatic, surfactant, cleansing agent, skin and hair conditioner, and foam booster in cosmetics.

Oleyl Epoxypropyldimonium Chloride

Can be vegetable/synthetic or animal. Ammonium compound of ▶ *oleyl alcohol*. Hair conditioner in cosmetics.

Oleyl Erucate

Can be vegetable or animal. Compound of ▶ *oleyl alcohol* and vegetable erucic acid. Emollient in cosmetics.

Oleyl Ethyl Phosphate

Can be vegetable/synthetic or animal. Phosphoric acid compound of ▶ *oleyl alcohol*. Surfactant and emulsifier in cosmetics.

Oleyl Glyceryl Ether
Can be vegetable or animal. Compound of ► *oleyl alcohol* and ► *glycerol.* Skin conditioner and emollient in cosmetics.

Oleyl Hydroxyethyl Imidazoline
Can be vegetable/synthetic or animal. Nitrogen and carbon compound of ► *oleic acid.* Antistatic and hair conditioner in cosmetics.

Oleyl Lactate
Can be vegetable/microbiological or animal. Compound of ► *oleyl alcohol* and ► *lactic acid.* Emollient in cosmetics.

Oleyl Lanolate
From living or killed animals. Chemically altered ► *lanolin.* Antistatic and emollient in cosmetics.

Oleyl Linoleate
Can be vegetable or animal. Compound of ► *oleyl alcohol* and ► *linoleic acid.* Emollient in cosmetics.

Oleyl Myristate
Can be vegetable or animal. Compound of ► *oleyl alcohol* and ► *myristic acid.* Emollient in cosmetics.

Oleyl Oleate
Can be vegetable or animal. Compound of ► *oleyl alcohol* and ► *oleic acid.* Emollient in cosmetics.

Oleyl Palmitamide
Can be vegetable or animal. Compound of ► *oleyl alcohol* and ► *palmitic acid.* Opacifier and viscosity controlling agent in cosmetics.

Oleyl Phosphate
Can be vegetable or animal. Phosphoric acid compound of ► *oleyl alcohol.* Surfactant and emulsifier in cosmetics.

Oleyl Stearate
Can be vegetable or animal. Compound of ► *oleyl alcohol* and ► *stearic acid.* Emollient in cosmetics.

Omega-3 Fatty Acids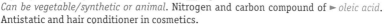
Can be vegetable or animal. A special group of essential ► *unsaturated fatty acids,* the most important being alpha-linolenic acid (ALA, see ► *linolenic acid*), ► *eicosapentaenoic acid* (EPA) and ► *docosahexaenoic acid* (DHA). Omega-3 fatty acids occur naturally in vegetable oils (ALA) as well as in animal fats, especially ► *fish oil* (EPA, DHA). The human body requires ALA, EPA and DHA, but is able to produce EPA and DHA from ALA. Used as ingredients in dietary supplements, for the prevention or complementary treatment of a number of disorders (e. g. cardiovascular disease, cancer, complications during pregnancy and lactation periods, and neurological or psychiatric disorders). EPA and especially DHA are most commonly used. Omega-3 fatty acids are regarded as having

a special part to play in nutrition, although actual intake requirements and their significance for health are still subject to debate.

Omega-6 Fatty Acids 🌱 🐄
Can be vegetable or animal. Group of essential ► *unsaturated fatty acids*. The most important are ► *linoleic acid* and ► *arachidonic acid*.

Omega-9 Fatty Acids 🌱 🐄
Can be vegetable or animal. Group of nonessential ► *unsaturated fatty acids*. Examples are ► *oleic acid* and vegetable erucic acid.

Omental Lipids 🐄
From killed animals. ► *Fat* from the peritoneum, from the abdomens of cattle. Emollient in cosmetics.

Organ Extracts 🐄
From killed animals. Extracts and distillates of animal organ tissue. Used especially as source materials for ► *homeopathic medicines,* but also in so-called organotherapy, a method by which the pure extracts are introduced to the body (supposed to have a tonic, regenerative effect and stimulate the immune system).

Some of the organ extracts from pigs:
Cartilago suis (cartilage), *Cerebrum suis* (brain), *Colon suis* (intestine), *Cor suis* (heart), *Corpus pineale suis* (pineal gland), *Cutis suis* (skin), *Diencephalon suis* (diencephalon, part of the brain), *Discus intervertebralis suis* (intervertebral disc), *Duodenum suis* (duodenum), *Embryo suis* (embryo), *Funiculus umbilicalis suis* (umbilical cord), *Glandula suprarenalis suis* (adrenal gland), *Hepar suis* (liver), *Medulla spinalis suis* (spinal cord), *Mucosa coli suis* (intestinal mucous membrane), *Mucosa ductus choledochi* (mucous membrane of the bile duct), *Mucosa ilei suis* (intestinal mucous membrane), *Mucosa jejuni suis* (intestinal mucous membrane), *Mucosa nasalis suis* (nasal mucous membrane), *Mucosa oculi suis* (mucous membrane of the eye), *Mucosa oesophagi suis* (mucous membrane of the esophagus), *Mucosa oris suis* (mucous membrane of the mouth), *Mucosa pulmonis suis* (mucous membrane of the lung), *Mucosa pylori suis* (mucous membrane of the stomach), *Mucosa recti suis* (mucous membrane of the rectum), *Mucosa vesicae felleae suis* (mucous membrane of the gall bladder), *Nervus opticus suis* (optical nerve), *Os suis* (bone), *Ovarium suis* (ovary), *Pankreas suis* (pancreas), *Placenta suis* (► *placenta*), *Placenta totalis suis* (whole placenta), *Prostata suis* (prostate gland), *Pulmo suis* (lung), *Pulpa dentis suis* (dental pulp), *Pyelon suis* (renal pelvis, part of the kidney), *Ren suis* (kidney), *Retina suis* (retina), *Splen suis* (spleen), *Testis suis* (testicle), *Thymus suis* (► *thymus[1]*), *Tonsilla suis* (tonsil), *Tuba uterina suis* (uterine tube), *Tunica mucosa vesicae urinariae suis* (mucous membrane of the bladder), *Ureter suis* (ureter), *Urethra suis* (urethra), *Uterus suis* (uterus), *Vena suis* (vein), *Ventriculus suis* (stomach wall), *Vesica fellea suis* (gall bladder), *Vesica urinaria suis* (bladder).

In the case of cattle extracts, similar terms are used, replacing *suis* for "pig" with *bovis* for "cattle," e.g.:
Cor lysat. bovis fetal. (fetal heart), *Diencephal. lysat. bovis fetal.* (fetal diencephalon), *Funicul. umbilical. lysat. bovis fetal.* (fetal umbilical cord), *Gland. suprarenal. lysat.*

bovis juv. (calf adrenal gland), *Hepar lysat. bovis fetal. et juv.* (fetal and calf liver), *Medull. spinal. lysat. bovis fetal.* (fetal spinal cord), *Pancreas lysat. bovis juv.* (calf pancreas), *Pulmo lysat. bovis fetal.* (fetal lung), *Ren lysat. bovis fetal. et juv.* (fetal and calf kidney), *Testes lysat. bovis juv.* (calf testicle), *Thym. lysat. bovis juv.* (► thymus[1]), *Vasa lysat. bovis fetal* (fetal blood vessel).

Ornithine

Can be vegetable or animal. An ► *amino acid*. Originally isolated from chicken manure. Obtained industrially from ► *arginine*. Skin conditioner in cosmetics. In nutritional and bodybuilding supplements. Ornithine aspartate is used in medication from treating brain damage caused by liver failure.

Ornithine Aspartate ► Ornithine

Ornithine HCl

Can be vegetable or animal. Compound of ► *ornithine*. Skin conditioner in cosmetics. In nutritional supplements.

Orotate ► Orotic Acid

Orotic Acid

(Vitamin B$_{13}$ [outdated])

Can be vegetable or animal. An acid, earlier considered to be a B vitamin. Occurs naturally in ► *milk*, yeasts and moulds. Industrial production from ► *arginine*. The salts of orotic acid are called "orotates." In nutritional supplements. Magnesium orotate is an active agent medication for treating muscle cramps and helping to prevent heart attacks. Zinc orotate is used for treating zinc deficiency.

Os Suis ► Organ Extract

Ostrea Shell Extract

From killed animals. Extract from the shells of European flat ► *oysters*. Skin conditioner and abrasive in cosmetics.

Ostrea Shell Powder

From killed animals. Ground shells of European flat ► *oysters*. Abrasive in cosmetics.

Otter ► Hair

Ovum

(Whole egg)

From living and killed animals (► *egg)*. The entire contents of chicken ► *eggs*, without the shell. Cooking and baking ingredient, ingredient in convenience products. Skin and hair conditioner in cosmetics.

Ovum Oil

From living and killed animals (► *egg)*. Oil from ► *egg yolks*. Emollient in cosmetics.

Ovum Powder

From living and killed animals (► *egg)*. Ground, dried whole ► *eggs*. Abrasive in cosmetics.

Ovum Shell Powder
From living and killed animals (► egg). Ground ► *egg* shells. Abrasive in cosmetics.

Ox Gall
From killed animals. Gall, or bile, is a yellow or green fluid formed in the livers of vertebrate animals, stored in der gall bladder and passed on as needed to the digestive tract, where it acts as an emulsifier for fat digestion. Obtained from the gall bladders of cattle. Main ingredient in gall soap for removing stains and cleansing textiles. Fat solvent in biological detergents. Used by artists and restorers/conservators as a wetting agent/ surfactant for degreasing surfaces and as a flow controlling agent in watercolour painting, gold leaf work, marbling and printing (e.g. lithography, etchings).

Ox Kidney Fat ► *Suet*

Oxidized Beeswax
From living animals. Chemically altered ► *beeswax*. Viscosity controlling agent in cosmetics.

Oxidized Keratin
From killed or living animals. Chemically altered ► *keratin*. Hair and skin conditioner in cosmetics.

Oysters
Killed animals. Animals that belong to the ► *bivalves*. Traditionally collected from the foreshore, are now "farmed" worldwide in huge numbers in aquacultures ("oyster banks"). Regarded by some as a delicacy or even as an ► *aphrodisiac*. The shells are used in cosmetics (► *ostrea shell powder*, ► *ostrea shell extract*) and as a homeopathic preparation (► *calcium carbonicum*).

P

Palmitamide DEA
Palmitamide MEA
Can be vegetable/synthetic or partly animal. Alcohol compounds of ► *palmitic acid*. Antistatics, viscosity controlling agents and foam boosters in cosmetics.

Palmitamidohexadecanediol
Can be vegetable/synthetic or partly animal. Alcohol compound of ► *palmitic acid*. Skin conditioner in cosmetics.

Palmitamidopropyl Betaine
Can be vegetable/synthetic or partly animal. Ammonium compound of ► *palmitic acid*. Antistatic, surfactant, cleansing agent, hair and skin conditioner, and foam booster in cosmetics.

Palmitamidopropyl Diethylamine
Palmitamidopropyl Dimethylamine
Can be vegetable/synthetic or partly animal. Ammonia compounds of ► *palmitic acid*. Antistatics in cosmetics.

Palmitamidopropyl Dimethylamine Lactate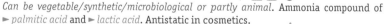
Can be vegetable/synthetic/microbiological or partly animal. Ammonia compound of ► *palmitic acid* and ► *lactic acid*. Antistatic in cosmetics.

Palmitamidopropyl Dimethylamine Propionate
Can be vegetable/synthetic/microbiological or partly animal. Ammonia compound of ► *palmitic acid* and ► *propionic acid*. Antistatic in cosmetics.

Palmitamidopropylamine Oxide
Can be vegetable/synthetic or partly animal. Ammonia compound of ► *palmitic acid*. Antistatic, surfactant, cleansing agent and hair conditioner, foam booster and hydrotrope in cosmetics.

Palmitamine
Can be vegetable/synthetic or partly animal. Ammonia compound of ► *palmitic acid*. Antistatic in cosmetics.

Palmitamine Oxide
Can be vegetable/synthetic or partly animal. Antistatic, surfactant, foam booster, hydrotrope, hair conditioner and cleansing agent in cosmetics.

Palmitates
Mostly vegetable, can also be animal. Salts and esters of ► *palmic acid.* Used especially in cosmetics. Some examples: ► *ascorbyl palmitate,* ► *cetearyl palmitate,* ► *cetyl palmitate,* ► *ethyl palmitate,* ► *glyceryl palmitate,* ► *magnesium palmitate,* ► *potassium palmitate,* ► *retinyl palmitate,* ► *sodium palmitate,* ► *zinc palmitate.*

Palmitic Acid
(Hexadecanoic acid)
Mostly vegetable, can also be animal. A ► *saturated fatty acid.* Occurs naturally in many vegetable and animal fats (e.g. palm oil, ► *cocoa butter* and cottonseed oil, or ► *tallow,* ► *butter* and ► *lard*). Obtained primarily from palm oil, but also from the fat of slaughtered animals. Emollient and emulsifier in cosmetics, also as ► *palmitates.* In lubricants and soaps. Constituent of the defoliant napalm.

Palmitoleamidopropyl Dimethylamine Lactate
Can be synthetic/vegetable/microbiological or animal. Ammonia compound of ► *palmitoleic acid* and ► *lactic acid.* Antistatic in cosmetics.

Palmitoleamidopropyl Dimethylamine Propionate
Can be synthetic/vegetable/microbiological or animal. Ammonia compound of ► *palmitoleic acid* and ► *propionic acid.* Antistatic in cosmetics.

Palmitoleic Acid
(9-cis-hexadecenoic acid)
Can be vegetable or animal. An ► *unsaturated fatty acid.* Occurs in all animal tissues, especially in the liver, also in ► *butterfat,* ► *lard* and ► *tallow.* Constituent of numerous vegetable oils (especially macadamia nut oil and sea buckthorn oil). Constituent of several compounds used in cosmetics, e.g. ► *glyceryl dipalmitoleate,* ► *palmitoleamidopropyl dimethylamine lactate* and ► *tripalmitolein.*

Palmitoyl Carnitine
Can be synthetic, vegetable or animal. Compound of ► *palmitic acid* and ► *carnitine.* Skin conditioner in cosmetics.

Palmitoyl Collagen Amino Acids
From killed animals. Chemically altered ► *amino acids* from ► *collagen.* Antistatic and cleansing agent in cosmetics.

Palmitoyl Glutamic Acid
Vegetable, can also be partly animal. Compound of ► *palmitic acid* and ► *glutamic acid.* Skin conditioner in cosmetics.

Palmitoyl Glycine
Can be animal or vegetable/synthetic/microbiological. Compound of ► *palmitic acid* and ► *glycine.* Hair conditioner and cleansing agent in cosmetics.

Palmitoyl Grape Seed
Mostly vegetable, can also be partly animal. Reaction product of grape seed extract and a ► *palmitic acid* compound. Skin conditioner in cosmetics.

Palmitoyl Hydrolyzed Collagen
From killed animals. Chemically/enzymatically altered ► *collagen*. Antistatic, emollient and surfactant in cosmetics.

Palmitoyl Hydrolyzed Milk Protein
From living and killed animals (► milk). Chemically/enzymatically altered ► *milk protein*. Antistatic and cleansing agent in cosmetics.

Palmitoyl Hydrolyzed Wheat Protein
Mostly vegetable, can also be partly animal. Compound of chemically/enzymatically altered wheat protein and a compound of ► *palmitic acid*. Surfactant and cleansing agent in cosmetics.

Palmitoyl Hydroxypropyltrimonium Amylopectin/ Glycerin Crosspolymer
Mostly vegetable/synthetic, can also be partly animal. Ammonium compound of ► *palmitic acid* and ► *glycerol*. Skin conditioner in cosmetics.

Palmitoyl Inulin
Mostly vegetable, can also be partly animal. Sugar compound of ► *palmitic acid*. Emollient and emulsifier in cosmetics.

Palmitoyl Keratin Amino Acids
From killed or living animals. Chemically altered ► *amino acids* from ► *keratin*. Antistatic and cleansing agent in cosmetics.

Palmitoyl Myristyl Serinate
Can be animal or synthetic/vegetable. Compound of ► *palmitic acid*, myristyl alcohol (from ► *myristic acid*) and ► *serine*. Skin conditioner in cosmetics.

Palmitoyl Oligopeptide
Can be vegetable or animal. Compound of ► *palmitic acid* and ► *amino acids*. Skin conditioner and cleansing agent in cosmetics.

Palmitoyl Pea Amino Acids
Palmitoyl Quinoa Amino Acids
Mostly vegetable, can also be partly animal. Compound of vegetable ► *amino acids* and ► *palmitic acid*. Hair and skin conditioner in cosmetics.

Palmitoyl PG-Trimonium Chloride
Mostly vegetable/synthetic, can also be partly animal. Ammonium compound of ► *palmitic acid*. Antistatic and hair conditioner in cosmetics.

Palmitoyl Silk Amino Acids
From killed animals. Chemically altered ► *amino acids* from ► *silk*. Hair conditioner and cleansing agent in cosmetics.

P

Palmitoyl Synthopeptide

Can be vegetable or animal. Compound of synthetic ► *amino acids* and ► *palmitic acid*. Skin conditioner in cosmetics.

Palmityl Alcohol ► *Cetyl Alcohol*

Palmityl Trihydroxyethyl Propylenediamine Dihydrofluoride

Can be vegetable/synthetic or partly animal. Compound of ► *palmitic acid* and ammonia. Oral care and antiplaque agent in cosmetics.

Pancreas (Lysat.) Bovis ► *Organ Extract*

Pancreas Suis ► *Organ Extract*

Pancreatin

From killed animals. Mixture of ► *enzymes* (► *amylase*, ► *lipase* and ► *proteases*), occurs naturally in pancreatic juice, produced in the pancreas. Plays an important part in digestive processes, especially the digestion of fats, but also of carbohydrates and proteins. Obtained from pancreases of pigs. Hair and skin conditioner in cosmetics. Used for cleaning false teeth, softening callused skin and in medication for substituting deficient enzymes due to diseases of the pancreas.

Pantethine

Can be vegetable, synthetic or animal. Variant of ► *pantothenic acid*. Emollient, hair conditioner in cosmetics.

Panthenol

(Dexpanthenol. D-panthenol. Provitamin B$_5$)

Can be vegetable, synthetic or animal. An alcohol. Precursor of ► *pantothenic acid*. Obtained from pantothenic acid. Can be of animal origin, e.g. from liver. Antistatic, hair and skin conditioner in cosmetics. Anti-inflammatory and soothing agent, e.g. in ointments, creams, and eye and nose drops.

Panthenyl Ethyl Ether. Panthenyl Ethyl Ether Acetate

Can be vegetable/synthetic or animal. Ether compounds of ► *panthenol*. Antistatics and hair conditioners in cosmetics.

Panthenyl Hydroxypropyl Steardimonium Chloride

Can be vegetable/synthetic or animal. Ammonium compound of ► *panthenol* and ► *stearic acid*. Antistatic and hair conditioner in cosmetics.

Panthenyl Triacetate

Can be vegetable or animal. Compound of ► *panthenol* and acetic acid. Antistatic and hair conditioner in cosmetics.

Pantothenic Acid

(Vitamin B$_5$)

Can be vegetable, synthetic or animal. A water-soluble ► *vitamin*. Part of ► *coenzyme A*, plays an important part in metabolism. Found in all vegetable and animal tissues, especially liver and muscle, ► *royal jelly*, yeasts, cereals and legumes. Can be obtained from

from liver. Industrial production from petroleum derivatives, also from ► *aspartic acid*. Antistatic, hair and skin conditioner in cosmetics. In some food supplements, e.g. as calcium pantothenate. Used for wound treatment. Used for producing ► *coenzyme A*.

Pantothenic Acid Polypeptide
Can be vegetable, synthetic or animal. Compound of ► *pantothenic acid* and ► *amino acids*. Antistatic, hair and skin conditioner in cosmetics.

Paper
Vegetable, can be partly animal. Thin material composed of pressed plant fibres, mostly cellulose. Can contain animal ► *glue*. Used especially for writing and printing (books, newspapers, posters, documents, letters, etc.), as well as painting and drawing. Diverse industrial uses (construction, packaging). Also in hygiene and cleaning products.

Parchment
From killed animals. Untanned animal skin, especially of calves, sheep and goats, treated with lime. Especially fine parchment is known as vellum. Parchment has been used since ancient times as writing material, having replaced papyrus. Now only used for deeds, religious writings, painting, bookbinding, calligraphy and conservation/restoration.

PCA Glyceryl Oleate
Can be vegetable or animal. Compound of ► *proline*, ► *glycerol* and ► *oleic acid*. Emollient in cosmetics.

Pea Palmitate
Mostly vegetable, can also be partly animal. Reaction product of pea extract and a compound of ► *palmitic acid*. Skin conditioner in cosmetics.

Pearl
From killed animals. Hard, often round deposits of ► *mother of pearl*, formed in the tissue of ► *bivalves*, e.g. as a response to foreign bodies, parasites or injuries. Pearls are either formed naturally or as "cultured pearls" created by transplanting pearl-producing tissue from a "donor" animal. Imitation pearls are made by compacting mother of pearl powder, shaping fragments of mother of pearl or coating ► *wax* pellets with ► *fish silver* or ► *guanine*. Used in jewellery, pearl necklaces, decorative objects, etc.

Pearl Essence ► Fish Silver

Pearlescence
(Iridescence)
Not an actual ingredient, but an optical effect that makes the colour of objects change depending on the angle of view or illumination. This occurs naturally, for instance with ► *pearls* and ► *mother of pearl*, or soap bubbles. This effect is deliberately achieved by using mother of pearl or pearls, but also using pearlescents in cosmetics, plastics and coatings. Examples of pearlescents that can be of animal origin are ► *guanine* and ► *glycol distearate*. Silicates and metal compounds are used as mineral pearlescents.

Pectin
Vegetable. A polysaccharide. Occurs naturally in all higher land plants, especially in

some fruits. Obtained especially from apples, citrus fruits and beets. Used as a gelling agent and binding agent in foods, especially in jellies and jams. Binding agent, emulsion stabilizer and viscosity controlling agent in cosmetics. Can be confused with ► *gelatin* due to the additional term "gelling agent" also used in the context of ingredient declaration on food packaging, but is in fact always purely vegetable.

PEG (Polyethylene Glycol)

(E 1521. Macrogol)
Synthetic. Water-soluble polymers based on ethylene oxide, can be liquid or solid. Product of the petrochemical industry. While PEG itself is synthetic, its compounds contain ► *fatty acids* and other substances that can be vegetable, animal or mineral. Used in cosmetics and pharmaceutical drugs, as well as in dietary supplements and laxatives.
For information on specific PEG compounds see the following entries. Because of the large number of such compounds, and in the interest of clarity and comprehensibility, those substances with denominations that differ merely by a number and whose functions are more or less identical have been contracted to single denominations, such as "PEG-n distearate." This means a slight change in the alphabetical order of the entries.

PEG-2 Lactamide

Can be synthetic/vegetable/microbiological or partly animal. ► *PEG* compound of ► *lactic acid.* Humectant in cosmetics.

PEG-2 Milk Solids

From living and killed animals (► milk). ► *PEG* compound of ► *milk* solids. Antistatic and emollient in cosmetics.

PEG-2 Oleammonium Chloride

Can be vegetable/synthetic or animal. ► *PEG* and ammonium compound of ► *oleic acid.* Antistatic, emulsifier and surfactant in cosmetics.

PEG-2 Oleate SE

Can be vegetable/synthetic or animal. ► *PEG* compound of ► *oleic acid.* Emulsifier in cosmetics.

PEG-2 Stearamide Carboxylic Acid

Can be vegetable/synthetic or animal. ► *PEG* and ammonia compound of ► *stearic acid.* Surfactant in cosmetics.

PEG-2 Stearate SE

Can be vegetable/synthetic or animal. ► *PEG* compound of ► *stearic acid.* Emulsifier and opacifier in cosmetics.

PEG-2 Stearmonium Chloride

Can be vegetable/synthetic or animal. ► *PEG* and ammonium compound of ► *stearic acid.* Antistatic and emulsifier in cosmetics.

PEG-3 Dioleoylamidoethylmonium Methosulfate

Can be vegetable/synthetic or animal. ► *PEG* and ammonium compound of ► *oleyl alcohol.* Antistatic and hair conditioner in cosmetics.

PEG-3 Dipalmitate
Mostly vegetable/synthetic, can also be partly animal. ► *PEG* compound of ► *palmitic acid*. Emulsifier in cosmetics.

PEG-3 Tallow Propylenedimonium Dimethosulfate
From killed animals. ► *PEG* compound of chemically altered ► *tallow*. Antistatic in cosmetics.

PEG-3/PPG-2 Glyceryl/Sorbitol Hydroxystearate/Isostearate
Can be vegetable/synthetic or animal. ► *PEG* and ► *PPG* compound of ► *glycerol* and ► *stearic acid*. Emulsifier in cosmetics.

PEG-4 Polyglyceryl-2 Distearate
PEG-4 Polyglyceryl-2 Stearate
Can be vegetable/synthetic or animal. ► *PEG* compounds of ► *glycerol* and ► *stearic acid*. Emulsifiers in cosmetics.

PEG-4 Stearamide
Can be vegetable/synthetic or animal. ► *PEG* and ammonia compound of ► *stearic acid*. Surfactant in cosmetics.

PEG-5 DEDM Hydantoin Oleate
Can be vegetable/synthetic or animal. ► *PEG* and ammonium compound of ► *oleic acid*. Antimicrobial agent in cosmetics.

PEG-5 Stearyl Ammonium Chloride
Can be vegetable/synthetic or animal. ► *PEG* and ammonium compound of ► *stearyl alcohol*. Antistatic and surfactant in cosmetics.

PEG-5 Stearyl Ammonium Lactate
Can be synthetic/vegetable/microbiological or animal. ► *PEG* and ammonium compound of ► *stearyl alcohol* and ► *lactic acid*. Antistatic and surfactant in cosmetics.

PEG-5 Tall Oil Sterol Ether
Synthetic/vegetable. ► *PEG* compound of ► *tallol*. Antistatic in cosmetics.

PEG-5 Tallow Benzonium Chloride
From killed animals. ► *PEG* compound of chemically altered ► *tallow*. Antistatic, surfactant in cosmetics.

PEG-5 Tricaprylyl Citrate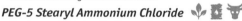
Mostly vegetable/synthetic, can also be partly animal. ► *PEG* compound of ► *capryl alcohol* and citric acid. Emulsifier in cosmetics.

PEG-5 Tricetyl Citrate
Mostly vegetable/synthetic, can also be partly animal. ► *PEG* compound of ► *cetyl alcohol* and citric acid. Emollient in cosmetics.

PEG-5 Tridecyl Citrate
Mostly vegetable/synthetic, can also be partly animal. ► *PEG* compound of ► *decyl alcohol* and citric acid. Emollient in cosmetics.

PEG-5 Tristearyl Citrate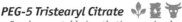
Can be vegetable/synthetic or animal. ► *PEG* compound of ► *stearyl alcohol* and citric acid. Emollient in cosmetics.

PEG-6 Isopalmitate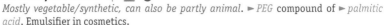
Mostly vegetable/synthetic, can also be partly animal. ► *PEG* compound of ► *palmitic acid.* Emulsifier in cosmetics.

PEG-7 Tallow Amine
From killed animals. Chemically altered ► *tallow.* Emulsifier in cosmetics.

PEG-8 Caprate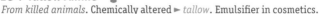
Mostly vegetable/synthetic, can also be partly animal. ► *PEG* compound of ► *capric acid.* Emulsifier in cosmetics.

PEG-8 Caprylate
Mostly vegetable/synthetic, can also be partly animal. ► *PEG* compound of ► *caprylic acid.* Emulsifier in cosmetics.

PEG-8 Caprylate/Caprate
Mostly vegetable/synthetic, can also be partly animal. ► *PEG* compound of ► *caprylic acid* and ► *capric acid.* Emulsifier in cosmetics.

PEG-8 Diisostearate
Can be vegetable/synthetic or animal. ► *PEG* compound of ► *stearic acid.* Emulsifier in cosmetics.

PEG-8 Hydrogenated Fish Glycerides
From killed animals. Chemically altered ► *fish oil.* Emollient and emulsifier in cosmetics.

PEG-10 Stearyl Benzonium Chloride
Can be vegetable/synthetic or animal. ► *PEG* compound of ► *stearyl alcohol.* Antistatic and surfactant in cosmetics.

PEG-11 Tallow Amine
From killed animals. Chemically altered ► *tallow.* Emulsifier in cosmetics.

PEG-13 Hydrogenated Tallow Amide
From killed animals. Chemically altered ► *tallow.* Emulsifier in cosmetics.

PEG-13 Mink Glycerides
From killed animals. Chemically altered ► *mink oil.* Emulsifier in cosmetics.

PEG-15 Stearmonium Chloride
Can be vegetable/synthetic or animal. ► *PEG* and ammonium compound of ► *stearic acid.* Antistatic and surfactant in cosmetics.

PEG-15 Tallow Amine
From killed animals. Chemically altered ► *tallow.* Antistatic in cosmetics.

PEG-15 Tallow Polyamine
From killed animals. Chemically altered ► *tallow.* Antistatic and emulsifier in cosmetics.

Veganissimo A to Z

PEG-20 Glyceryl Isostearate

Can be vegetable/synthetic or animal. ► *PEG* compound of ► *glycerol* and ► *stearic acid.* Emulsifier in cosmetics.

PEG-20 Hydrogenated Castor Oil Triisostearate

Can be vegetable/synthetic or animal. ► *PEG* compound of ► *stearic acid* and vegetable ricinoleic acid. Emulsifier and viscosity controlling agent in cosmetics.

PEG-20 Methyl Glucose Distearate

Can be vegetable/synthetic or animal. ► *PEG* and sugar compound of ► *stearic acid.* Emollient and emulsifier in cosmetics.

PEG-20 Methyl Glucose Sesquistearate

Can be vegetable/synthetic or animal. ► *PEG* and sugar compound of ► *stearic acid.* Emollient and emulsifier in cosmetics.

PEG-20 Methyl Glucose Sesquicaprylate/Sesquicaprate

Can be vegetable/synthetic or partly animal. ► *PEG* and sugar compound of ► *caprylic acid* and ► *stearic acid.* Emollient and emulsifier in cosmetics.

PEG-20 Tallow Ammonium Ethosulfate

From killed animals. ► *PEG* compound of chemically altered ► *tallow.* Antistatic in cosmetics.

PEG-20 Tallowate

From killed animals. ► *PEG* compound of chemically altered ► *tallow.* Emulsifier in cosmetics.

PEG-25 Glyceryl Trioleate

Can be vegetable/synthetic or animal. ► *PEG* compound of ► *glycerol* and ► *oleic acid.* Emulsifier in cosmetics.

PEG-40 Sorbitan Perisostearate

Can be vegetable/synthetic or animal. ► *PEG* compound of the sugar alcohol sorbitol and ► *stearic acid.* Surfactant and emulsifier in cosmetics.

PEG-40 Sorbitan Peroleate

Can be vegetable/synthetic or animal. ► *PEG* compound of the sugar alcohol sorbitol and ► *oleic acid.* Emulsifier and surfactant in cosmetics.

PEG-40 Sorbitol Hexaoleate

Can be vegetable/synthetic or animal. ► *PEG* compound of the sugar alcohol sorbitol and ► *oleic acid.* Surfactant in cosmetics.

PEG-45 Stearate Phosphate

Can be vegetable/synthetic or animal. ► *PEG* and phosphoric acid compound of ► *stearic acid.* Surfactant in cosmetics.

PEG-50 Shea Butter

Synthetic/vegetable. ► *PEG* compound of shea butter (► *Butyrospermum parkii butter*). Emulsifier in cosmetics.

PEG-50 Sorbitol Hexaoleate

Can be vegetable/synthetic or animal. ► *PEG* compound of the sugar alcohol sorbitol and ► *oleic acid*. Emulsifier in cosmetics.

PEG-60 Shea Butter Glycerides

Synthetic/vegetable. ► *PEG* compound of shea butter (► *Butyrospermum parkii butter*). Emollient and emulsifier in cosmetics.

PEG-60 Sorbitan Tetrastearate
PEG-60 Sorbitol Tetrastearate

Can be vegetable/synthetic or animal. ► *PEG* compounds of the sugar alcohol sorbitol and ► *stearic acid*. Emulsifiers in cosmetics.

PEG-75 Cocoa Butter Glycerides

Synthetic/vegetable. ► *PEG* compound of ► *cocoa butter*. Emulsifier in cosmetics.

PEG-75 Shea Butter Glycerides

Synthetic/vegetable. ► *PEG* compound of shea butter (► *Butyrospermum parkii butter*). Emulsifier in cosmetics.

PEG-75 Shorea Butter Glycerides

Synthetic/vegetable. ► *PEG* compound of ► *Shorea robusta butter*. Cosmetic emulsifier.

PEG-n Beeswax

From living animals. Chemically altered ► *beeswax*. Emulsifiers in cosmetics.

PEG-n Caprylic/Capric Glycerides

Mostly vegetable/synthetic, can also be partly animal. ► *PEG* compounds of ► *caprylic acid* and ► *capric acid*. Emulsifiers in cosmetics.

PEG-n Dioleate

Can be vegetable/synthetic or animal. ► *PEG* compounds of ► *oleic acid*. Emulsifiers in cosmetics. PEG-75 dioleate also acts as a surfactant.

PEG-n Distearate

Can be vegetable/synthetic or animal. ► *PEG* compounds of ► *stearic acid*. Emulsifiers in cosmetics. PEG-150 distearate also acts as surfactant and viscosity controlling agent, PEG-250 distearate is also a cleansing agent and surfactant.

PEG-n Hydrogenated Castor Oil Isostearate

Can be vegetable/synthetic or animal. ► *PEG* compounds of castor oil (vegetable) and ► *stearic acid*. Emulsifiers and viscosity regulators in cosmetics.

PEG-n Isostearate

Can be vegetable/synthetic or animal. ► *PEG* compounds of ► *stearic acid*. Emulsifiers in cosmetics. PEG-10 isostearate also acts as a surfactant.

PEG-n Glyceryl Oleate

(Macrogol glyceryl oleate)

Can be vegetable/synthetic or animal. ► *PEG* compounds of ► *glycerol* and ► *oleic acid*. Emulsifiers in cosmetics. PEG-30 glyceryl oleate also a surfactant. Excipients in medicines.

PEG-n Glyceryl Ricinoleate
(Macrogol glyceryl ricinoleate)
Can be vegetable/synthetic or partly animal. ► *PEG* compounds of ► *glycerol* and ricinoleic acid. Emulsifiers in cosmetics. Excipients in pharmaceutical drugs.

PEG-n Glyceryl Tallowate
From killed animals. Chemically altered ► *tallow*. Emulsifiers/surfactants in cosmetics.

PEG-n Glyceryl Stearate
(Macrogol glyceryl stearate)
Can be vegetable/synthetic or animal. ► *PEG* compounds of ► *glycerol* and ► *stearic acid*. Emulsifiers and surfactants in cosmetics. Excipients in pharmaceutical drugs.

PEG-n Hydrogenated Castor Oil Isostearate
Can be vegetable/synthetic or animal. ► *PEG* compounds of ► *stearic acid* and castor oil. Emulsifiers and viscosity controlling agents in cosmetics.

PEG-n Hydrogenated Lanolin
From living or killed animals. Chemically altered ► *lanolin*. Emulsifiers and emollients in cosmetics.

PEG-n Hydrogenated Tallow Amine
From killed animals. Chemically altered ► *tallow*. Emulsifiers/surfactants in cosmetics.

PEG-n Lanolate
From living or killed animals. Chemically altered ► *fatty acids* from ► *lanolin*. Emulsifiers in cosmetics.

PEG-n Lanolin
From living or killed animals. Chemically altered ► *lanolin*. Emulsifiers in cosmetics. PEG-10 lanolin is also an emollient.

PEG-n Oleamide
Can be vegetable/synthetic or animal. ► *PEG* and ammonia compounds of ► *oleic acid*. Emulsifiers in cosmetics. PEG-3 oleamide is also a surfactant.

PEG-n Oleamine
Can be vegetable/synthetic or animal. ► *PEG* and ammonia compounds of ► *oleic acid*. Emulsifiers in cosmetics. PEG-30 oleamine is also a surfactant.

PEG-n Oleate
Can be vegetable/synthetic or animal. ► *PEG* compounds of ► *oleic acid*. Emulsifiers and surfactants in cosmetics.

PEG-n Palmitate
Mostly vegetable/synthetic, can also be partly animal. ► *PEG* compounds of ► *palmitic acid*. Emulsifiers and surfactants in cosmetics.

PEG-n Propylene Glycol Stearate
Can be vegetable/synthetic or animal. ► *PEG* compounds of ► *stearic acid*. Emulsifiers in cosmetics.

PEG-n Sorbitan Beeswax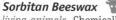
From living animals. Chemically altered ► *beeswax.* Emulsifiers and surfactants in cosmetics.

PEG-n Sorbitan Oleate
Can be vegetable/synthetic or animal. ► *PEG* compounds of the sugar alcohol sorbitol and ► *oleic acid.* Emulsifiers in cosmetics.

PEG-n Sorbitan Stearate
Can be vegetable/synthetic or animal. ► *PEG* compounds of the sugar alcohol sorbitol and ► *stearic acid.* Emulsifiers and surfactants in cosmetics.

PEG-n Sorbitan Tetraoleate
Can be vegetable/synthetic or animal. ► *PEG* compounds of the sugar alcohol sorbitol and ► *oleic acid.* Emulsifiers in cosmetics.

PEG-n Stearamine
Can be vegetable/synthetic or animal. ► *PEG* and ammonia compounds of ► *stearic acid.* Antistatics and emulsifiers in cosmetics. PEG-50 stearamine is also a surfactant.

PEG-n Stearate
Can be vegetable/synthetic or animal. ► *PEG* compounds of ► *stearic acid.* Emulsifiers and surfactants in cosmetics, except PEG-3 stearate (a humectant). PEG-1 stearate is also used as an opacifier, and PEG-8 stearate and PEG-20 stearate as humectants.

PEG-n Tallate
Synthetic/vegetable. ► *PEG* compounds of ► *tallol.* Emulsifiers in cosmetics.

PEG-n Tallow Amide
From killed animals. ► *PEG* compounds of chemically altered ► *tallow.* Emulsifiers in cosmetics.

PEG-n Tallow Aminopropylamine
From killed animals. ► *PEG* compounds of chemically altered ► *tallow.* Emulsifiers in cosmetics.

PEG-n Trihydroxystearin
Can be vegetable/synthetic or animal. ► *PEG* compounds of ► *stearic acid.* Emulsifiers and surfactants in cosmetics.

Pellis Lipida
From killed animals. ► *Fat* from the skins of killed animals. Emollient in cosmetics.

Pelt ► *Fur*

Pentadesma Butyracea Butter
Vegetable. Oily extract from the nut of the West African butter tree. Not to be confused with animal ► *butter.* Emollient in cosmetics.

Pentaerythrityl Dioleate
Can be vegetable or animal. Compound of the sugar alcohol erythritol and ► *oleic acid.* Emollient in cosmetics.

Pentaerythrityl Distearate
Can be vegetable or animal. Compound of the sugar alcohol erythritol and ▸ *stearic acid.* Emulsifier in cosmetics.

Pentaerythrityl Isostearate/Caprate/Caprylate/Adipate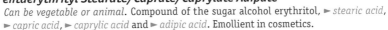
Pentaerythrityl Stearate/Caprate/Caprylate Adipate
Can be vegetable or animal. Compound of the sugar alcohol erythritol, ▸ *stearic acid,* ▸ *capric acid,* ▸ *caprylic acid* and ▸ *adipic acid.* Emollient in cosmetics.

Pentaerythrityl Stearate
Can be vegetable or animal. Compound of the sugar alcohol erythritol and ▸ *stearic acid.* Emollient in cosmetics.

Pentaerythrityl Stearate/Isostearate/Adipate/Hydroxystearate
Can be vegetable or animal. Compound of the sugar alcohol erythritol, ▸ *stearic acid* and ▸ *adipic acid.* Skin conditioner and viscosity controlling agent in cosmetics.

Pentaerythrityl Tetracaprylate/Caprate
Can be vegetable or partly animal. Compound of the sugar alcohol erythritol, ▸ *capric acid* and ▸ *caprylic acid.* Emollient in cosmetics.

Pentaerythrityl Tetraisostearate
Can be vegetable or animal. Compound of the sugar alcohol erythritol and ▸ *stearic acid.* Emollient, emulsifier and surfactant in cosmetics.

Pentaerythrityl Tetraoleate
Can be vegetable or animal. Compound of the sugar alcohol erythritol and ▸ *oleic acid.* Emollient and viscosity controlling agent in cosmetics.

Pentaerythrityl Tetrastearate
Can be vegetable or animal. Compound of the sugar alcohol erythritol and ▸ *stearic acid.* Emollient and viscosity controlling agent.

Pentaerythrityl Trioleate
Can be vegetable or animal. Compound of the sugar alcohol erythritol and ▸ *oleic acid.* Emollient in cosmetics.

Pentahydrosqualene
Mostly from killed animals, can also be vegetable. Compound of ▸ *squalene.* Emollient in cosmetics.

Pepsin
From killed animals. An ▸ *enzyme* that breaks down ▸ *proteins* as part of the digestive process. One of the constituents of ▸ *rennet.* Obtained from the mucous membranes of pig stomachs. Skin and hair conditioner in cosmetics. In nutritional supplements.

Phenylalanine
Synthetic or vegetable/microbiological. An essential ▸ *amino acid.* Occurs naturally in many vegetable and animal tissues. Industrially synthesized from petroleum products or derived from glucose using bacterial cultures. Antistatic in cosmetics. In nutritional

supplements. In infusions for parenteral nutrition. Used as a source material for producing the artificial sweetener aspartame.

Phosphatidylcholine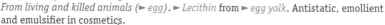
From living and killed animals (► egg). ► *Lecithin* from ► *egg yolk.* Antistatic, emollient and emulsifier in cosmetics.

Phospholipase A₂
Mostly from living or killed animals, can also be microbiological. ► *Enzymes* that play a part in fat metabolism and break down ► *phospholipids.* Found in the body tissues of mammals as well as in snake, scorpion and bee venom. Most often obtained from pancreases of killed pigs. Can also be obtained from animal venom or yeast cultures. Used for producing ► *lysolecithin.*

Phospholipids
Can be animal, vegetable or microbiological. Phosphoric acid compounds classified as ► *lipids* that play an important part in the cell membranes of all organisims. Examples of phospholipids are ► *lecithin* and ► *sphingosine.* Skin conditioner in cosmetics.

Phthalic Anhydride/Glycerin/Glycidyl Decanoate Copolymer
Can be vegetable/synthetic or partly animal. Polymer compound of ► *glycerol* and ► *capric acid.* Antistatic, film forming agent and viscosity controlling agent in cosmetics.

Phytomenadion ► Vitamin K

Phytonadione ► Vitamin K

Phytosphingosine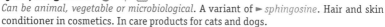
Can be animal, vegetable or microbiological. A variant of ► *sphingosine.* Hair and skin conditioner in cosmetics. In care products for cats and dogs.

Pig Bristles ► China Bristles

Pigskin Extract ► Sus Extract

Pisces. Pisces Extract
From killed animals. Extract from whole ► *fish* of various species. Skin conditioner in cosmetics.

Piscum Cartilage Extract
From killed animals. Extract from fish cartilage. Skin conditioner in cosmetics.

Piscum Iecur Oil
From killed animals. Oil from the livers of various fish species. Emollient in cosmetics.

Piscum Ovum Extract
From killed animals. Extract from fish eggs. Skin conditioner in cosmetics.

PLA ► Polyllactic Acid

Placenta
Mostly from killed animals, can also be from living animals or humans. Organ that develops in the uterus of placental mamals during pregnancy for the purpose of transferring

substances between mother and embryo, and is expelled after birth. Obtained mostly from killed pregnant animals, e.g. cows, sheep and pigs. Used as ► *organ extract*, in food supplements, cosmetics and ► *homeopathic medicines*. Also used as a source of cosmetic ingredients: ► *hydrolyzed human placental protein*, ► *hydrolyzed placental protein*, ► *placental enzymes*, ► *placental lipids*, ► *placental protein*.

Placenta (Lysat.) Bovis ► *Organ Extracts*

Placenta Suis ► *Organ Extracts*

Placental Enzymes
Mostly from killed animals, can also be from living animals. ► *Enzymes* from mammalian ► *placenta*. Skin conditioner in cosmetics.

Placental Lipids
Mostly from killed animals, can also be from living animals. ► *Lipids* from mammalian ► *placenta*. Skin conditioner in cosmetics.

Placental Protein
Mostly from killed animals, can also be from living animals. ► *Proteins* from mammalian ► *placenta*. Humectant in cosmetics.

Placuna Placenta ► *Capiz*

Plain Caramel ► *Caramel Colouring*

Plasma ► *Blood Plasma*

Plasma Proteins ► *Serum Proteins*

Pollen
From living and killed animals. Powder produced by the flowers of seed-bearing plants for reproductive purposes (transmission from plant to plant either airborne or carried by animals). Gathered by ► *bees* and used for feeding their larvae. Obtained by humans using pollen traps (meshed wire devices in the beehive entrance that strip the pollen off the legs of the bees returning home; legs and wings can be torn off in the process). Skin conditioner in cosmetics. Used as a nutritional supplement.

Pollen Extract
From living and killed animals. Extract from ► *pollen*. Emollient and skin protecting substance in cosmetics.

Polyalkylene Glycol Ethers
(Fatty alcohol ethoxylates [FAEO])
Can be vegetable/synthetic or animal. ► *Nonionic surfactants*, comprising► *PEG* compounds of ► *cetyl alcohol*, ► *lauryl alcohol*, ► *oleyl alcohol* or ► *stearyl alcohol*. Emulsifiers and surfactants in cosmetics (► *ceteareth-n*, ► *ceteth-n*, ► *laureth-n*, ► *oleth-n*, ► *steareth-n*). In many industrial applications, e.g. textile processing, paints, coatings and adhesives.

Polycaprolactone
Synthetic, can theoretically also be animal. Alcohol compound of ► *caproic acid*. Derived

P

industrially from petroleum products. Stabilizer in cosmetics. Excipient in pharmaceutical drugs. Used in plastic production, e.g. in biodegradable packaging materials. Is further processed to the synthetic polyamind fibre.

Polyethylene Glycol. Polyethylene Glycol Ethers ► PEG

Polyethylglutamate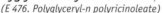
Can be vegetable/synthetic/microbiological or partly animal. Alcohol compound of ► *glutamic acid*. Binding agent in cosmetics.

Polyglycerin-3
Can be vegetable or animal. Polymer compound of ► *glycerol*. Humectant in cosmetics.

Polyglycerol Esters of Fatty Acids
(E 475)
Can be vegetable or animal. Compounds of ► *fatty acids* and ► *glycerol*. Emulsifiers and foam inhibitor in foods.

Polyglycerol Polyricinoleate
(E 476. Polyglyceryl-n polyricinoleate)
Can be vegetable or partly animal. Compounds of ► *glycerol* and ricinoleic acid (vegetable). Emulsifiers in reduced-fat sandwich spreads, salad dressings and chocolate products. Emulsifiers and viscosity controlling agents in cosmetics.

Polyglyceryl-2 Caprylate
Can be vegetable or partly animal. Compound of ► *glycerol* and ► *caprylic acid*. Emulsifier in cosmetics.

Polyglyceryl-2 Dipolyhydroxystearate
Can be vegetable or animal. Compound of ► *glycerol* and ► *stearic acid*. Skin conditioner in cosmetics.

Polyglyceryl-2 Isopalmitate
Can be vegetable or partly animal. Compound of ► *glycerol* and ► *palmitic acid*. Emulsifier in cosmetics.

Polyglyceryl-2 Lanolin Alcohol Ether
From living or killed animals. Compound of ► *glycerol* and chemically altered ► *lanolin*. Emulsifier in cosmetics.

Polyglyceryl-2-PEG-4 Stearate
Can be vegetable/synthetic or animal. Compound of ► *glycerol* and ► *stearic acid*. Emulsifier in cosmetics.

Polyglyceryl-2 Sesquiisostearate
Can be vegetable or animal. Compound of ► *glycerol* and ► *stearic acid*. Emulsifier in cosmetics.

Polyglyceryl-2 Sesquioleate
Can be vegetable or animal. Compound of ► *glycerol* and ► *oleic acid*. Emulsifier in cosmetics.

Polyglyceryl-2 Sesquistearate
Can be vegetable or animal. Compound of ► *glycerol* and ► *stearic acid*. Emulsifier in cosmetics.

Polyglyceryl-2 Sorbitan Pentacaprylate
Polyglyceryl-2 Sorbitan Tetracaprylate
Can be vegetable or partly animal. Compounds of ► *glycerol* and ► *caprylic acid* with the sugar alcohol sorbitol. Emulsifiers in cosmetics.

Polyglyceryl-2 Tetraisostearate
Polyglyceryl-2 Tetrastearate
Polyglyceryl-2 Triisostearate
Can be vegetable or animal. Compounds of ► *glycerol* and ► *stearic acid*. Emulsifiers in cosmetics.

Polyglyceryl-3 Beeswax
From living animals. Polymer compound of ► *glycerol* and ► *beeswax*. Emulsifier in cosmetics.

Polyglyceryl-3 Cetyl Ether
Can be vegetable or animal. Compound of ► *glycerol* and ► *cetyl alcohol*. Emulsifier in cosmetics.

Polyglyceryl-3 Cocoate
Can be vegetable or partly animal. Compound of ► *glycerol* and coconut ► *fatty acids*. Emulsifier in cosmetics.

Polyglyceryl-3 Dicaprate
Can be vegetable or animal. Compound of ► *glycerol* and ► *capric acid*. Emulsifier in cosmetics.

Polyglyceryl-3 Dicocoate
Can be vegetable or partly animal. Compound of ► *glycerol* and coconut ► *fatty acids*. Emollient and emulsifier in cosmetics.

Polyglyceryl-3 Methylglucose Distearate
Can be vegetable or partly animal. Compound of ► *glycerol* and ► *stearic acid*. Emulsifier in cosmetics.

Polyglyceryl-3 Stearate SE
Can be vegetable or animal. Compound of ► *glycerol* and ► *stearic acid*. Emulsifier in cosmetics.

Polyglyceryl-3 Triisostearate
Can be vegetable or animal. Compound of ► *glycerol* and ► *stearic acid*. Emollient and emulsifier in cosmetics.

Polyglyceryl-4 Dilaurate
Can be vegetable or partly animal. Compound of ► *glycerol* and ► *lauric acid*. Emollient and emulsifier in cosmetics.

P

Polyglyceryl-4 Lauryl Ether
Can be vegetable or partly animal. Compound of ► *glycerol* and ► *lauryl alcohol.* Emollient and emulsifier in cosmetics.

Polyglyceryl-4-PEG-2 Cocamide
Can be vegetable/synthetic or partly animal. ► *PEG* compound of ► *glycerol* and coconut fatty acids. Emulsifier and surfactant in cosmetics.

Polyglyceryl-10 Decalinoleate
Can be vegetable or partly animal. Compound of ► *glycerol* and ► *linoleic acid.* Emulsifier in cosmetics.

Polyglyceryl-10 Decaoleate
Can be vegetable or animal. Compound of ► *glycerol* and ► *oleic acid.* Emulsifier in cosmetics.

Polyglyceryl-10 Decastearate
Can be vegetable or animal. Compound of ► *glycerol* and ► *stearic acid.* Emulsifier and opacifier in cosmetics.

Polyglyceryl-10 Didecanoate
Can be vegetable or partly animal. Compound of ► *glycerol* and ► *capric acid.* Emollient and emulsifier in cosmetics.

Polyglyceryl-10 Heptaoleate
Can be vegetable or animal. Compound of ► *glycerol* and ► *oleic acid.* Emulsifier in cosmetics.

Polyglyceryl-10 Heptastearate
Can be vegetable or animal. Compound of ► *glycerol* and ► *stearic acid.* Emulsifier in cosmetics.

Polyglyceryl-10 Mono/Dioleate
Can be vegetable or animal. Compound of ► *glycerol* and ► *oleic acid.* Emulsifier in cosmetics.

Polyglyceryl-10 Pentalaurate
Can be vegetable or animal. Compound of ► *glycerol* and ► *lauric acid.* Emollient and emulsifier in cosmetics.

Polyglyceryl-10 Pentalinoleate
Can be vegetable or partly animal. Compound of ► *glycerol* and ► *linoleic acid.* Emollient and emulsifier in cosmetics.

Polyglyceryl-10 Trioleate
Can be vegetable or animal. Compound of ► *glycerol* and ► *oleic acid.* Emulsifier in cosmetics.

Polyglyceryl-n Caprate
Can be vegetable or animal. Compounds of ► *glycerol* and ► *capric acid.* Emulsifiers in cosmetics.

Polyglyceryl-n Diisostearate

Can be vegetable or animal. Compounds of ► *glycerol* and ► *stearic acid*. Emulsifiers in cosmetics.

Polyglyceryl-n Distearate

Can be vegetable or animal. Compounds of ► *glycerol* and ► *stearic acid*. Emulsifiers in cosmetics.

Polyglyceryl-n Dioleate

Can be vegetable or animal. Compounds of ► *glycerol* and ► *oleic acid*. Emulsifiers in cosmetics.

Polyglyceryl-n Dipalmitate

Can be vegetable or partly animal. Compounds of ► *glycerol* and ► *palmitic acid*. Emollients and emulsifiers in cosmetics.

Polyglyceryl-n Hexaoleate

Can be vegetable or animal. Compounds of ► *glycerol* and ► *oleic acid*. Emulsifiers in cosmetics. Polyglyceryl-10 hexaoleate is also used as an emollient.

Polyglyceryl-n Isostearate

Can be vegetable or animal. Compounds of ► *glycerol* and ► *stearic acid*. Skin conditioners in cosmetics.

Polyglyceryl-n Laurate

Can be vegetable or partly animal. Compounds of ► *glycerol* and ► *lauric acid*. Emulsifiers in cosmetics.

Polyglyceryl-n Myristate

Can be vegetable or partly animal. Compounds of ► *glycerol* and ► *myristic acid*. Emulsifiers in cosmetics.

Polyglyceryl-n Oleate

Can be vegetable or animal. Compounds of ► *glycerol* and ► *oleic acid*. Emulsifiers in cosmetics.

Polyglyceryl-n Oleyl Ether

Can be vegetable or animal. Compounds of ► *glycerol* and ► *oleyl alcohol*. Emulsifiers in cosmetics.

Polyglyceryl-n Palmitate

Can be vegetable or partly animal. Compounds of ► *glycerol* and ► *palmitic acid*. Emollients and emulsifiers in cosmetics.

Polyglyceryl-n Pentaoleate

Can be vegetable or animal. Compounds of ► *glycerol* and ► *oleic acid*. Emulsifiers in cosmetics. Polyglyceryl-4-pentaoleate is also used as an emollient.

Polyglyceryl-n Pentaricinoleate

Can be vegetable or partly animal. Compounds of ► *glycerol* and vegetable ricinoleic acid. Emollients and emulsifiers in cosmetics.

Polyglyceryl-n Pentastearate
Can be vegetable or animal. Compounds of ► *glycerol* and ► *stearic acid.* Emulsifiers in cosmetics. Polyglyceryl-4 pentastearate is also used as an emollient.

Polyglyceryl-n Ricinoleate
Can be vegetable or partly animal. Compounds of ► *glycerol* and vegetable ricinoleic acid. Emulsifiers in cosmetics.

Polyglyceryl-n Stearate
Can be vegetable or animal. Compounds of ► *glycerol* and ► *stearic acid.* Emulsifiers in cosmetics.

Polyglyceryl-n Tetraoleate
Can be vegetable or animal. Compounds of ► *glycerol* and ► *oleic acid.* Emulsifiers in cosmetics. Polyglyceryl-6 tetraoleate is also used as an emollient.

Polyglyceryl-n Tristearate
Can be vegetable or animal. Compounds of ► *glycerol* and ► *stearic acid.* Polyglyceryl-4 tristearate also used as an emollient.

Polyglyceryl Dimer Soyate
Can be vegetable or partly animal. Compound of ► *glycerol* and ► *fatty acids* from soy. Emulsifier in cosmetics.

Polyglyceryl Sorbitol
Can be vegetable or partly animal. Compound of ► *glycerol* with the sugar alcohol sorbitol. Humectant in cosmetics.

Polyhydroxystearic Acid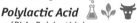
Can be vegetable or animal. Chemical variant of ► *stearic acid.* Emulsifier in cosmetics.

Polylactic Acid
(PLA. Polylactide)
Mostly microbiological/vegetable, can also be animal. Thermoplastic (remouldable under heat), biodegradable plastics, comprising many mutually chemically bonded ► *lactic acid* molecules. Made by chemical transformation (polymerization) of ► *lactide.* In many products, e.g. textiles, packaging, foils, plastic containers. Medical use in degradable sutures and implants.

Polylactide ► *Polylactic Acid*

Polylysine
Polylysine HBR
Microbiological. Polymer compounds of ► *lysine.* Hair conditioner in cosmetics.

Polyoxyethylene Sorbitan Fatty Acid Esters ► *Polysorbates*

Polyoxyethylene (20) Sorbitan Monolaurate ► *Polysorbate 20*

Polyoxyethylene (20) Sorbitan Monooleate ► *Polysorbate 80*

Polyoxyethylene (20) Sorbitan Monopalmitate ► *Polysorbate 40*

Polyoxyethylene (20) Sorbitan Monostearate ► *Polysorbate 60*

Polyoxyethylene (20) Sorbitan Tristearate ► *Polysorbate 65*

Polypeptides

Can be vegetable, microbiological or animal. Compounds of several ► *amino acids.* Can be obtained from plants, animal tissues ("slaughterhouse waste") or yeast cultures. In some cosmetic ingredients, e.g. ► *alanine/histidine/lysine polypeptide copper HCl,* ► *arginine/lysine polypeptide,* ► *ascorbic acid polypeptide,* ► *cholecalciferol polypeptide,* ► *myristoyl glycine/histidine/lysine polypeptide,* ► *pantothenic acid polypeptide,* ► *saccharomyces polypeptides.*

Polypropylene Glycol ► *PPG*

Polysorbates

(Polyoxyethylene sorbitan fatty acid esters)

Mostly vegetable/synthetic, can also be partly animal. Polymer compounds of the sugar alcohol sorbitol and ► *fatty acids* (see the following entries).

Polysorbate 20

(E 432. Polyoxyethylene (20) sorbitan monolaurate. Tween® 20)

Mostly vegetable/synthetic, can theoretically also be partly animal. ► *Polysorbate* of ► *lauric acid.* Emulsifier and stabilizer in foods.

Polysorbate 40

(E 434. Polyoxyethylene (20) sorbitan monopalmitate. Tween® 40)

Mostly vegetable/synthetic, can also be partly animal. ► *Polysorbate* of ► *palmitic acid.* Emulsifier and stabilizer in foods.

Polysorbate 60

(E 435. Polyoxyethylene (20) sorbitan monostearate. Tween® 60)

Can be vegetable/synthetic or animal. ► *Polysorbate* of ► *stearic acid.* Emulsifier and stabilizer in foods.

Polysorbate 65

(E 436. Polyoxyethylene (20) sorbitan tristearate. Tween® 65)

Can be vegetable/synthetic or animal. ► *Polysorbate* of ► *stearic acid.* Emulsifier and stabilizer in foods.

Polysorbate 80

(E 433. Polyoxyethylene (20) sorbitan monooleate. Tween® 80)

Can be vegetable/synthetic or animal. ► *Polysorbate* of ► *oleic acid.* Emulsifier and stabilizer in foods.

Ponceau 4R ► *Cochineal Red A*

Porcelain

(China)

Can be entirely mineral or mineral/from killed animals. Ceramic material, made from kaolin (porcelain clay) and other minerals. Can also contain ► *bone ash* (► *bone china*). Used for making tableware, dolls/figurines, tiles and bathroom ceramics (toilets, basins, etc.). Industrial use as building material and in electric insulators. In dental crowns.

Potassium Abietoyl Hydrolyzed Collagen
From killed animals. Chemically/enzymatically altered ► *collagen.* Cosmetic surfactant.

Potassium Ascorbyl Tocopheryl Phosphate
Can be vegetable/microbiological/synthetic or partly animal. Potassium and phosphoric acid compound of ► *vitamin C* and ► *vitamin E.* Skin protective substance in cosmetics.

Potassium Bitartrate
(E 336. Potassium hydrogen tartrate. Monopotassium tartrate. Cream of tartar. Dipotassium tartrate)
Vegetable/microbiological, animal substances may be involved in processing. Salt deposits, consisting mostly of potassium hydrogen tartrate, formed by crystallization during fermentation and storage of ► *wine.* Raising agent in baked goods (cream of tartar baking powder). Remedy for indigestion. Excipient in industrial processes.

Potassium Caseinate
From living and killed animals (► milk). Potassium salt of ► *casein.* Antistatic in cosmetic products.

Potassium Cetyl Phosphate
Mostly vegetable/synthetic, can theoretically also be animal. Potassium and phosphoric acid compound of ► *cetyl alcohol.* Surfactant in cosmetics.

Potassium Coco Hydrolyzed Animal Protein
► *Potassium Cocoyl Hydrolyzed Animal Protein*

Potassium Cocoyl Glutamate
Vegetable, can theoretically also be partly animal. Potassium salt compound of ► *glutamic acid* and coconut ► *fatty acids.* Surfactant in cosmetics.

Potassium Cocoyl Hydrolyzed Animal Protein
From killed or living animals. Collective term for potassium compounds of chemically/enzymatically altered animal ► *proteins* and coconut ► *fatty acids.* Includes the following substances: ► *potassium cocoyl hydrolyzed casein,* ► *potassium cocoyl hydrolyzed collagen,* ► *potassium cocoyl hydrolyzed keratin,* ► *potassium cocoyl hydrolyzed silk.*

Potassium Cocoyl Hydrolyzed Casein
From living and killed animals (► milk). Chemically/enzymatically altered ► *casein.* Antistatic in cosmetics.

Potassium Cocoyl Hydrolyzed Collagen
From killed animals. Chemically/enzymatically altered ► *collagen.* Antistatic and surfactant in cosmetics.

Potassium Cocoyl Hydrolyzed Keratin
From killed or living animals. Chemically/enzymatically altered ► *keratin.* Antistatic in cosmetics.

Potassium Cocoyl Hydrolyzed Silk
From killed animals. Chemically/enzymatically altered ► *proteins* from ► *silk.* Antistatic in cosmetics.

Potassium Deceth-4 Phosphate
Can be vegetable/synthetic or partly animal. Potassium and phosphoric acid compound of ► *decyl alcohol.* Emulsifier in cosmetics.

Potassium DNA
Can be vegetable, animal or microbiological. Potassium salt of ► *DNA.* Skin conditioner in cosmetics.

Potassium Glutamate ► *Glutamate*

Potassium Guanylate ► *Dipotassium Guanylate*

Potassium Hyaluronate
From killed animals or microbiological. Potassium salt of ► *hyaluronic acid.* Film forming agent in cosmetics.

Potassium Inosinate ► *Dipotassium Inosinate*

Potassium Lactate
(E 326)
Can be mineral/microbiological/vegetable or partly animal. Potassium salt of ► *lactic acid.* Humectant and acidity regulator in foods. Antimicrobial agent in cosmetics.

Potassium Lauroyl Collagen Amino Acids
From killed animals. Chemically altered ► *collagen.* Antistatic and surfactant in cosmetic products.

Potassium Lauroyl Glutamate
Mineral/vegetable, can theoretically also be partly animal. Potassium compound of ► *lauryl alcohol* and ► *glutamic acid.* Hair conditioner and cleansing agent in cosmetics.

Potassium Lauroyl Hydrolyzed Collagen
From killed animals. Chemically/enzymatically altered ► *collagen.* Antistatic and surfactant in cosmetics.

Potassium Myristoyl Glutamate
Mineral/vegetable, can theoretically also be partly animal. Potassium compound of myristyl alcohol (from ► *myristic acid*) and ► *glutamic acid.* Hair conditioner and cleansing agent in cosmetics.

Potassium Myristoyl Hydrolyzed Collagen
From killed animals. Chemically/enzymatically altered ► *collagen.* Antistatic and surfactant in cosmetics.

Potassium Oleate
Can be mineral/vegetable or animal. Potassium salt of ► *oleic acid.* Emulsifier and surfactant in cosmetics.

P

Potassium Oleoyl Hydrolyzed Collagen

From killed animals. Chemically/enzymatically altered ► *collagen*. Antistatic and surfactant in cosmetics.

Potassium Palmitate

Mostly mineral/vegetable, can also be partly animal. Potassium salt of ► *palmitic acid*. Emulsifier and surfactant in cosmetics.

Potassium Sodium Tartrate ► *Sodium Potassium Tartrate*

Potassium Stearate

Can be mineral/vegetable or animal. Potassium salt of ► *stearic acid*. Emulsifier, surfactant and cleansing agent in cosmetics.

Potassium Stearoyl Hydrolyzed Collagen

From killed animals. Chemically/enzymatically altered ► *collagen*. Antistatic, surfactant, hair conditioner and skin protecting substance in cosmetics.

Potassium Tallate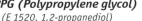

Mineral/vegetable. Potassium salt of ► *tallol*. Antistatic, emulsifier and surfactant in cosmetics.

Potassium Tallowate

From killed animals. Chemically altered ► *tallow*. Emulsifier and surfactant in cosmetics. In liquid and medicinal soaps.

Potassium Tartrate

(E 336)

Vegetable/microbiological, animal substances may be involved in processing. Potassium salt of ► *tartaric acid*. Raising agent, complexing agent, acidifier and acidity regulator in foods.

Potassium Tartrates

(E 336)

Vegetable/microbiological, animal substances may be involved in processing. Potassium salts of ► *tartaric acid*: ► *potassium tartrate*, ► *potassium bitartrate*.

Potassium Undecylenoyl Hydrolyzed Collagen

From killed animals. Chemically/enzymatically altered ► *collagen*. Antidandruff agent, antistatic, surfactant, hair and skin conditioner in cosmetics.

PPG (Polypropylene glycol)

(E 1520. 1,2-propanediol)

Synthetic. Polymers based on propylene. Product of the petrochemical industry. While PPG itself is synthetic, its chemical compounds often have constituents from ► *fats* and other substances that can either be vegetable, animal or mineral. PPG compounds are often used in cosmetics. Industrial use as surfactant and wetting agent.

For information on specific PPG compounds see the following entries. Because of the large number of such compounds, and in the interest of clarity and comprehensibility, those substances with denominations that differ merely by a number and whose functions are more or less identical have been contracted to single denominations, such as "PPG-n Ceteth-n." This means a slight change in the order of the entries.

PPG-1 Trideceth-6

Mostly vegetable/synthetic, can also be partly animal. ► *PPG* compound of ► *decyl alcohol*. Emollient and emulsion stabilizer in cosmetics.

PPG-2 Hydrogenated Tallowamine

From killed animals. ► *PPG* compound of ► *tallow*. Emollient, skin conditioner and antistatic in cosmetics.

PPG-2 Isoceteth-20 Acetate

Mostly vegetable/synthetic, can also be partly animal. ► *PPG* compound of acetic acid and ► *cetyl alcohol*. Emulsifier and skin conditioner in cosmetics.

PPG-2 Isostearate

Can be vegetable/synthetic or animal. ► *PPG* compound of ► *stearic acid*. Emollient and skin conditioner in cosmetics.

PPG-2 Tallowamine

From killed animals. ► *PPG* compound of ► *tallow*. Emulsifier, antistatic and hair conditioner in cosmetics.

PPG-3-Deceth-2 Carboxylic Acid

Mostly vegetable/synthetic, can also be partly animal. ► *PPG* compound of ► *decyl alcohol*. Emollient and cleansing agent in cosmetics.

PPG-3-Isosteareth-9

Can be vegetable/synthetic or animal. ► *PPG* compound of ► *stearic acid*. Emulsifier in cosmetics.

PPG-5-Ceteth-10 Phosphate

Mostly vegetable/synthetic, can also be partly animal. ► *PPG* compound of ► *cetyl alcohol*. Surfactant and emulsifier in cosmetics.

PPG-5 Lanolate

From living or killed animals. ► *PPG* compound of ► *fatty acids* from ► *lanolin*. Emulsifier and emollient in cosmetics.

PPG-5 Lanolin Wax. PPG-5 Lanolin Wax Glyceride

From living or killed animals. ► *PPG* compounds of lanolin wax (► *lanolin cera*). Emollients, hair conditioners and emulsifiers in cosmetics.

PPG-8 Polyglyceryl-2 Ether

Can be vegetable/synthetic or partly animal. ► *PPG* compound of ► *glycerol*. Emollient and emulsion stabilizer in cosmetics.

PPG-9 Diglyceryl Ether

Can be vegetable/synthetic or partly animal. ► *PPG* compound of ► *glycerol*. Emollient and skin conditioner in cosmetics.

PPG-10 Cetyl Ether Phosphate
Mostly vegetable/synthetic, can also be partly animal. ► *PPG* compound of ► *cetyl alcohol.* Emollient, cleansing agent, emulsifier and surfactant in cosmetics.

PPG-12-Laneth-50
From living or killed animals. ► *PPG* compound of ► *lanolin alcohol.* Emulsifier in cosmetics.

PPG-12-PEG-50 Lanolin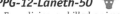
From living or killed animals. ► *PPG* compound of ► *lanolin.* Emollient, hair conditioner and emulsifier in cosmetics.

PPG-15 Isostearate. PPG-15 Stearate
Can be vegetable/synthetic or animal. ► *PPG* compounds of ► *stearic acid.* Emollients in cosmetics.

PPG-15 Stearyl Ether Benzoate
Can be vegetable/synthetic or animal. ► *PPG* compound of ► *stearyl alcohol.* Emollient in cosmetics.

PPG-17 Dioleate
Can be vegetable/synthetic or animal. ► *PPG* compound of ► *oleic acid.* Emollient, skin conditioner in cosmetics.

PPG-20 Methyl Glucose Ether Distearate
Can be vegetable/synthetic or animal. ► *PPG* compound of ► *stearic acid.* Humectant, skin conditioner in cosmetics.

PPG-20-PEG-20 Hydrogenated Lanolin
From living or killed animals. ► *PPG* compound of ► *lanolin.* Emulsifier, skin conditioner and emollient in cosmetics.

PPG-24-PEG-21 Tallowaminopropylamine
From killed animals. ► *PPG* compound of ► *tallow.* Emulsifier, antistatic and hair conditioner in cosmetics.

PPG-30 Isocetyl Ether
Mostly vegetable/synthetic, can also be partly animal. ► *PPG* compound of ► *cetyl alcohol.* Emollient, skin conditioner in cosmetics.

PPG-n-Ceteareth-n
Can be vegetable/synthetic or animal. ► *PPG* compounds of ► *cetostearyl alcohol.* Emulsifiers in cosmetics.

PPG-n-Ceteth-n
Mostly vegetable/synthetic, can also be partly animal. A large number of ► *PPG* compounds of ► *cetyl alcohol.* Emulsifiers in cosmetics, depending on the compounds also emulsion stabilizers, skin conditioners and surfactants.

PPG-n Cetyl Ether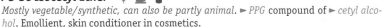
Mostly vegetable/synthetic, can also be partly animal. ► *PPG* compounds of ► *cetyl*

alcohol. Skin conditioners and emollients in cosmetics, depending on the compound also emulsifiers or surfactants.

PPG-n-Deceth-n

Mostly vegetable/synthetic, can also be partly animal. ► *PPG* compounds of ► *decyl alcohol*. Emollients, skin conditioners and emulsion stabilizers in cosmetics. PPG-2-deceth-10 is used only as an emulsifier.

PPG-n-Decyltetradeceth-n

Mostly vegetable/synthetic, can also be partly animal. ► *PPG* compounds of ► *decyl alcohol*. Emulsifiers in cosmetics.

PPG-n-Glycereth-n

Can be vegetable/synthetic or partly animal. ► *PPG* compounds of ► *glycerol*. Emulsifiers in cosmetics, PEG-24-glycereth-24 also used as a cleansing agent.

PPG-n Glyceryl Ether

Can be vegetable/synthetic or partly animal. ► *PPG* compound of ► *glycerol*. Emulsifiers and emollients in cosmetics. PPG-55 glyceryl ether also used as a solvent in cosmetics.

PPG-n-Isodeceth-n

Mostly vegetable/synthetic, can also be partly animal. ► *PPG* compounds of ► *decyl alcohol*. Emulsifiers in cosmetics, some are also skin conditioners and emulsion stabilizers.

PPG-n Lanolin Alcohol Ether

From living or killed animals. ► *PPG* compounds of ► *lanolin alcohol*. Emollients, hair conditioners and emulsifiers in cosmetics.

PPG-n Oleate

Can be vegetable/synthetic or animal. ► *PPG* compounds of ► *oleic acid*. Emollients in cosmetics.

PPG-n Oleyl Ether

Can be vegetable/synthetic or animal. ► *PPG* compounds of ► *oleyl alcohol*. Emollients in cosmetics.

PPG-n-PEG-n Lanolin Oil

From living or killed animals. ► *PPG* compounds of ► *lanolin oil*. Emollients, hair conditioners and emulsifiers in cosmetics.

PPG-n-Steareth-n

Can be vegetable/synthetic or animal. ► *PPG* compounds of ► *stearyl alcohol*. Emollients in cosmetics. PPG-23-steareth-34 also used as an emulsifier.

PPG-n Stearyl Ether

Can be vegetable/synthetic or animal. ► *PPG* compounds of ► *stearyl alcohol*. Emollients in cosmetics.

PPG-n Trideceth-n

Mostly vegetable/synthetic, can also be partly animal. ► *PPG* compounds of ► *decyl alcohol*. Emollients, emulsifiers and emulsion stabilizers in cosmetics.

Prednisolone. Prednisone ► *Corticosteroids*

Pristane
Can be animal or synthetic. An oily liquid. Occurs naturally, especially in shark liver oil (► *squali iecur oil*), also in vegetable and mineral oils. Industrially obtained from shark livers or petroleum derivatives. Emollient and moisturizer in cosmetics. In lubricants and corrosion inhibitors.

Procollagen
From killed animals. A biological precursor of ► *collagen*. Film forming agent, skin and hair conditioner in cosmetics.

Progesterone
Vegetable, can theoretically also be animal. A ► *steroid* hormone that plays an important part as a female sexual hormone. Progesterone is produced especially in ovaries and ► *placenta* of female mammals. Derived industrially from vegetable steroids, e.g. from soybeans or yams. Used in medication, e.g. for treating hormonal disorders and as hormone substitution (e.g. in menopause, after surgery, and for diseases of the uterus), and as preparation for pregnancies via in vitro fertilization. In some oral contraceptives and injections for long-term contraception.

Proline
(L-proline)
Can be vegetable or animal. A nonessential ► *amino acid*. Produced biochemically from ► *glutamic acid* or ► *hydrolyzed protein*. Antistatic, skin and hair conditioner in cosmetics. The therapeutically and economically significant ACE inhibitor ► *captopril* is synthesized from L-proline.

Propionic Acid
(E280)
Synthetic. An organic acid. Occurs naturally in essential oils and during bacterial degradation of vegetable and animal substances, e.g. in cheese production. Industrial production from petroleum derivatives. Used as a food preservative, as are its salts calcium propionate, potassium propionate and sodium propionate. Constituent of various cosmetic ingredients.

Propionyl Collagen Amino Acids
From killed animals. Chemically altered ► *collagen*. Hair conditioner and detangling agent in cosmetics.

Propolis
From living animals. Mixture of tree resins and digestive juices of ► *bees*. Used by bees as a building material for sealing small cracks and reinforcing the hive. Antiseborrheic, moisturizer and smoothing agent in cosmetics. Antimicrobial agent in toothpastes, shampoos, deodorants, etc. In natural remedies and food supplements. Ingredient in violin varnish.

Propyl Gallate ► *Gallates*

Propylene Glycol Caprylate
Mostly vegetable/synthetic, can also be partly animal. ► *Glycol* compound of ► *caprylic acid*. Skin conditioner and emollient in cosmetics.

Propylene Glycol Ceteth-3 Acetate
Mostly vegetable/synthetic, can also be partly animal. ► *Glycol* compound of ► *cetyl alcohol*. Skin conditioner and emollient in cosmetics.

Propylene Glycol Ceteth-3 Propionate
Mostly vegetable/synthetic, can also be partly animal. ► *Glycol* compound of ► *cetyl alcohol* and ► *propionic acid*.

Propylene Glycol Dicaprate
Mostly vegetable/synthetic, can also be partly animal. ► *Glycol* compound of ► *capric acid*. Emollient in cosmetics.

Propylene Glycol Dicaproate
Mostly vegetable/synthetic, can also be partly animal. ► *Glycol* compound of ► *caproic acid*. Emollient in cosmetics.

Propylene Glycol Dicaprylate
Mostly vegetable/synthetic, can also be partly animal. ► *Glycol* compound of ► *caprylic acid*. Emollient and viscosity controlling agent in cosmetics.

Propylene Glycol Dicaprylate/Dicaprate
Mostly vegetable/synthetic, can also be partly animal. ► *Glycol* compound of ► *caprylic acid* and ► *capric acid*. Emollient in cosmetics.

Propylene Glycol Diisostearate
Can be vegetable/synthetic or animal. ► *Glycol* compound of ► *stearic acid*. Emollient in cosmetics.

Propylene Glycol Dioleate
Can be vegetable/synthetic or animal. ► *Glycol* compound of ► *oleic acid*. Emollient in cosmetics. Additive in food packaging.

Propylene Glycol Distearate
Can be vegetable/synthetic or animal. ► *Glycol* compound of ► *stearic acid*. Emollient, viscosity controlling agent, pearlescent, opacifier in cosmetics. Food packaging additive.

Propylene Glycol Hydroxystearate
Can be vegetable/synthetic or animal. ► *Glycol* compound of ► *stearic acid*. Emollient, skin conditioner, emulsifier, opacifier and pearlescent in cosmetics.

Propylene Glycol Isoceteth-3 Acetate
Mostly vegetable/synthetic, can also be partly animal. ► *Glycol* compound of ► *cetyl alcohol*. Emollient in cosmetics.

Propylene Glycol Isodeceth-n
Mostly vegetable/synthetic, can also be partly animal. ► *Glycol* compound of ► *decyl alcohol*. Emulsifier in cosmetics.

P

Propylene Glycol Isostearate
Can be vegetable/synthetic or animal. ▸ *Glycol* compound of ▸ *stearic acid*. Emollient, emulsifier, pearlescent and opacifier in cosmetics.

Propylene Glycol Oleate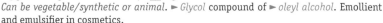
Can be vegetable/synthetic or animal. ▸ *Glycol* compound of ▸ *oleic acid*. Emollient and emulsifier in cosmetics. Additive in food packaging.

Propylene Glycol Oleate SE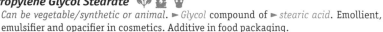
Can be vegetable/synthetic or animal. ▸ *Glycol* compound of ▸ *oleic acid*. Emulsifier and opacifier in cosmetics.

Propylene Glycol Oleth-5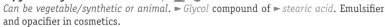
Can be vegetable/synthetic or animal. ▸ *Glycol* compound of ▸ *oleyl alcohol*. Emollient and emulsifier in cosmetics.

Propylene Glycol Stearate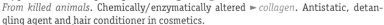
Can be vegetable/synthetic or animal. ▸ *Glycol* compound of ▸ *stearic acid*. Emollient, emulsifier and opacifier in cosmetics. Additive in food packaging.

Propylene Glycol Stearate SE
Can be vegetable/synthetic or animal. ▸ *Glycol* compound of ▸ *stearic acid*. Emulsifier and opacifier in cosmetics.

Propyl Gallate ▸ *Gallates*

Propyltrimonium Hydrolyzed Collagen
From killed animals. Chemically/enzymatically altered ▸ *collagen*. Antistatic, detangling agent and hair conditioner in cosmetics.

Protease
(Peptidase. Proteinase)
Can be from killed animals or microbiological. ▸ Enzymes that break down ▸ *proteins*. Are present in all living cells and play an important part in cellular metabolism in the whole body. Also produced in the stomachs, pancreases and intestines of animals (▸ *pepsin*, chymotrypsine and ▸ *trypsine*) for the purpose of protein digestion. Industrial production from pig pancreases or bacterial or yeast cultures. Skin conditioner in cosmetics. In detergents for the purpose of degrading protein contaminants. Active agents in pharmaceutial drugs, e.g. ▸ *pancreatin*.

Protein
Can be animal, vegetable or microbiological. Collective term for substances in all organisms with molecules made up of various ▸ *amino acids*. Molecules with up to 100 amino acid building blocks (monomeres) are called ▸ *polypeptides*; those with more than 100 monomeres are proteins. Proteins play an important dietary role, supplying energy and essential amino acids, and fulfil many functions in the body, e.g. in energy balance and cell metabolism, in hormones and transmitters, in connective tissues. They are essential constituents of many animal substances used in industrial processes (including the food and cosmetics industries), e.g. ▸ *casein*, ▸ *elastin*, ▸ *gelatin*, ▸ *keratin* and ▸ *silk*.

Protein Hydrolysate ► *Hydrolyzed Animal Protein*

Provitamins
Can be animal or vegetable. Precursors of ► *vitamins*, must be converted in the body to the active forms of the respective vitamins in order for the body to be able to utilize them. Also see the following entries.

Provitamin A ► *Carotene*

Provitamin B₅ ► *Panthenol*

Provitamin D₂ ► *Ergosterol*

Provitamin D₃ ► *7-Dehydrocholesterol*

Pulmonary Surfactant
Can be from killed animals or vegetable/synthetic. Surface-active substance in the lung. Obtained from lungs of cattle or pigs, can also be derived from ► *phospholipids*, ► *fatty acids* and ► *amino acids*. In medication for infant respiratory distress syndrome.

Pyridoxal 5-Phosphate ► *Vitamin B₆*

Pyridoxine ► *Vitamin B₆*

Pyridoxine-5'-Phosphate ► *Vitamin B₆*

Pyridoxine Dicaprylate
Mostly synthetic/vegetable, can be partly microbiological or animal. Compound of ► *vitamin B₆* and ► *caprylic acid*. Antistatic, hair and skin conditioner in cosmetics.

Pyridoxine Dilaurate
Synthetic/vegetable/microbiological, can theoretically also be partly animal. Compound of ► *vitamin B₆* and ► *lauric acid*. Antistatic, humectant, hair and skin conditioner in cosmetics.

Pyridoxine Dipalmitate
Mostly synthetic/vegetable, can be partly microbiological or animal. Compound of ► *vitamin B₆* and ► *palmitic acid*. Antistatic, hair and skin conditioner in cosmetics.

Pyridoxine Glycyrrhetinate
Synthetic/vegetable/microbiological. Compound of ► *vitamin B₆* and ► *glycyrrhetinic acid*. Skin conditioner in cosmetics.

Pyridoxine HCl ► *Vitamin B₆*

Pyridoxine Hydrochloride ► *Vitamin B₆*

Pyridoxine Tripalmitate
Mostly synthetic/vegetable, can be partly microbiological or animal. Compound of ► *vitamin B₆* and ► *palmitic acid*. Antistatic, hair and skin conditioner in cosmetics.

Pyrogenium
From killed animals. Extract of decomposed beef. In ► *homeopathic medicines*.

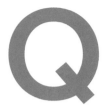

Q10. Q₁₀. Q-10 ► *Ubiquinone*

Quark 🐄
(Curd cheese. Fromage blanc [French]. Kwark [Dutch]. Topfen [Austrian]. Twaróg [Polish])
From living and killed animals (► milk). A type of ► *cheese* made by souring and curdling ► *milk* with ► *lactic acid bacteria*, and then draining off the ► *whey*. ► *Rennet* is also used for curdling. Used for making cheeses, as a food in its own right and as an ingredient in foods. Traditionally used as an external remedy for fever and local inflammations/injuries.

Quaternary Ammonium Compounds 🧪 🐄 🌱
Can be synthetic/animal or synthetic/vegetable. Water-soluble ammonium compounds and ► *cationic surfactants* with antimicrobial or preserving properties. Quarternary ammonium compounds can contain chemically altered animal fats. The compounds include ► *cetylpyridinium chloride* and ► *cetrimonium bromide*, as well as the following substances labelled as "Quaternium." Used for instance as surfactants in cosmetics, laundry detergents and fabric softeners. In surface disinfectants, pesticides and wood preservatives.

Quaternium-16 🐄
From killed animals. ► *Quaternary ammonium compound*, contains chemically altered ► *tallow*. Antistatic and hair conditioner in cosmetics.

Quaternium-18 🐄
From killed animals. ► *Quaternary ammonium compound*, contains chemically altered ► *tallow*. Antistatic, surfactant and hair conditioner in cosmetics.

Quaternium-18 Bentonite 🐄
Quaternium-18/Benzalkonium Bentonite
Quaternium-18 Hectorite
From killed animals. ► *Quaternary ammonium compounds*, contain chemically altered ► *tallow*. Viscosity controlling agent and gelling agent in cosmetics.

Quaternium-18 Methosulfate 🐄
From killed animals. ► *Quaternary ammonium compound*, contains chemically altered ► *tallow*. Antistatic in cosmetics.

Quaternium-26

From killed animals. ► *Quaternary ammonium compound,* contains chemically altered ► *mink oil.* Antistatic and hair conditioner in cosmetics.

Quaternium-27

From killed animals. ► *Quaternary ammonium compound,* contains chemically altered ► *tallow.* Antistatic and hair conditioner in cosmetics.

Quaternium-33

From living or killed animals. ► *Quaternary ammonium compound,* contains chemically altered ► *lanolin.* Antistatic and hair conditioner in cosmetics.

Quaternium-53

From killed animals. ► *Quaternary ammonium compound,* contains chemically altered ► *tallow.* Antistatic and hair conditioner in cosmetics.

Quaternium-60

From living or killed animals. ► *Quaternary ammonium compound,* contains chemically altered ► *lanolin.* Antistatic and hair conditioner in cosmetics.

Quaternium-77
Quaternium-78

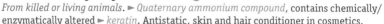

Can be vegetable/synthetic or animal. ► *Quaternary ammonium compounds* of ► *stearic acid* and ► *palmitic acid.* Antistatics and hair conditioners in cosmetics.

Quaternium-79 Hydrolyzed Keratin

From killed or living animals. ► *Quaternary ammonium compound,* contains chemically/enzymatically altered ► *keratin.* Antistatic, skin and hair conditioner in cosmetics.

Quaternium-79 Hydrolyzed Milk Protein

From living and killed animals (► milk). ► *Quaternary ammonium compound,* contains chemically/enzymatically altered ► *milk protein.* Antistatic, skin and hair conditioner in cosmetics.

Quaternium-79 Hydrolyzed Silk

From killed animals. ► *Quaternary ammonium compound,* contains chemically/enzymatically altered ► *silk.* Antistatic, skin and hair conditioner in cosmetics.

Quaternium-83

From killed animals. ► *Quaternary ammonium compound,* contains chemically altered ► *tallow.* Antistatic and hair conditioner in cosmetics.

Quaternium-n Hydrolyzed Collagen

From killed animals. ► *Quaternary ammonium compounds,* contain chemically/enzymatically altered ► *collagen.* Antistatics, skin and hair conditioners in cosmetics.

Quercus Infectoria Gall Extract

Both vegetable and animal. Extract from ► *oak apples.* Antiseborrheic and astringent in cosmetics.

Quorn ► Mycoprotein

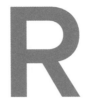

Rabbit-Skin Glue
(Rabbit size)
From killed animals. Adhesive from the skin of rabbits and hares. Obtained by boiling the skins. Used in oil painting (as sizing for canvases), in bookbinding and in conservation/restoration, as well as for joinery and musical instruments.

Ramipril
Microbiological or synthetic. An ACE inhibitor (pharmaceutical drug that lowers blood pressure), chemically related to ► *captropil*. Produced from ► *alanine*.

Rana Bufo ► *Bufo*

Reconstituted Meat
From killed animals. Industrial product composed of meat fragments and leftovers ("slaughterhouse waste"). Used for producing cheap foods. Often in convenience products, e.g. chicken nuggets, meat salads, also an ingredient in commercial kitchens.

Rennet
From killed animals or microbiological. A product that coagulates milk protein (► *casein*). Consists mainly of the ► *enzyme* chymosin and in lesser quantites ► *pepsin*. Obtained from the maws (fourth stomach) of killed calves. Can also be produced using genetically modified bacteria or moulds. A similar substance is obtained from yeast cultures ("microbial rennet"). Used as a coagulant for curdling ► *milk* in ► *cheese* production.

Rennin ► *Rennet*

Reptilase ► *Batroxobin*

Retinol
(Vitamin A₁)
Mostly synthetic, can also be from living or killed animals. An aliphatic alcohol and the most important form of ► *vitamin A*. Has many functions in the body, especially in the skin and eyes. Occurs naturally, especially in animal tissues, ► *egg yolk* and ► *milk*. Is produced in the body from provitamin A (► *carotene*). Industrial production from petroleum products. Skin conditioner in cosmetics. ► *Retinyl palmitate* is used in medicines.

Retinol Acetate ► *Retinyl Acetate*

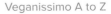

Retinol Linoleate ▸ *Retinyl Linoleate*

Retinol Palmitate ▸ *Retinyl Palmitate*

Retinol Propionate ▸ *Retinyl Propionate*

Retinyl Acetate
(Retinol acetate)
Mostly synthetic, can also be from living or killed animals. Compound of ▸ *retinol* and acetic acid. Skin conditioner in cosmetics.

Retinyl Palmitate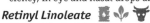
(Retinol palmitate)
Mostly synthetic/vegetable, can also be from living or killed animals. Compound of ▸ *retinol* and ▸ *palmitic acid*. Is the most abundant natural form of ▸ *vitamin A* in animal tissues. Industrial production primarily from synthetic retinol and palmitic acid. Skin conditioner in cosmetics. Active agent in medication, e.g. for treating vitamin A deficiency, in eye and nasal drops and tear substitutes.

Retinyl Linoleate
(Retinol linoleate)
Mostly synthetic/vegetable, can also be from living or killed animals. Compound of ▸ *retinol* and ▸ *linoleic acid*. Skin conditioner in cosmetics.

Retinyl Propionate
(Retinol propionate)
Mostly synthetic, can also be partly animal. Compound of ▸ *retinol* and ▸ *propionic acid*. Skin conditioner in cosmetics.

Riboflavin
(E 101. Lactoflavin. Vitamin B$_2$)
Mostly synthetic or microbiological, can also be animal. Water-soluble ▸ *vitamin*. Can be obtained from ▸ *whey* or yeast, but is usually produced synthetically or from genetically modified organisms. Yellow colouring agent in foods. In vitamin supplements. Colourant and skin conditioner in cosmetics.

Riboflavin Tetraacetate
Mostly synthetic or microbiological, can also be animal. Acetic acid compound of ▸ *riboflavin*. Skin conditioner in cosmetics.

Riboflavin-5'-Phosphate
(E 101/E 101a. Flavin mononucleotide)
Mostly synthetic or microbiological, can also be animal. Derivative of ▸ *riboflavin*. Yellow food colour.

Ribonucleic Acid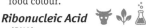
(RNA)
Can be animal, vegetable or microbiological. A nucleic acid, similar to ▸ *DNA*. A central function consists of expressing genetic information in proteins in all living cells. Can be from living or killed animals, plants, yeasts or bacteria. Skin conditioner in cosmetics.

R

Ricinoleamidopropyl Dimethylamine Lactate

Mostly vegetable/synthetic/microbiological, can also be partly animal. Ammonia compound of ► *lactic acid*. Antistatic and hair conditioner in cosmetics.

RNA ► *Ribonucleic Acid*

Rock Salmon

From killed animals. Filleted dorsal tissue of spiny dogfish (► *sharks*). Used as food.

Roe

From killed animals. Fish eggs cut out of the bellies of female ► *fish*. Is regarded as a "delicacy" (► *caviar*). Used as a cosmetic ingredient (► *hydrolyzed roe*).

Rosin Hydrolyzed Collagen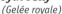

From killed animals. Chemically/enzymatically altered ► *collagen*. Film forming agent, hair fixative, skin and hair conditioner in cosmetics.

Royal Jelly
(Gelée royale)

From living and killed animals. Secretion from the glands of worker ► *bees*. Used for feeding the larvae—especially the queen larvae—of a bee colony. Obtained by specialized beekeepers, who repeatedly remove the queens from the hives and replace them with new queen larvae, for whom royal jelly is produced. The continuous replacement of the larvae and removal of the jelly stimulates an unnaturally constant production. Skin conditioner in cosmetics. Used as a dietary supplement. Royal jelly is used, similarly to ► *propolis*, as a source material for pharmaceutical products. According to Canadian law, royal jelly is not a food, but a natural health product.

Royal Jelly Extract

From living animals. Extract from ► *royal jelly*. Skin conditioner in cosmetics.

Royal Jelly Powder

From living animals. Dried ► *royal jelly*. Skin conditioner in cosmetics.

R

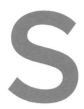

Sable

From killed animals. ► *Fur* from the pelt of sables, a species of marten. From hunted or farmed animals. In coats, jackets and other items of clothing. The hairs are also used in ► *brushes*.

Saccharin

(E 954)

Synthetic. Artificial sweetener (petroleum product). Not related to saccharose (► *sugar*).

Saccharose ► *Sugar*

Sal Butter ► *Shorea Robusta Butter*

Salmo Oil ► *Salmon Oil*

Salmo Ovum Extract

From killed animals. Extract from salmon eggs (► *roe*). Skin conditioner in cosmetics.

Salmon Calcitonin ► *Calcitonin*

Salmon Oil

(Salmo oil)

From killed animals. ► *Fish oil* from the bodies of salmon. Emollient and skin conditioner in cosmetics. In nutritional supplements as a source of ► *omega-3 fatty acids*.

Salts of Fatty Acids

► *Sodium, Potassium and Calcium Salts of Fatty Acids*

Sarcosine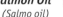

(N-methylglycine)

Can be from killed animals, synthetic or microbiological. A (non-proteinogenic) ► *amino acid* that derives from ► *glycine*. Occurs naturally in muscle and connective tissue, but also in plant tissues. Obtained from cartilage or ► *gelatin*, for example. Synthetic production from chloroacetic acid and ammonia. Also from genetically modified microorganisms. Skin conditioner in cosmetics.

Sardines

Killed animals. Herring-like ► *fish*. Used as food (canned sardines).

Saturated Fatty Acids

Can be animal or vegetable. ► *Fatty acids* that have no "double bonds" (the neighbouring carbon atoms are only simply bonded with each another, unlike ► *unsaturated fatty acids*). Saturated fatty acids are found especially in animal fats (e.g. ► *butterfat*, ► *lard* and ► *tallow*), but also in solid vegetable fats (e.g. palm fat, coconut fat). Examples for unsaturated fatty acids: ► *capric acid*, ► *caproic acid*, ► *palmitic acid* and ► *stearic acid*.

Scyllii Pellis Extract

From killed animals. Extract from the skin of catsharks (► *sharks*). From commercial fishing. Skin conditioner in cosmetics.

Sepia

From killed animals. Dye from the secretion ("ink") of the ink sacs of cephalopods, especially those of the common cuttlefish (*Sepia officinalis*). Sepia was used earlier as a dye and in ink for drawing and painting, and still is to some extent, for instance in watercolour painting. Some foods, especially black pasta, are dyed with sepia. Skin conditioner in cosmetics. The ink of the common cuttlefish is used for ► *homeopathic medicines*.

Sepia Extract

From killed animals. Extract from the nidamental gland (responsible for forming the egg cases) of the common cuttlefish, *Sepia officinalis*. Skin conditioner in cosmetics.

Sepia Officinalis ► *Sepia*

Serica

(Fibroin)

From killed animals. The fibrous ► *protein* of ► *silk*. Humectant, skin and hair conditioner and smoothing agent in cosmetics.

Serica Powder

(Silk powder)

From killed animals. Finely ground ► *silk*. Humectant, skin and hair conditioner and smoothing agent in cosmetics.

Sericin

(Silk glue)

From killed animals. The sticky outer layer of ► *silk*. Antistatic, skin and hair conditioner and smoothing agent in cosmetics.

Serine

Can be animal or synthetic. A nonessential ► *amino acid*, present in almost all ► *proteins*. Obtained from tissues containing ► *keratin* tissues or via processing of petroleum derivatives. Antistatic, hair and skin conditioner in cosmetics.

Serum

(Blood serum)

From killed animals. The liquid fraction of ► *blood* without the clotting factors, comprising water and proteins (► *serum protein*). From cattle or calf blood. Skin conditioner and skin protective substance in cosmetics.

Serum Albumin ► Serum Protein

Serum Protein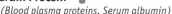
(Blood plasma proteins. Serum albumin)
From killed animals. ► *Proteins* from blood ► *serum*. Humectant, hair and skin conditioner in cosmetics.

Sharks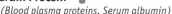
Killed animals. Cartilaginous fishes, exploited economically either directly or indirectly ("bycatch") in considerable numbers (according to some estimations, as many as 100 million individual animals per year). Many species are on the brink of extinction as a result. Used as food (e.g. ► *shark fin*, ► *rock salmon*) and for obtaining fats (e.g. ► *squali iecur oil*) and alcohols (e.g. ► *batyl alcohol*, ► *chimyl alcohol*).

Shark Fin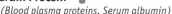
From killed animals. The dorsal or pectoral fins of various shark species. Often the fins are cut off the living animals and the mutilated animals are then thrown back into the sea to die. Millions of sharks die this way each year. Used as food, especially as shark fin soup. Regarded as an ► *aphrodisiac*, especially in China.

Shark Liver Oil ► Squali Iecur Oil

Shea Butter ► Butyrospermum Parkii Butter

Sheep's Cheese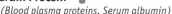
From living and killed animals (► *milk*). ► *Cheese* made from the ► *milk* of sheep. Used as food and food ingredient.

Sheepskin ► Fur

Shell Cordovan ► Horse Leather

Shellac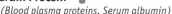
(E 904. Gum lac)
From living and killed animals. Dark brown resin from the excretions of lac scale insects, collected from the branches the insects live on. Used earlier for producing gramophone records. Still used in paints, lacquers and polishes for furniture and musical instruments. Also in technical appliances as an insulator or adhesive. Emollient, film forming agent, viscosity controlling agent and hair fixative in cosmetics. Adhesive in cigarettes. Glazing agent for foods (e.g. confectionery, fresh fruit) and coffee beans. In ► *chewable mass* for chewing gum. Coating agent and ink for medicinal pills and tablets.

Shellac Cera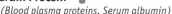
(Shellac wax)
From living and killed animals. ► *Wax* from ► *shellac*. Emollient, film forming agent, hair and skin conditioner, and binding agent in cosmetics.

Shellfish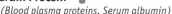
From killed animals. Culinary term for aquatic invertebrate animals with exoskeletons. Its most general meaning encompasses ► *bivalves*, aquatic snails and ► *crustaceans*.

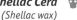

Shorea Butter ► *Shorea Robusta Butter*

Shorea Robusta Butter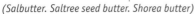
(Salbutter. Saltree seed butter. Shorea butter)
Vegetable. Fat from the fruits and seeds of the sal tree. Not to be confused with animal ► *butter*. Emollient in cosmetics. Used in foods, e.g. as a partial substitute for ► *cocoa butter* in chocolate products.

Shorea Stenoptera Butter ► *Illipé Butter*

Shortening
Can be both vegetable and from killed animals. Special semisolid fat with a relatively high melting point. Often contains at least some animal fats, such as ► *suet* or ► *lard*. Used in baked goods, for frying and deep-frying.

Silanetriol Arginate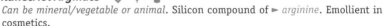
Can be mineral/vegetable or animal. Silicon compound of ► *arginine*. Emollient in cosmetics.

Silanetriol Glutamate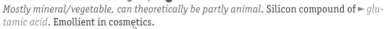
Mostly mineral/vegetable, can theoretically be partly animal. Silicon compound of ► *glutamic acid*. Emollient in cosmetics.

Silanetriol Lysinate
Mineral/microbiological. Silicon compound of ► *lysine*. Emollient in cosmetics.

Silk
From killed animals. Shiny, elastic fibres from the spun cocoons of silkworms. The fibres consist of the protein fibroin (► *serica*); the sticky outer layer (silk glue) consists of ► *sericin*. In order to avoid the cocoons being torn, the silkworm pupae are killed with hot water or steam before they they can emerge as moths. The threads are then unwound from the cocoons in one piece. In fashion items, clothing, sewing and embroidery thread. Used as a painting surface (silk painting). Used earlier in silk-screen printing and dental floss, has now been replaced by synthetic fibres in both cases.

Silk Amino Acids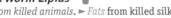
From killed animals. ► *Amino acids* from ► *silk*. Humectant, hair and skin conditioner in cosmetics.

Silk Glue ► *Sericin*

Silk Powder ► *Serica Powder*

Silk Proteins
From killed animals. ► *Proteins* from ► *silk*, mostly fibroin (► *serica*) but also ► *sericin*.

Silk Worm Lipids
From killed animals. ► *Fats* from killed silkworms, obtained from ► *silk* production. Skin conditioner in cosmetics.

Simplesse® ► *Fat Substitutes*

S

Sine Adipe Colostrum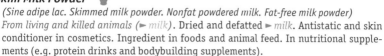
From living and killed animals (► milk*).* Fat-free ► *colostrum.* Skin conditioner in cosmetics.

Sine Adipe Lac ► Skim Milk Powder

Skim Milk. Skimmed Milk
From living and killed animals (► milk*).* Defatted ► *milk* (< 0.5% fat). Used as food and ingredient in foods and animal feed.

Skim Milk Powder
(Sine adipe lac. Skimmed milk powder. Nonfat powdered milk. Fat-free milk powder)
From living and killed animals (► milk*).* Dried and defatted ► *milk.* Antistatic and skin conditioner in cosmetics. Ingredient in foods and animal feed. In nutritional supplements (e.g. protein drinks and bodybuilding supplements).

Snail Cream
(Elicina®)
From living animals. Extract from the slime of snails of the species *Helix aspersa Müller.* Contains, among other substances, ► *allantoin,* ► *elastin* and ► *collagen.* According to the producer, the slime is collected from living animals on snail farms and processed for use as a cosmetics ingredient. Is supposed to improve skin elasticity and scar healing.

Snake Venom ► Venom

Soap
Can be from killed animals or vegetable. Sodium or potassium salts of ► *fatty acids* (e.g. ► *potassium tallowate* ► *sodium tallowate*). Soaps act especially as ► *surfactants,* and are used for personal hygiene and cleaning surfaces. Produced from vegetable (coconut, olive oil, palm) or animal fats (► *tallow,* ► *lard,* bone fat) with the aid of sodium or potassium lyes (hydroxides). Most solid soaps (e.g. hand and body soaps) consist primarily of sodium salts of fatty acids. Liquid and soft soaps consist mostly of inferior fats (e.g. "slaughterhouse waste") treated with potassium hydroxide. Liquid detergents, shower gels and shampoos are generally not "soaps" in the narrower sense of the word, but contain water, mixed surfactants and a variety of excipients (fragrances, colourants, conditioners, etc.).

Sodium-5'-Inosinate ► Disodium Inosinate

Sodium-5'-Ribonucleotide ► Disodium-5'-Ribonucleotide

Sodium, Potassium and Calcium Salts of Fatty Acids
(E 470a. Salts of fatty acids)
Mostly vegetable, but can also be animal. Mixed mineral salts of ► *fatty acids.* Emulsifier, stabilizer, anticaking agent and glazing agent in foods.

Sodium Aluminum Chlorohydroxy Lactate
Can be mineral/microbiological/vegetable or partly animal. Sodium salt of ► *lactic acid.* Antiperspirant and deodorant in cosmetics.

Sodium Aluminum Lactate
Can be mineral/microbiological/vegetable or partly animal. Sodium salt of ► *lactic acid.* Buffering agent and astringent in cosmetics.

Sodium Ascorbyl/Cholesteryl Phosphate
From living or killed animals, can also be synthetic. Compound of ► *vitamin C* and ► *cholesterol.* Antioxidant and skin conditioner in cosmetics.

Sodium Beeswax
From living animals. Chemically altered ► *beeswax.* Emulsifier and skin conditioner in cosmetics.

Sodium Behenoyl Lactylate
Can be mineral/vegetable/microbiological or partly animal. Sodium salt of ► *lactic acid.* Surfactant and emulsifier in cosmetics.

Sodium C8-16 Isoalkylsuccinyl Lactoglobulin Sulfonate
From living and killed animals (► *milk).* Chemically altered whey protein (► *lactoglobulin*). Surfactant, hair and skin conditioner in cosmetics.

Sodium Caproamphoacetate
Mostly mineral/vegetable, can also be partly animal. Compound of sodium, acetic acid and ► *capric acid.* Surfactant, hair conditioner, cleansing and foaming agent in cosmetics.

Sodium Caproamphohydroxypropylsulfonate
Mostly mineral/vegetable, can also be partly animal. Sodium and sulphur compound of ► *capric acid.* Surfactant, foaming agent and cleansing agent in cosmetics.

Sodium Caproamphopropionate
Mineral/vegetable, can also be partly animal. Sodium compound of ► *capric acid* and ► *propionic acid.* Surfactant, hair conditioner, cleansing and foaming agent in cosmetics.

Sodium Caproyl Lactylate
Mostly mineral/vegetable/microbiological, can also be partly animal. Sodium compound of ► *capric acid* and ► *lactic acid.* Emulsifier in cosmetics.

Sodium Caprylate
Mostly mineral/vegetable, can also be partly animal. Sodium salt of ► *caprylic acid.* Emulsifier and surfactant in cosmetics.

Sodium Capryleth-n Carboxylate
Mostly mineral/synthetic/vegetable, can also be partly animal. Polymer compounds of ► *capryl alcohol.* Surfactants in cosmetics.

Sodium Caryloamphoacetate
Mostly mineral/synthetic/vegetable, can also be partly animal. Sodium compound of ► *caprylic acid.* Cosmetic surfactant, foaming and cleansing agent, hair conditioner.

Sodium Caryloamphohydroxypropylsulfonate
Mostly mineral/vegetable, can also be partly animal. Sodium and sulphur compound of ► *caprylic acid.* Surfactant and emulsifier in cosmetics.

Sodium Capryloamphopropionate
Mostly mineral/vegetable, can be partly animal. Sodium compound of ► *caprylic acid* and ► *propionic acid.* Cosmetic surfactant, foaming and cleansing agent, hair conditioner.

Sodium Caprylyl Sulfonate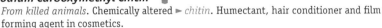
Mostly mineral/vegetable, can also be partly animal. Sodium and sulphur compound of ► *caprylic acid.* Surfactant and emulsifier in cosmetics.

Sodium Carboxyethyl Tallow Polypropylamine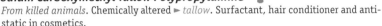
From killed animals. Chemically altered ► *tallow.* Surfactant, hair conditioner and anti-static in cosmetics.

Sodium Carboxymethyl Chitin
From killed animals. Chemically altered ► *chitin.* Humectant, hair conditioner and film forming agent in cosmetics.

Sodium Carboxymethyl Tallow Polypropylamine
From killed animals. Chemically altered ► *tallow.* Surfactant, hair conditioner and anti-static in cosmetics.

Sodium Caseinate
From living and killed animals (► milk). Sodium salt of ► *casein.* Antistatic and hair conditioner in cosmetics.

Sodium Cetearyl Sulfate
Can be mineral/vegetable or partly animal. Compound of ► *palmitic acid* and ► *stearic acid.* Surfactant, cleansing agent and foaming agent in cosmetics.

Sodium Ceteth-13 Carboxylate
Mostly synthetic/vegetable, can also be partly animal. Polymer compound of ► *cetyl alcohol.* Emulsifier and surfactant in cosmetics.

Sodium Cetyl Sulfate
Mostly mineral/vegetable, can also be partly animal. Sodium and sulphur compound of ► *cetyl alcohol.* Emulsifier and surfactant in cosmetics.

Sodium Chitosan Methylene Phosphonate
Mostly from killed animals, can also be vegetable/mineral. Chemically altered ► *chitosan.* Chelating agent in cosmetics.

Sodium Cholesteryl Sulfate
From living or killed animals, can also be synthetic. Chemically altered ► *cholesterol.* Skin conditioner in cosmetics.

Sodium Chondroitin Sulfate
From killed animals. Chemically altered ► *chondroitin.* Antistatic and hair conditioner in cosmetics.

Sodium Coco/Hydrogenated Tallow Sulfate
From killed animals. Chemically altered ► *tallow.* Surfactant, cleansing agent and foaming agent in cosmetics.

Sodium Cocoyl Collagen Amino Acids 🐮
From killed animals. Chemically altered ► *amino acids* from ► *collagen*. Antistatic, surfactant and hair conditioner in cosmetics.

Sodium Cocoyl Glutamate 🌿 🐮
Vegetable, can theoretically also be partly animal. Compound of ► *glutamic acid* and coconut ► *fatty acids*. Surfactant and cleansing agent in cosmetics.

Sodium Cocoyl Hydrolyzed Collagen 🐮
From killed animals. Chemically/enzymatically altered ► *collagen*. Antistatic, surfactant and hair conditioner in cosmetics.

Sodium Cocoyl Hydrolyzed Keratin 🐮
From killed or living animals. Chemically/enzymatically altered ► *keratin*. Antistatic, surfactant and hair conditioner in cosmetics.

Sodium Cocoyl Lactylate 💎 🌿 🧪 🐮
Mostly mineral/vegetable/microbiological, can also be partly animal. Compound of coconut ► *fatty acids* and ► *lactic acid*. Surfactant, emulsifier and cleansing agent in cosmetics.

Sodium Cocoyl Sarcosinate 🐮 🧫 🧪
Can be from killed animals, synthetic or microbiological. Chemically altered ► *sarcosine*. Surfactant, foaming agent, cleansing agent and skin conditioner in cosmetics.

Sodium Diceteareth-10 Phosphate 💎 🌿 🐮
Mostly mineral/vegetable, can also be partly animal. Polymer compound of ► *cetostearyl alcohol*. Emulsifier in cosmetics.

Sodium Dioleth-8 Phosphate 💎 🌿 🐮
Can be mineral/vegetable or animal. Polymer compound of ► *oleyl alcohol*. Emulsifier in cosmetics.

Sodium DNA 🐮 🌿
Can be animal or vegetable. Sodium compound of ► *DNA*. Used as a skin conditioner in cosmetics.

Sodium Glutamate ► *Glutamates*

Sodium Glycereth-1 Polyphosphate 💎 🌿 🐮
Can be mineral/vegetable or partly animal. Polymer compound of ► *glycerol*. Surfactant, chelating agent and viscosity controlling agent in cosmetics.

Sodium Glycerophosphate 💎 🌿 🐮
Can be mineral/vegetable or partly animal. Sodium and phosphoric acid compound of ► *glycerol*. Oral care and antiplaque substance in cosmetics.

Sodium Glyceryl Oleate Phosphate 💎 🌿 🐮
Can be mineral/vegetable or animal. Sodium and phosphoric acid compound of ► *glycerol* and ► *oleic acid*. Surfactant and emulsifier in cosmetics.

Sodium Heparin ► *Heparin*

Sodium Hyaluronate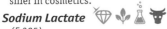
Can be from killed animals or microbiological. Sodium salt of ► *hyaluronic acid*. Humectant in cosmetics.

Sodium Hyaluronate Crosspolymer
Sodium Hyaluronate Dimethylsilanol
Can be from killed animals or microbiological. Sodium compounds of ► *hyaluronic acid*. Humectants and skin conditioners in cosmetics.

Sodium Hydrogenated Tallow Glutamate
From killed animals. Chemically altered ► *tallow*. Surfactant and cleansing agent in cosmetics.

Sodium Hydrolyzed Casein
From living and killed animals (► milk*).* Chemically/enzymatically altered ► *casein*. Hair and skin conditioner in cosmetics.

Sodium Hydroxymethylglycinate
Mostly from killed animals, can also be synthetic or microbiological. Sodium compound of ► *glycine*. Preservative in cosmetics.

Sodium Inosinate ► *Disodium Inosinate*

Sodium Isostearate
Can be mineral/vegetable or animal. Sodium salt of ► *stearic acid*. Cleansing agent and surfactant in cosmetics.

Sodium Isosteareth-n Carboxylate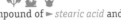
Can be mineral/vegetable or animal. Polymer compounds of ► *stearyl alcohol*. Emulsifiers in cosmetics.

Sodium Isostearoamphoacetate
Can be mineral/vegetable or animal. Acetic acid compound of ► *stearic acid*. Surfactant, cleansing agent and hair conditioner and foaming agent in cosmetics.

Sodium Isostearoamphopropionate
Can be vegetable/synthetic or animal. Compound of ► *stearic acid* and ► *propionic acid*. Surfactant, cleansing agent, hair conditioner and foaming agent in cosmetics.

Sodium Isostearoyl Lactate
Can be mineral/vegetable or animal. Sodium salt of ► *stearic acid* and ► *lactic acid*. Cleansing agent, emulsifier and surfactant in cosmetics.

Sodium Isostearoyl Lactylate
Can be mineral/vegetable or animal. Compound of ► *stearic acid* and ► *lactic acid*. Emulsifier in cosmetics.

Sodium Lactate
(E 325)
Can be mineral/vegetable/microbiological or partly animal. Sodium salt of ► *lactic acid*. Acidity regulator/buffering agent and humectant in foods and cosmetics.

Sodium Lactate Methylsilanol
Can be mineral/vegetable/microbiological or partly animal. Sodium compound of ► *lactic acid*. Skin conditioner in cosmetics.

Sodium Laneth Sulfate
From living or killed animals. Chemically altered ► *lanolin*. Surfactant and emulsion stabilizer in cosmetics.

Sodium Lauroyl Collagen Amino Acids
From killed animals. Chemically altered ► *amino acids* from ► *collagen*. Antistatic and hair conditioner in cosmetics.

Sodium Lauroyl Glutamate
Mostly mineral/vegetable, can theoretically also be partly animal. Sodium compound of ► *glutamic acid*. Antistatic, surfactant and hair conditioner in cosmetics.

Sodium Lauroyl Hydrolyzed Collagen
From killed animals. Chemically/enzymatically altered ► *collagen*. Antistatic, surfactant and hair conditioner in cosmetics.

Sodium Lauroyl Hydrolyzed Silk
From killed animals. Chemically/enzymatically altered ► *silk*. Antistatic and hair conditioner in cosmetics.

Sodium Lauroyl Sarcosinate
Can be from killed animals, synthetic or microbiological. Chemically altered ► *sarcosine*. Antistatic, surfactant, viscosity controlling agent, emulsifier, hair and skin conditioner, cleansing agent and foaming agent in cosmetics.

Sodium Lauroyl Silk Amino Acids
From killed animals. Chemically altered ► *amino acids* from ► *silk*. Skin conditioner and surfactant in cosmetics.

Sodium Lauryl Sulfate
Mineral/vegetable, can theoretically be partly animal. Sodium and sulphuric acid compound of ► *lauryl alcohol*. ► *Anionic surfactant* and foaming agent in detergents. Denaturant, emulsifier, surfactant and foaming agent in cosmetics.

Sodium Methyl Oleoyl Taurate
Can be vegetable/synthetic or animal. Sodium compound of ► *oleic acid* and ► *taurine*. Antistatic, surfactant, foaming agent and cleansing agent in cosmetics.

Sodium Methyl Palmitoyl Taurate
Mostly vegetable/synthetic, can also be partly animal. Sodium compound of ► *palmitic acid* and ► *taurine*. Used as a surfactant, cleansing agent and foaming agent in cosmetics.

Sodium Methyl Stearoyl Taurate
Can be vegetable/synthetic or animal. Compound of ► *stearic acid* and ► *taurine*. Surfactant, cleansing agent and foaming agent in cosmetics.

S

Sodium Myristoyl Glutamate
Mostly mineral/vegetable, can also be partly animal. Sodium salt of ► *glutamic acid.*
Surfactant and cleansing agent in cosmetics.

Sodium Myristoyl Hydrolyzed Collagen
From killed animals. Chemically/enzymatically altered ► *collagen.* Antistatic and hair
conditioner in cosmetics.

Sodium Myristoyl Sarcosinate
Can be from killed animals, synthetic or microbiological. Chemically altered ► *sarcosine.*
Antistatic, surfactant, viscosity controlling agent, cleansing agent, foaming agent and
hair conditioner in cosmetics.

Sodium Oleate
Can be mineral/vegetable or animal. Sodium salt of ► *oleic acid.* Emulsifier, surfactant,
viscosity controlling agent and cleansing agent in cosmetics.

Sodium Oleoyl Hydrolyzed Collagen
From killed animals. Chemically/enzymatically altered ► *collagen.* Antistatic and hair
conditioner in cosmetics.

Sodium Oleoyl Isethionate
Can be mineral/synthetic/vegetable or animal. Sodium compound of ► *oleic acid.* Used
as an antistatic, surfactant, foaming agent, cleansing agent and hair conditioner in
cosmetics.

Sodium Oleoyl Lactylate
Can be mineral/vegetable/microbiological or animal. Sodium compound of ► *oleic acid*
and ► *lactic acid.* Emulsifier in cosmetics.

Sodium Oleth Sulfate
Can be mineral/synthetic/vegetable or animal. Sodium and sulphur compound of ► *oleyl
alcohol.* Emulsifier, foaming agent and cleansing agent in cosmetics.

Sodium Oleth-n Phosphate
Can be mineral/synthetic/vegetable or animal. Sodium and phosphoric acid compounds
of ► *oleyl alcohol.* Emulsifiers, surfactants, foaming agents and cleansing agents in
cosmetics.

Sodium Oleyl Sulfate
Can be mineral/vegetable or animal. Sodium and sulphur compound of ► *oleyl alcohol.*
Emulsifier, foaming agent and cleansing agent in cosmetics.

Sodium Palmitate
Mostly mineral/vegetable, can also be animal. Sodium salt of ► *palmitic acid.* Emulsifier,
surfactant, viscosity controlling agent and cleansing agent in cosmetics.

Sodium Palmitoyl Chondroitin Sulfate
From killed animals. Chemically altered ► *chondroitin.* Hair and skin conditioner in
cosmetics.

Sodium Palmitoyl Hydrolyzed Collagen

From killed animals. Chemically/enzymatically altered ► *collagen*. Hair and skin conditioner in cosmetics.

Sodium Phthalate Stearyl Amide

Can be mineral/vegetable or animal. Sodium compound of ► *stearyl alcohol*. Emulsifier in cosmetics.

Sodium Polyglutamate

Mineral/vegetable, can theoretically be partly animal. Sodium salt of ► *glutamic acid*. Humectant, and hair and skin conditioner in cosmetics.

Sodium Potassium Tartrate

(E 337. Potassium sodium tartrate. Rochelle salt. Seignette's salt)
Mineral/vegetable/microbiological, animal substances may be involved in processing. Sodium and potassium salts of ► *tartaric acid*. Raising agent, complexing agent, acidifier and acidity regulator in foods. Buffering agent in cosmetics.

Sodium Riboflavin Phosphate

Mostly mineral/synthetic or microbiological, can also be animal. Sodium and phosphoric acid compound of ► *vitamin B₂*. Skin conditioner in cosmetics.

Sodium RNA

Vegetable or animal. Sodium salt of ► *ribonucleic acid*. Skin conditioner in cosmetics.

Sodium Sarcosinate

Can be from killed animals, synthetic or microbiological. Sodium salts of ► *sarcosine*. Viscosity controlling agent and hair conditioner in cosmetics.

Sodium Soy Hydrolyzed Collagen

From killed animals. Chemically/enzymatically altered ► *collagen*. Antistatic, surfactant and hair conditioner in cosmetics.

Sodium Stearate

Can be mineral/vegetable or animal. Sodium salt of ► *stearic acid*. Emulsifier and surfactant in cosmetics. Main constituent of many ► *soaps*.

Sodium Steareth-4 Phosphate

Can be mineral/synthetic/vegetable or animal. Polymer compound of ► *stearyl alcohol*. Emulsifier in cosmetics.

Sodium Stearoamphoacetate

Mineral/vegetable or animal. Sodium and acetic acid compound of ► *stearic acid*. Antistatic, surfactant, hair conditioner, foaming and cleansing agent in cosmetics.

Sodium Stearoyl Casein

From living and killed animals (► milk). Chemically altered ► *casein*. Hair and skin conditioner in cosmetics.

Sodium Stearoyl Chondroitin Sulfate

From killed animals. Chemically altered ► *chondroitin*. Hair and skin conditioner.

Sodium Stearoyl DNA
Can be mineral/vegetable or animal. Sodium salts of ► *stearic acid* and ► *DNA*. Skin conditioner in cosmetics.

Sodium Stearoyl Glutamate
Mineral/vegetable or animal. Sodium compound of ► *stearic acid* and ► *glutamic acid*. Emulsifier, cleansing agent, hair and skin conditioner in cosmetics.

Sodium Stearoyl Hyaluronate
Can be from killed animals or microbiological. Sodium salts of ► *stearic acid* and ► *hyaluronic acid*. Hair and skin conditioner in cosmetics.

Sodium Stearoyl Hydrolyzed Collagen
From killed animals. Chemically/enzymatically altered ► *collagen*. Antistatic and hair conditioner in cosmetics.

Sodium Stearoyl Hydrolyzed Corn Protein
Can be vegetable or animal. Sodium compound of ► *stearic acid* and chemically/enzymatically altered corn protein. Hair and skin conditioner in cosmetics.

Sodium Stearoyl Hydrolyzed Silk
From killed animals. Chemically/enzymatically altered ► *silk*. Hair and skin conditioner in cosmetics.

Sodium Stearoyl Hydrolyzed Soy Protein
Sodium Stearoyl Hydrolyzed Wheat Protein
Can be vegetable or animal. Sodium compounds of ► *stearic acid* and chemically/enzymatically altered vegetable proteins (soy and wheat, respectively). Hair and skin conditioners in cosmetics.

Sodium Stearoyl Lactalbumin
From living and killed animals (► *milk).* Sodium salts of ► *stearic acid* and ► *albumin* from ► *milk*. Hair and skin conditioner in cosmetics.

Sodium Stearoyl Lactylate ► *Sodium stearoyl-2-lactylate*

Sodium Stearoyl-2-lactylate
(E 481. Lactate. Sodium stearoyl lactylate)
Can be vegetable or animal. Sodium salt of ► *stearoyl lactylic acid*. Emulsifier and flour treatment agent in foods. Emulsifier in cosmetics.

Sodium Stearoyl Oat Protein
Sodium Stearoyl Pea Protein
Sodium Stearoyl Soy Protein
Can be vegetable or animal. Sodium compounds of ► *stearic acid* and vegetable proteins. Hair and skin conditioners in cosmetics.

Sodium Stearyl Betaine
Can be mineral/synthetic/vegetable or animal. Sodium and ammonium compound of ► *stearyl alcohol*. Surfactant, foam booster and cleansing agent in cosmetics.

Sodium Stearyl Sulfate

Can be mineral/vegetable or animal. Sodium compound of ► *stearyl alcohol*. Surfactant, cleansing agent and emulsifier in cosmetics.

Sodium Tallow Sulfate

From killed animals. Chemically altered ► *tallow*. Used as a surfactant and emulsifier in cosmetics.

Sodium Tallowamphoacetate

From killed animals. Chemically altered ► *tallow*. Surfactant in cosmetics.

Sodium Tallowate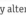

From killed animals. Chemically altered ► *tallow*. Emulsifier, surfactant, cleansing agent and foam booster in cosmetics.

Sodium Tartrate
Sodium Tartrates

(E 335. (i) Monosodium tartrate. (ii) Disodium tartrate)
Vegetable/microbiological, animal substances may be involved in processing. Sodium salts of ► *tartaric acid*. Obtained from tartaric acid. Raising agents, complexing agents, acidifiers and acidity regulators in foods.

Sodium Trideceth Sulfate

Mostly mineral/synthetic/vegetable, can also be partly animal. Sodium compound of ► *decyl alcohol*. Used as an emulsifier, surfactant, cleansing agent and foaming agent in cosmetics.

Sodium Trideceth-n Carboxylate

Can be synthetic/mineral/vegetable or partly animal. Polymer compounds of ► *decyl alcohol*. Surfactants, foaming agent and cleansing substances in cosmetics.

Sodium Tridecyl Sulfate

Can be mineral/vegetable or partly animal. Sodium and sulphur compound of ► *decyl alcohol*. Emulsifier, surfactant and foaming agent in cosmetics.

Sodium Tridecylbenzenesulfonate

Can be mineral/vegetable or partly animal. Sodium and sulphur compound of ► *decyl alcohol*. Surfactant, cleansing agent and foaming agent in cosmetics.

Sodium/TEA-Lauroyl Collagen Amino Acids

From killed animals. Chemically altered ► *collagen*. Antistatic, surfactant and hair conditioner in cosmetics.

Sodium/TEA-Lauroyl Hydrolyzed Collagen

From killed animals. Chemically/enzymatically altered ► *collagen*. Antistatic and surfactant in cosmetics.

Sodium/TEA-Lauroyl Hydrolyzed Keratin

From killed or living animals. Chemically/enzymatically altered ► *keratin*. Antistatic, surfactant and hair conditioner in cosmetics.

Veganissimo A to Z

Sodium/TEA-Lauroyl Keratin Amino Acids

From killed or living animals. Chemically altered ► *keratin*. Antistatic, surfactant and hair conditioner in cosmetics.

Sodium/TEA-Undecylenoyl Collagen Amino Acids

From killed animals. Chemically altered ► *collagen*. Antistatic, surfactant and hair conditioner in cosmetics.

Sodium/TEA-Undecylenoyl Hydrolyzed Collagen

From killed animals. Chemically/enzymatically altered ► *collagen*. Antistatic, surfactant, cleansing agent skin and hair conditioner in cosmetics.

Soluble Collagen

From killed animals. Water-soluble ► *collagen*. Antistatic, film forming agent, humectant, hair and skin conditioner in cosmetics.

Soluble Proteoglycan

From killed animals. ► *Protein* and saccharide compound obtained from cartilage. Hair and skin conditioner in cosmetics.

Sorbeth-n Isostearate

Can be vegetable/synthetic or partly animal. Polymer compounds of the sugar alcohol sorbitol and ► *stearic acid*. Emulsifiers in cosmetics.

Sorbitan Caprylate

Mostly vegetable, can also be partly animal. ► *Sorbitan fatty acid ester* of ► *caprylic acid*. Emulsifier in cosmetics.

Sorbitan Diisostearate

Can be vegetable or animal. ► *Sorbitan fatty acid ester* of ► *stearic acid*. Emulsifier in cosmetics.

Sorbitan Dioleate

Can be vegetable or animal. ► *Sorbitan fatty acid ester* of ► *oleic acid*. Emulsifier in cosmetics.

Sorbitan Distearate

Can be vegetable or animal. ► *Sorbitan fatty acid ester* of ► *stearic acid*. Emollient in cosmetics.

Sorbitan Fatty Acid Esters

Can be vegetable or animal. Reaction products of the sugar alcohol sorbitol with ► *fatty acids*. Emulsifiers in foods (► *sorbitan monolaurate*, ► *sorbitan monooleate*, ► *sorbitan monopalmitate*, ► *sorbitan monostearate*, ► *sorbitan tristearate*) and ingredients in cosmetic products (see remaining entries between ► *sorbitan caprylate* and ► *sorbitan trioleate*).

Sorbitan Isostearate

Can be vegetable or partly animal. ► *Sorbitan fatty acid ester* of ► *stearic acid*. Emulsifier in cosmetics.

Sorbitan Laurate ► *Sorbitan Monolaurate*

Sorbitan Monolaurate 🌱 🐄
(E 493. Sorbitan laurate. Sorbitan fatty acid ester)
Vegetable, can theoretically also be partly animal. ► *Sorbitan fatty acid ester* of ► *lauric acid*. Emulsifier in foods and cosmetics.

Sorbitan Monooleate 🌱 🐄
(E 494. Sorbitan oleate. Sorbitan fatty acid ester)
Can be vegetable or animal. ► *Sorbitan fatty acid ester* of ► *oleic acid*. Emulsifier in foods and cosmetics.

Sorbitan Monopalmitate 🌱 🐄
(E 495. Sorbitan palmitate. Sorbitan fatty acid ester)
Mostly vegetable, can also be partly animal. ► *Sorbitan fatty acid ester* of ► *palmitic acid*. Emulsifier in foods and cosmetics.

Sorbitan Monostearate 🌱 🐄
(E 491. Sorbitan stearate. Sorbitan fatty acid ester)
Can be vegetable or animal. ► *Sorbitan fatty acid ester* of ► *stearic acid*. Emulsifier in foods and cosmetics.

Sorbitan Oleate ► *Sorbitan Monooleate*

Sorbitan Palmitate ► *Sorbitan Monopalmitate*

Sorbitan Sesquiisostearate 🌱 🐄
Can be vegetable or animal. ► *Sorbitan fatty acid ester* of ► *stearic acid*. Emulsifier in cosmetics.

Sorbitan Sesquioleate 🌱 🐄
Can be vegetable or animal. ► *Sorbitan fatty acid ester* of ► *oleic acid*. Emulsifier in cosmetics.

Sorbitan Sesquistearate 🌱 🐄
Can be vegetable or animal. ► *Sorbitan fatty acid ester* of ► *stearic acid*. Emulsifier in cosmetics.

Sorbitan Stearate ► *Sorbitan Monostearate*

Sorbitan Triisostearate 🌱 🐄
Can be vegetable or animal. ► *Sorbitan fatty acid ester* of ► *stearic acid*. Emulsifier in cosmetics.

Sorbitan Trioleate 🌱 🐄
Can be vegetable or animal. ► *Sorbitan fatty acid ester* of ► *oleic acid*. Emulsifier in cosmetics.

Sorbitan Tristearate 🌱 🐄
(E 492. Sorbitan tristearate. Sorbitan fatty acid ester)
Can be vegetable or animal. ► *Sorbitan fatty acid ester* of ► *stearic acid*. Emulsifier in foods and cosmetics.

Sourdough ▸ *Backferment*

Soybean Palmitate

Mostly vegetable, can also be partly animal. Reaction product of soy fatty acids and ▸ *palmitic acid*. Emollient, refatting substance in cosmetics.

Spanish Fly

(Lytta vesicatoria. Cantharis vesicatoria)

From killed animals. Dried, powdered insects from the family of the blister beetles. Used earlier as a lethal poison. Still used as *Cantharis vesicatoria* in ▸ *homeopathic medicines*. Also regarded as an ▸ *aphrodisiac*.

Sperm Oil ▸ *Spermaceti*

Spermaceti

(Sperm oil)

From killed animals. ▸ *Wax* from the heads of killed sperm whales. Used earlier in medicines, skin creams, shampoos and candles, and for treating leather. Products from whaling are banned in Canada (with exemptions for Aboriginal peoples); substances from vegetable fats are now used instead, e.g. ▸ *cetyl palmitate* or jojoba oil.

Sphingolipids

Can be from killed animals or vegetable. ▸ *Lipids* and important constituents of cell membranes, especially in nerve tissue (playing an important part in signal transmission). Their main constituent is ▸ *sphingosine*. Can also be obtained from plants. Emollient, skin conditioner and skin protective substance in cosmetics.

Sphingosine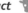

Can be from killed animals or vegetable/microbiological. Alcohol that occurs naturally in animal ▸ *fats*, especially in the brain, spinal cord and pancreas. Main constituent of ▸ *sphingolipids* in cell membranes. Also obtained biotechnologically from vegetable fats with the aid of microorganisms. Various derivatives are used in cosmetics: ▸ *ceramides*, ▸ *hydroxycaproyl phytosphingosine*, ▸ *hydroxycapryloyl phytosphingosine*, ▸ *hydroxylauroyl phytosphingosine*, ▸ *lactoyl phytosphingosine*, ▸ *phytosphingosine*.

Spinal Cord Extract

From killed animals. Extract from animal spinal cords. Skin conditioner in cosmetics.

Spinal Lipid Extract

From killed animals. ▸ *Fat* from animal spinal cords. Emollient in cosmetics.

Spleen Extract

From killed animals. Extract from animal spleens. Skin conditioner in cosmetics.

Spleen Hydrolysate

From killed animals. Chemically/enzymatically altered ▸ *proteins* from animal spleens. Skin conditioner in cosmetics.

Split Leather

From killed animals. ▸ *Leather* cut horizontally to obtain several layers from one piece,

S

often with additional coating (e.g. polyurethane) and embossing. Cheap leather, e.g. in furniture, footwear, belts.

Sponges 🐮
(Spongia)
From killed animals. Plant-like animals that live anchored to the sea floor. Due to their absorbency they are used as bath sponges, cleaning sponges and natural tampons, as well as in watercolour painting. Used as "spongia tosta" (toasted over coals) in ► *homeopathic medicines*.

Spongia. Spongia Tosta ► Sponges

Squalane 🐮 🌿
(Perhydrosqualene)
Can be from killed animals or vegetable. A hydrocarbon compound. Occurs naturally (along with ► *squalene*) in ► *fish liver oil* and many vegetable oils. Obtained from shark liver oil (► *squali iecur oil*) or olive oil. Emollient, hair and skin conditioner, and refatting substance in cosmetics.

Squalene 🐮 🌿
Can be from killed animals or vegetable. A hydrocarbon compound. Occurs naturally (along with ► *squalane*) in ► *Lebertran* and many vegetable oils. Obtained from shark liver oil (► *squali iecur oil*) or olive oil. Antistatic, emollient, hair conditioner and refatting substance in cosmetics.

Squali Iecur Oil 🐮
(Shark liver oil)
From killed animals. Oil from the fresh livers of various shark species. Contains the alkylglycerols ► *batyl alcohol*, ► *chimyl alcohol* and selachyl alcohol, also ► *pristane*. From commercial fishing. Emollient, refatting agent and skin conditioner in cosmetics. In food supplements for stimulating the immune system. As complementary treatment for cancer and radiation therapy.

Squid 🐮
Killed animals. Order of cephalopods (marine invertebrates). From commercial fishing. Used as food, especially in the Mediterranean Basin. Used for obtaining ► *sepia*.

Squirrel Hair ► Brushes

Stearalkonium Bentonite 🐮
From killed animals. A ► *quarternary ammonium compound*. Contains chemically altered ► *tallow*. Viscosity controlling agent and gelling agent in cosmetics.

Stearalkonium Chloride 🐮
From killed animals. A ► *quarternary ammonium compound*. Contains chemically altered ► *tallow*. Preservative, antistatic and surfactant in cosmetics.

Stearalkonium Dimethicone Copolyol Phthalate 🌿 🧪 🐮
Can be vegetable/synthetic or partly animal. A ► *quarternary ammonium compound*. Hair conditioner in cosmetics.

Stearalkonium Hectorite

From killed animals. A ► *quarternary ammonium compound*. Contains chemically altered ► *tallow*. Viscosity controlling agent and gelling agent in cosmetics.

Stearamide

Can be vegetable/synthetic or animal. Ammonia compound of ► *stearic acid*. Opacifier, viscosity controlling agent and foam booster in cosmetics.

Stearamide AMP

Can be vegetable/synthetic or animal. Ammonia compound of ► *stearic acid*. Viscosity controlling agent and foam booster in cosmetics.

Stearamide DEA

Can be vegetable/synthetic or animal. Ammonia compound of ► *stearic acid*. Antistatic, viscosity controlling agent and foam booster in cosmetics.

Stearamide DEA-Distearate

Can be vegetable/synthetic or animal. Ammonia compound of ► *stearic acid*. Opacifier, viscosity controlling agent and foam booster in cosmetics.

Stearamide DIBA-Stearate

Can be vegetable/synthetic or animal. Ammonia compound of ► *stearic acid*. Opacifier, viscosity controlling agent and foam booster in cosmetics.

Stearamide MEA

Can be vegetable/synthetic or animal. Ammonia compound of ► *stearic acid*. Antistatic, viscosity controlling agent and foam booster in cosmetics.

Stearamide MEA-Stearate

Can be vegetable/synthetic or animal. Ammonia compound of ► *stearic acid*. Antistatic, opacifier and viscosity controlling agent in cosmetics.

Stearamide MIPA

Can be vegetable/synthetic or animal. Ammonia compound of ► *stearic acid*. Antistatic, viscosity controlling agent and foam booster in cosmetics.

Stearamidoethyl Diethanolamine

Can be vegetable/synthetic or animal. Ammonia compound of ► *stearic acid*. Antistatic and skin conditioner in cosmetics.

Stearamidoethyl Diethylamine

Can be vegetable/synthetic or animal. Ammonia compound of ► *stearic acid*. Antistatic and hair conditioner in cosmetics.

Stearamidoethyl Diethylamine Phosphate

Can be vegetable/synthetic or animal. Ammonia compound of ► *stearic acid*. Antistatic and hair conditioner in cosmetics.

Stearamidoethyl Ethanolamine

Can be vegetable/synthetic or animal. Ammonia compound of ► *stearic acid*. Antistatic and emulsifier in cosmetics.

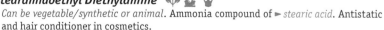

Stearamidoethyl Ethanolamine Phosphate
Can be vegetable/synthetic or animal. Ammonia compound of ► *stearic acid*. Antistatic in cosmetics.

Stearamidopropyl Betaine
Can be vegetable/synthetic or animal. Ammonium compound of ► *stearic acid*. Antistatic, surfactant, hair and skin conditioner, cleansing agent and foaming agent in cosmetics.

Stearamidopropyl Cetearyl Dimonium Tosylate
Can be vegetable/synthetic or animal. Ammonium compound of ► *stearic acid*. Antistatic in cosmetics.

Stearamidopropyl Dimethicone
Can be vegetable/synthetic or animal. Ammonia and silicone compound of ► *stearic acid*. Corrosion inhibitor and film forming agent in cosmetics.

Stearamidopropyl Dimethylamine
Can be vegetable/synthetic or animal. Ammonia compound of ► *stearic acid*. Antistatic, emulsifier, surfactant and hair conditioner in cosmetics.

Stearamidopropyl Dimethylamine Lactate
Can be vegetable/synthetic/microbiological or animal. Ammonia compound of ► *stearic acid* and ► *lactic acid*. Antistatic and hair conditioner in cosmetics.

Stearamidopropyl Dimethylamine Stearate
Can be vegetable/synthetic or animal. Ammonia compound of ► *stearic acid*. Emulsifier and hair conditioner in cosmetics.

Stearamidopropyl Ethyldimonium Ethosulfate
Can be vegetable/synthetic or animal. Ammonium compound of ► *stearic acid*. Antistatic and hair conditioner in cosmetics.

Stearamidopropyl Morpholine
Can be vegetable/synthetic or animal. Ammonia compound of ► *stearic acid*. Antistatic in cosmetics.

Stearamidopropyl Morpholine Lactate
Can be synthetic/vegetable/microbiological or animal. Ammonia compound of ► *stearic acid* and ► *lactic acid*. Antistatic in cosmetics.

Stearamidopropyl PG-Dimonium Chloride Phosphate
Stearamidopropyl Pyrrolidonylmethyl Dimonium Chloride
Stearamidopropyl Trimonium Methosulfate
Can be vegetable/synthetic or animal. Ammonium compounds of ► *stearic acid*. Antistatics and hair conditioners in cosmetics.

Stearamidopropylamine Oxide
Can be vegetable/synthetic or animal. Ammonia compound of ► *stearic acid*. Antistatic, surfactant, hair conditioner, foam booster and hydrotrope in cosmetics.

Stearamine
Can be vegetable/synthetic or animal. Ammonia compound of ► *stearic acid*. Antistatic in cosmetics.

Stearamine Oxide
Can be vegetable/synthetic or animal. Ammonia compound of ► *stearic acid*. Antistatic, surfactant, hydrotrope, cleansing agent, hair conditioner and foam booster in cosmetics.

Stearates
Can be vegetable or animal. Salts and esters of ► *stearic acid*. Used especially in cosmetics. Some examples: ► *aluminum stearate*, ► *cetearyl stearate*, ► *cetyl stearate*, ► *ethyl stearate*, ► *glyceryl stearate*, ► *magnesium stearate*, ► *potassium stearate*, ► *sodium stearate*, ► *zinc stearate*.

Steardimonium Hydroxypropyl Hydrolyzed Casein
From living and killed animals (► milk). Chemically/enzymatically altered ► *casein*. Antistatic in cosmetics.

Steardimonium Hydroxypropyl Hydrolyzed Collagen
From killed animals. Chemically/enzymatically altered ► *collagen*. Used as an antistatic in cosmetics.

Steardimonium Hydroxypropyl Hydrolyzed Keratin
From killed or living animals. Chemically/enzymatically altered ► *keratin*. Antistatic in cosmetics.

Steardimonium Hydroxypropyl Hydrolyzed Rice Protein
Can be vegetable/synthetic or animal. Ammonium compound of ► *stearic acid* and rice protein. Antistatic in cosmetics.

Steardimonium Hydroxypropyl Hydrolyzed Silk
From killed animals. Chemically/enzymatically altered ► *silk*. Used as an antistatic in cosmetics.

Steardimonium Hydroxypropyl Hydrolyzed Vegetable Protein
Can be vegetable/synthetic or animal. Ammonium compound of ► *stearic acid* and vegetable protein. Antistatic in cosmetics.

Steardimonium Hydroxypropyl Hydrolyzed Wheat Protein
Can be vegetable or animal. Ammonium compound of ► *stearic acid* and wheat protein. Antistatic in cosmetics.

Steareth-10 Allyl Ether/Acrylates Copolymer
Can be vegetable/synthetic or animal. Polymer compound of ► *stearic acid*. Film forming agent in cosmetics.

Steareth-2 Phosphate
Can be vegetable/synthetic or animal. ► *PEG* compound of ► *stearic acid*. Emulsifier in cosmetics.

S

Steareth-5 Stearate
Can be vegetable/synthetic or animal. ► *PEG* compound of ► *stearic acid*. Emulsifier and skin conditioner in cosmetics.

Steareth-n
Can be vegetable/synthetic or animal. ► *PEG* compounds of ► *stearic acid*. Emulsifiers and surfactants in cosmetics, some also used as cleansing, gelling or refatting agents.

Stearic Acid
(E 570. Octadecanoic acid)
Can be from killed animals or vegetable. A ► *saturated fatty acid*. Occurs naturally in almost all animal and vegetable ► *fats* (especially ► *tallow*, ► *butter* and ► *lard*, or ► *cocoa butter*, coconut fat and palm oil). Obtained from both the fat of slaughtered animals and vegetable fats. Emulsifier, emulsion stabilizer, refatting and cleansing agent in cosmetics, also in the form of ► *stearates*. In lubricants and ► *soaps*, especially as ► *sodium stearate*). In candles (► *stearin*), modelling compounds and anticaking agents.

Stearin
Can be vegetable or animal. Solid mixture of ► *stearic acid* and ► *palmitic acid*. Obtained from palm oil or ► *tallow*. Used for making candles and ► *soaps*.

Stearone
Can be mineral/vegetable or animal. Chemically altered ► *stearic acid*. Viscosity controlling agent in cosmetics.

Stearoxy Dimethicone
Stearoxymethicone/Dimethicone Copolymer
Can be mineral/vegetable or animal. Silicone compounds of ► *stearyl alcohol*. Emollients and skin conditioners in cosmetics.

Stearoxytrimethylsilane
Can be mineral/vegetable or animal. Silicon compound of ► *stearyl alcohol*. Emollient and skin conditioner in cosmetics.

Stearoyl Glutamic Acid
Can be vegetable or animal. Compound of ► *stearic acid* and ► *glutamic acid*. Skin conditioner in cosmetics.

Stearoyl Inulin
Can be vegetable or animal. A polysaccharide compound of ► *stearic acid*. Emollient and emulsifier in cosmetics.

Stearoyl Lactylic Acid
Can be vegetable/microbiological or animal. Compound of ► *stearic acid*, ► *lactic acid* and ► *polylactic acid*. Emulsifier in cosmetics. Its salts ► *sodium stearoyl-2 lactylate* and ► *calcium stearoyl-2 lactylate* are used as food additives.

Stearoyl Leucine
Can be vegetable, microbiological or animal. Compound of ► *stearic acid* and ► *leucine*. Emulsifier, hair and skin conditioner and surfactant in cosmetics.

Stearoyl PG-Trimonium Chloride
Can be vegetable/synthetic or animal. Ammonium compound of ► *stearic acid*. Antistatic and hair conditioner in cosmetics.

Stearoyl Sarcosine
Can be from killed animals, synthetic or microbiological. Chemically altered ► *sarcosine*. Antistatic, surfactant and hair conditioner in cosmetics.

Steartrimonium Bromide
(Stearyl trimethyl ammonium bromide [STAB]. Trimethyl octadecyl ammonium bromide)
Can be vegetable/synthetic or animal. ► *Quaternary ammonium compound* of ► *stearyl alcohol*. Antistatic, hair conditioner and preservative in cosmetics. ► *Cationic surfactant* in detergents. Surfactant in diverse industrial production processes.

Steartrimonium Chloride
(Stearyl trimethyl ammonium chloride [STAC]. Trimethyl octadecyl ammonium chloride)
Can be vegetable/synthetic or animal. ► *Quaternary ammonium compound* of ► *stearyl alcohol*. Preservative in cosmetics. Active agent in topical antiseptics. Used as a ► *cationic surfactant* in detergents, also as a surfactant in a variety of industrial production processes.

Steartrimonium Hydroxyethyl Hydrolyzed Collagen
From killed animals. Chemically/enzymatically altered ► *collagen*. Antistatic, hair and skin conditioner in cosmetics.

Steartrimonium Methosulfate
Can be vegetable/synthetic or animal. ► *Quaternary ammonium compound* of ► *stearyl alcohol*. Antistatic in cosmetics.

Steartrimonium Saccharinate
Can be vegetable/synthetic or animal. ► *Quaternary ammonium compound* of ► *stearyl alcohol*. Antistatic and hair conditioner in cosmetics.

Stearyl Acetate
Can be vegetable/synthetic or animal. acetic acid compound of ► *stearyl alcohol*. Emollient, skin conditioner in cosmetics.

Stearyl Acetyl Glutamate
Can be vegetable/synthetic or animal. Compound of ► *stearyl alcohol* and ► *glutamic acid*. Emulsifier, hair and skin conditioner and surfactant in cosmetics.

Stearyl Alcohol
(Octadecanol. Octadecyl alcohol)
Can be vegetable or animal. A ► *fatty alcohol* derived from ► *stearic acid*. Emollient, emulsion stabilizer, opacifier, viscosity controlling agent, foam booster and refatting agent in cosmetics. In medicinal creams and ointments, also as a constituent of ► *cetostearyl alcohol*. Used for producing ► *surfactants*. In lubricants.

Stearyl Beeswax
From living animals. Chemically altered ► *beeswax*. Emollient in cosmetics.

Stearyl Behenate
Can be vegetable or animal. Compound of ► *stearyl alcohol* and vegetable behenic acid. Emollient, skin conditioner in cosmetics.

Stearyl Benzoate
Can be vegetable/synthetic or animal. Compound of ► *stearyl alcohol* and benzoic acid. Emollient in cosmetics.

Stearyl Betaine
Can be vegetable/synthetic or animal. Ammonium compound of ► *stearyl alcohol*. Antistatic, surfactant, hair and skin conditioner and foaming agent in cosmetics.

Stearyl Caprylate
Can be vegetable or animal. Compound of ► *stearyl alcohol* and ► *caprylic acid*. Emollient and skin conditioner in cosmetics.

Stearyl Citrate
Can be vegetable/microbiological or animal. Citric acid compound of ► *stearyl alcohol*. Emollient and skin conditioner in cosmetics.

Stearyl Dimethicone
Can be mineral/vegetable or animal. Silicone compound of ► *stearyl alcohol*. Emollient, skin conditioner in cosmetics.

Stearyl Erucamide
Can be vegetable or animal. Compound of ► *stearyl alcohol* and vegetable erucic acid. Opacifier and viscosity controlling agent in cosmetics.

Stearyl Erucate
Can be vegetable or animal. Compound of ► *stearyl alcohol* and vegetable erucic acid. Emollient in cosmetics.

Stearyl Ethylhexanoate
Can be vegetable or animal. Compound of ► *stearyl alcohol* and ► *caproic acid*. Emollient and skin conditioner in cosmetics.

Stearyl Ethylhexyldimonium Chloride
Can be vegetable/synthetic or animal. Ammonium compound of ► *stearyl alcohol*. Antistatic and hair conditioner in cosmetics.

Stearyl Ethylhexyldimonium Methosulfate
Can be vegetable/synthetic or animal. Ammonium compound of ► *stearyl alcohol*. Antistatic and hair conditioner in cosmetics.

Stearyl Glycol
Can be vegetable/synthetic or animal. ► *Glycol* compound of ► *stearyl alcohol*. Emollient in cosmetics.

Stearyl Glycol Isostearate
Can be vegetable/synthetic or animal. ► *Glycol* compound of ► *stearyl alcohol* and ► *stearic acid*. Emollient in cosmetics.

Stearyl Glycyrrhetinate

Can be vegetable or animal. Compound of ► *stearyl alcohol* and *glycyrrhetinic acid*. Skin conditioner and soothing agent in cosmetics.

Stearyl Heptanoate

Can be vegetable or animal. Compound of ► *stearyl alcohol* and vegetable enanthic acid. Emollient and skin conditioner in cosmetics.

Stearyl Hydroxyethyl Imidazoline

Can be vegetable/synthetic or animal. Nitrogen and carbon compound of ► *stearyl alcohol*. Antistatic and hair conditioner in cosmetics.

Stearyl Hydroxyethylimidonium Chloride

Can be vegetable/synthetic or animal. Ammonium compound of ► *stearyl alcohol*. Antistatic, hair conditioner.

Stearyl Lactate

Can be vegetable/microbiological or animal. Compound of ► *stearyl alcohol* and ► *lactic acid*. Emollient and skin conditioner in cosmetics.

Stearyl Linoleate

Can be vegetable or animal. Compound of ► *stearyl alcohol* and ► *linoleic acid*. Emollient and opacifier in cosmetics.

Stearyl Methicone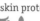

Can be vegetable/synthetic or animal. Silicone compound of ► *stearyl alcohol*. Emollient, skin conditioner and skin protective substance in cosmetics.

Stearyl Stearate
Stearyl Stearoyl Stearate

Can be animal or vegetable. Compounds of ► *stearyl alcohol* and ► *stearic acid*. Emollients, skin conditioners and viscosity controlling agents in cosmetics.

Stearyl Tartrate

(E 483. Stearyl palmityl tartrate)

Can be vegetable/microbiological or animal. Mixture of mono- and diglycerides of ► *saturated fatty acids* and ► *tartaric acid*. Emulsifier and flour treatment agent in foods (only in desserts and baked goods with the exception of bread).

Stearyl/Aminopropyl Methicone Copolymer

Can be vegetable/synthetic or animal. Silicone compound of ► *stearyl alcohol*. Emollient in cosmetics.

Stearylvinyl Ether/MA Copolymer

Can be vegetable/synthetic or animal. Polymer compound of ► *stearyl alcohol*. Antistatic, film forming agent and viscosity controlling agent in cosmetics.

Steroids

Can be animal or vegetable/synthetic. Hydrocarbon compounds that possess a common basic structure and belong to the ► *lipids*. Occur naturally in fungi, plants and animals and fulfil a number of important functions. The most important animal steroid is ► *cholesterol*, from which the steroid hormones, e.g. the ► *corticosteroids* and the sexual hormones (► *estrogen*, ► *progesterone*, ► *testosterone*), and ► *vitamin D₃* derive.

Stock ► *Bouillon*

Stomach Extract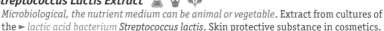

From killed animals. Extract from animal stomachs. Skin conditioner in cosmetics.

Streptococcus Lactis Extract

Microbiological, the nutrient medium can be animal or vegetable. Extract from cultures of the ► *lactic acid bacterium Streptococcus lactis*. Skin protective substance in cosmetics.

Streptococcus Thermophilus (Str. Thermophilus) ► *Yogurt Cultures*

Struthio Oil

From killed animals. Oil from fatty tissues of ostriches. Hair conditioner in cosmetics.

Sturgeon Roe ► *Caviar*

Succinic Acid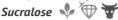

(E 363. Butanedioic acid)
Synthetic/vegetable/microbiological. An organic, hydrocarbon-based acid. Plays an important part in biochemical processes. Occurs naturally in many plants, fungi and algae, present as succinic acid salts (succinates) in the metabolism of all organisms. Obtained from petroleum products or from microorganisms. Acidifier in foods. As "succinates" in many cosmetic ingredients, e.g. combined with ► *fatty alcohols*.

Sucralose

(E 955. Trichlorgalactosaccharose. Trichlorosucrose)
Vegetable/mineral, may have been treated with animal substances. A noncaloric artificial sweetener, produced by chemically altering ► *sugar* with chlorides, about 600 times as sweet as sugar. Sweetener in diet foods.

Sucrose ► *Sugar*

Sucrose Acetate Isobutyrate

Can be synthetic/vegetable, may have been treated with animal substances. Compound of ► *sugar* and ► *butyric acid*. Film forming agent and plasticizer in cosmetics.

Sucrose Benzoate

Synthetic/vegetable, can theoretically have been treated with animal substances. Compound of ► *sugar* and benzoic acid. Film forming agent, plasticizer.

Sucrose Benzoate/Sucrose Acetate Isobutyrate Copolymer
Sucrose Benzoate/Sucrose Acetate Isobutyrate/Butyl Benzyl Phthalate Copolymer
Sucrose Benzoate/Sucrose Acetate Isobutyrate/Butyl Benzyl Phthalate/ Methyl Methacrylate Copolymer

Synthetic/vegetable, may be produced with animal substances. Mixed polymers of ► *sugar*, ► *butyric acid* and benzoic acid. Film forming, viscosity controlling agent in cosmetics.

Sucrose Cocoate

Vegetable, may have been treated with animal substances. ► *Sucrose ester* of coconut ► *fatty acids*. Antistatic, emulsifier and skin conditioner in cosmetics.

Sucrose Dilaurate

Vegetable, may have been treated with animal substances. ► *Sucrose ester* of ► *lauric acid*. Emulsifier and skin conditioner in cosmetics.

Sucrose Distearate

Can be vegetable or partly animal. ► *Sucrose ester* of ► *stearic acid*. Emollient, skin conditioner and emulsifier in cosmetics.

Sucrose Esters ► *Sucrose Esters of Fatty Acids*

Sucrose Esters of Fatty Acids

(E 473)

Can be vegetable or animal. Reaction product of ► *sugar* and one or more ► *fatty acids*. One of the ► *sugar surfactants*. Emulsifier and flour treatment agent in foods. Sucrose esters of fatty acids are also used in cosmetics, especially as emulsifiers and skin conditioners (e.g. in the form of ► *sucrose cocoate*, ► *sucrose distearate*, ► *sucrose oleate*, ► *sucrose palmitate*).

Sucroglycerides

(E 474)

Can be vegetable or partly animal. Mixture of ► *glycerides* and ► *sucrose esters of fatty acids*. Emulsifier and flour treatment agent in foods.

Sucrose Laurate

Vegetable, may have been treated with animal substances. ► *Sucrose ester* of ► *lauric acid*. Emulsifier, surfactant and skin conditioner in cosmetics.

Sucrose Myristate

Mostly vegetable, can also be animal. ► *Sucrose ester* of ► *myristic acid*. Emulsifier in cosmetics.

Sucrose Octaacetate

Vegetable/microbiological, may have been treated with animal substances. Compound of ► *sugar* and acetic acid. Denaturant in cosmetics.

Sucrose Oleate

Can be vegetable or animal. ► *Sucrose ester* of ► *oleic acid*. Emulsifier and skin conditioner in cosmetics.

Sucrose Palmitate

Mostly vegetable, can also be partly animal. ► *Sucrose ester* of ► *palmitic acid*. Emulsifier, surfactant and skin conditioner in cosmetics.

Sucrose Polybehenate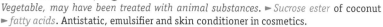

Vegetable, may have been treated with animal substances. ► *Sucrose ester* of vegetable behenic acid. Emollient and emulsifier in cosmetics.

S

Sucrose Polycottonseedate
Vegetable, may have been treated with animal substances. ► *Sucrose ester* of ► *fatty acids* from cottonseed. Emollient and emulsifier in cosmetics.

Sucrose Polylaurate
Vegetable, may have been treated with animal substances. ► *Sucrose ester* of ► *lauric acid*. Emulsifier and skin conditioner in cosmetics.

Sucrose Polylinoleate
Vegetable, may have been treated with animal substances. ► *Sucrose ester* of ► *linoleic acid*. Emulsifier and skin conditioner in cosmetics.

Sucrose Polyoleate
Can be vegetable or animal. ► *Sucrose ester* of ► *oleic acid*. Emulsifier and skin conditioner in cosmetics.

Sucrose Polysoyate
Vegetable, may have been treated with animal substances. ► *Sucrose ester* of fatty acids from soy. Emollient and emulsifier in cosmetics.

Sucrose Polystearate
Can be vegetable or animal. ► *Sucrose ester* of ► *stearic acid*. Emulsifier and skin conditioner in cosmetics.

Sucrose Ricinoleate
Vegetable, may have been treated with animal substances. ► *Sucrose ester* of vegetable ricinoleic acid. Emulsifier and skin conditioner in cosmetics.

Sucrose Stearate
Can be vegetable or animal. ► *Sucrose ester* of ► *stearic acid*. Emulsifier and skin conditioner in cosmetics.

Sucrose Tetrastearate Triacetate
Can be vegetable or animal. ► *Sucrose ester* of ► *stearic acid* and acetic acid. Emulsifier and skin conditioner in cosmetics.

Sucrose Tribehenate
Vegetable, may have been treated with animal substances. ► *Sucrose ester* of vegetable behenic acid. Emulsifier and skin conditioner in cosmetics.

Sucrose Tristearate
Can be vegetable or animal. ► *Sucrose ester* of ► *stearic acid*. Emulsifier and skin conditioner in cosmetics.

Suede
From killed animals. Collective term for ► *leather* with a rubbed, or "napped" surface. In clothing, footwear, accessories, etc.

Suet
From killed animals. Body ► *fat*, especially that surrounding the kidneys, usually from cattle, but also from sheep. Used for producing ► *tallow* and in margarine production.

Used as a frying and baking fat, especially in English cooking. Also used for deep-frying, e.g. in Belgium for potato chips (fries).

Sugar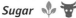

(Sucrose. Saccharose. Table sugar)
Vegetable, can also be treated with animal substances. Collective term for all sweet-tasting carbohydrates. Especially used to refer to table sugar (sucrose). Obtained from the juice of the sugarcane (in the tropics), sugar beet (in Europe and to a lesser extent in North America) or sugar palm (southeast Asia) by rinsing, centrifuging, drying and other separation methods. Cane sugar is available in various grades of quality and purity, for instance from whole cane sugar through brown muscovado and golden raw cane sugar to pure white refined sugar; beet sugar is always refined. Refined sugar is purified and bleached. During these processes, animal ► *activated carbon* can be used in addition to mineral substances. This method is not used for processing beet sugar, but certainly can be implemented in the case of refined cane sugar. In the case of refined sugar in processed foods, the labelling often does not disclose the sugar's origin, so it is not possible to know whether cane or beet sugar has been used. Sugar is used for sweetening foods and beverages, as well as a humectant, skin conditioner and soothing agent in cosmetics. Also used as a source material for additional ingredients in foods, cosmetics and detergents (e.g. ► *sucrose esters of fatty acids*, ► *sucroglycerides*, ► *caramel colouring*, ► *sugar surfactants* and the entries following ► *sucrose*).

Sugar Surfactants

Mostly vegetable, can also be partly animal. ► *Nonionic surfactants* in which the hydrophilic group of the surfactant molecule consists of carbhydrates, e.g. ► *sugar*. The hydrophobic group consists of ► *fatty alcohols* or ► *fatty acids*. Used in detergents, cosmetics and foods. Some examples: ► *caprylyl/capryl glucoside*, ► *decyl glucoside*, ► *sorbitan fatty acid esters*, ► *sucrose esters of fatty acids*.

Sulfated Glyceryl Oleate

Can be vegetable or partly animal. Sulphur compound of ► *glycerol* and ► *oleic acid*. Surfactant and cleansing agent in cosmetics.

Sulfite Ammonia Caramel ► *Caramel Colouring*

Surfactants

Can be animal, vegetable or synthetic. Substances with molecules that possess a hydrophobic (water-repelling) and a hydrophilic (water-attracting) group and reduce the surface tension of fluids. They facilitate the formation of dispersions or act as solubilizers. Surfactants are subdivided according to the charge of their hydrophilic groups into ► *anionic surfactants*, ► *cationic surfactants*, ► *nonionic surfactants* and ► *amphoteric surfactants*. Obtained from ► *fats*, ► *fatty acids* or ► *fatty alcohols*, as well as from petroleum products. Used to achieve a more even distribution in the application of cosmetic products. In detergents they increase the solubility of fat and dirt particles. In detergent labelling, they are generally listed simply as "surfactants," so that their origin cannot be ascertained. Surfactants are also used in many industrial processes, e.g. plastics production and metal-working.

S

Surimi
(Fish paste)
From killed animals. A processed foodstuff originally from Japan, consisting of fish muscle protein and additives. In seafood salads and imitation seafoods, such as imitation crab leg meat or shrimps.

Sus Extract
(Pigskin extract)
From killed animals. Extract fom the skin of pigs. Skin conditioner in cosmetics.

Sweet Whey Powder ► *Whey Powder*

Sweetbread ► *Thymus (1)*

Synthetic Beeswax
Can be synthetic vegetable or partly animal. A complex reaction product of various acids and alcohols that simulates the composition of natural ► *beeswax*. Consists mainly of hydrocarbons and fatty acid esters derived from vegetable or animal ► *fatty acids*. Binding agent, emulsion stabilizer and viscosity controlling agent in cosmetics.

S

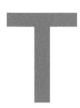

T

Tallamide DEA
Synthetic/vegetable. Ammonia compound of ► *fatty acids* from ► *tallol.* Antistatic, viscosity controlling agent and foam booster in cosmetics.

Tall Oil ► Tallol

Tall Oil Acid
Vegetable. ► *Fatty acids* from ► *tallol.* Emollient, cleansing agent and emulsifier in cosmetics.

Tall Oil Benzyl Hydroxyethyl Imidazolinium Chloride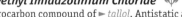
Vegetable/synthetic. Hydrocarbon compound of ► *tallol.* Antistatic and hair conditioner and cosmetics.

Tall Oil Glycerides
Vegetable. ► *Glycerides* from ► *tallol.* Emollient and skin conditioner in cosmetics.

Tall Oil Hydroxyethyl Imidazoline
Vegetable/synthetic. Hydrocarbon compound of ► *tallol.* Antistatic and hair conditioner in cosmetics.

Tall Oil Sterol
Vegetable. ► *Steroid* compounds from ► *tallol.* Emollient, refatting agent and skin conditioner in cosmetics.

Tallol
(Tall oil. Liquid rosin)
Vegetable. An oily, yellow-black liquid, and byproduct of cellulose production from the pulp of coniferous woods (*"tall"* = Swedish for "pine"). Consists principally of ► *fatty acids* and resin acids. Used in adhesives, printing inks, rubber and construction materials. Emollient and solvent in cosmetics. Source material for emulsifiers and surfactants in cosmetics (with "tall" or "tallate" in the name). Can potentially be confused with substances from ► *tallow;* ia also used an an alternative to ► *tallow fatty acids,* for instance in soap production.

Tallow
From killed animals. Solid body ► *fat* from ruminants, mostly cattle, but also sheep or

deer (► *deer tallow*). Is rendered from (melted out of) fatty tissues, primarily from "slaughterhouse waste." Used as a cooking and baking ingredient (especially ► *suet*). In many cosmetic ingredients (usually with "tallow" or "tallowate" in the name), e.g. as emulsifiers, surfactants and conditioners. Source material for ► *stearin*, e.g. for making candles and ► *soaps*, and ► *oleic acid*. Also in wax paper, oil pastels, paints, rubber (erasers) and lubricants. Can be used for producing biofuels. Ingredient in some leather-care products. In animal feed and birdseed products.

Tallow Acid
From killed animals. Chemically altered ► *tallow*. Emollient, cleansing agent, skin conditioner, refatting substance and emulsifier in cosmetics.

Tallow Alcohol
From killed animals. Chemically altered ► *tallow*. Emollient, refatting substance and emulsifier in cosmetics.

Tallow Amide
From killed animals. Chemically altered ► *tallow*. Emulsifier, emulsion stabilizer, surfactant, viscosity controlling agent and foam booster in cosmetics.

Tallow Amine
From killed animals. Chemically altered ► *tallow*. Emulsifier and surfactant in cosmetics.

Tallow Betaine
From killed animals. Chemically altered ► *tallow*. Surfactant, cleansing agent, hair and skin conditioner, and foam booster in cosmetics.

Tallow Dihydroxyethyl Betaine
From killed animals. Chemically altered ► *tallow*. Surfactant, foaming agent and cleansing agent in cosmetics.

Tallow Fatty Acids
From killed animals. Mixed ► *fatty acids* from ► *tallow*, especially ► *oleic acid*, ► *palmitic acid* and ► *stearic acid*. Constituent in many cosmetic ingredients, used for making soap, as fatty acids in foods, e.g. in margarine (also see ► *tallow*).

Tallow Glyceride(s)
From killed animals. ► *Glycerides* from ► *tallow*. Emollients, skin conditioners and emulsifiers in cosmetics.

Tallow Hydroxyethyl Imidazoline
From killed animals. Chemically altered ► *tallow*. Surfactant and hair conditioner in cosmetics.

Tallow Trihydroxyethyl Ammonium Acetate
From killed animals. Chemically altered ► *tallow*. Antistatic in cosmetics.

Tallowalkonium Chloride
From killed animals. Chemically altered ► *tallow*. Antistatic, preservative and surfactant in cosmetics.

Tallowamide DEA. Tallowamide MEA
From killed animals. Chemically altered ► *tallow.* Antistatics, emulsifiers, emulsion stabilizers, viscosity controlling agents and foam boosters in cosmetics.

Tallowamidopropyl Betaine
From killed animals. Chemically altered ► *tallow.* Surfactant, skin and hair conditioner, cleansing agent and foaming agent in cosmetics.

Tallowamidopropyl Dimethylamine
From killed animals. Chemically altered ► *tallow.* Surfactant in cosmetics.

Tallowamidopropyl Hydroxysultaine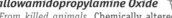
From killed animals. Chemically altered ► *tallow.* Surfactant, hair and skin conditioner, and foam booster in cosmetics.

Tallowamidopropylamine Oxide
From killed animals. Chemically altered ► *tallow.* Antistatic, surfactant, hydrotrope, cleansing agent and foam booster in cosmetics.

Tallowamine Oxide
From killed animals. Chemically altered ► *tallow.* Antistatic, emulsifier, surfactant, foaming agent, hydrotrope, cleansing agent and foam booster in cosmetics.

Tallowaminopropylamine
From killed animals. Chemically altered ► *tallow.* Emulsifier in cosmetics.

Tallowdimonium Propyltrimonium Dichloride
From killed animals. Chemically altered ► *tallow.* Antistatic, emulsifier and surfactant in cosmetics.

Talloweth-6
From killed animals. Chemically altered ► *tallow.* Emulsifier in cosmetics.

Tallowoyl Ethyl Glucoside
From killed animals. Chemically altered ► *tallow.* Cleansing agent and surfactant in cosmetics.

Tallowtrimonium Chloride
From killed animals. Chemically altered ► *tallow.* Antistatic, preservative, surfactant and hair conditioner in cosmetics.

Tannic Acid
Vegetable, can be partly animal. Derivative of ► *gallic acid* from oak apples, bark and other vegetable matter, especially oak bark. Astringent in cosmetics.

Tarantula Hispanica
From killed animals. Tincture of whole wolf spiders. In ► *homeopathic medicines.*

Tartaric Acid
(E 334)
Vegetable/microbiological, animal substances may be involved in processing. Isolated from

cream of tartar (► *potassium bitartrate*) with the aid of sulphuric acid. L(+)-tartaric acid is used as an acidifier in foods and a buffering agent in cosmetics.

Tartaric Acid Esters of Mono- and Diglycerides of Fatty Acids
(E 472 d)
Can be vegetable or animal. Reaction product of ► *tartaric acid* and ► *fatty acids*. Emulsifier and carrier substance in foods.

Tartrates
Vegetable/microbiological, can be treated with animal substances. Salts and esters of ► *tartaric acid*, e.g. ► *calcium tartrate*, ► *potassium bitartrate*, ► *potassium tartrate*, ► *sodium tartrates*, ► *sodium potassium tartrate*, ► *stearyl tartrate*.

Taurine
Synthetic. An organic acid that is chemically similar to ► *amino acids*, without actually being an amino acid. Occurs naturally in animal tissues and legumes. Was first isolated from ► *ox gall*. Industrial production now exclusively via synthesis from petroleum derivatives. In "energy drinks" and animal food (especially for cats). Buffering agent in cosmetics.

TEA-Abietoyl Hydrolyzed Collagen
From killed animals. Chemically/enzymatically altered ► *collagen*. Used as an antistatic, surfactant, cleansing agent, skin protecting substance and hair conditioner in cosmetics.

TEA-Cocoyl Glutamate
Synthetic/vegetable, can theoretically also be partly animal. Chemically altered compound of coconut ► *fatty acids* and ► *glutamic acid*. Surfactant, hair conditioner and cleansing agent in cosmetics.

TEA-Cocoyl Hydrolyzed Collagen
From killed animals. Chemically/enzymatically altered ► *collagen*. Antistatic, surfactant, skin and hair conditioner, and cleansing agent in cosmetics.

TEA-Cocoyl Sarcosinate
Vegetable/synthetic/from killed animals or vegetable/synthetic/microbiological. Chemically altered compound of coconut ► *fatty acids* and ► *sarcosine*. Surfactant, cleansing agent, hair conditioner and foaming agent in cosmetics.

TEA-Hydrogenated Tallow Glutamate
From killed animals. Chemically altered ► *tallow*. Surfactant, hair conditioner and cleansing agent in cosmetics.

TEA-Isostearate
Can be vegetable/synthetic or animal. Chemically altered ► *stearic acid*. Emulsifier, surfactant and hair conditioner in cosmetics.

TEA-Isostearoyl Hydrolyzed Collagen
From killed animals. Chemically/enzymatically altered ► *collagen*. Surfactant, hair and skin conditioner and cleansing agent in cosmetics.

TEA-Lactate

Mostly synthetic/vegetable/microbiological, can also be partly animal. Chemically altered ► *lactic acid.* Humectant and skin conditioner in cosmetics.

TEA-Laneth-5 Sulfate

From living or killed animals. Chemically altered ► *lanolin.* Emulsifier and skin conditioner in cosmetics.

TEA-Lauroyl Collagen Amino Acids

From killed animals. Chemically altered ► *amino acids* from ► *collagen.* Surfactant, skin and hair conditioner in cosmetics.

TEA-Lauroyl Hydrolyzed Collagen

From killed animals. Chemically/enzymatically altered ► *collagen.* Surfactant and skin conditioner in cosmetics.

TEA-Lauroyl Keratin Amino Acids

From killed or living animals. Chemically altered ► *amino acids* from ► *keratin.* Antistatic, surfactant, skin and hair conditioner, and cleansing agent in cosmetics.

TEA-Lauroyl Sarcosinate

Synthetic/animal or synthetic/vegetable/microbiological. Chemically altered ► *sarcosine.* Antistatic, surfactant, cleansing agent and foaming agent in cosmetics.

TEA-Myristoyl Hydrolyzed Collagen

From killed animals. Chemically/enzymatically altered ► *collagen.* Antistatic, surfactant, cleansing agent, foaming agent.

TEA-Oleate

Can be vegetable/synthetic or animal. Chemically altered ► *oleic acid.* Emulsifier, surfactant and cleansing agent in cosmetics.

TEA-Oleoyl Hydrolyzed Collagen

From killed animals. Chemically/enzymatically altered ► *collagen.* Antistatic, surfactant and skin conditioner in cosmetics.

TEA-Oleoyl Sarcosinate

Synthetic/animal or synthetic/vegetable/microbiological. Compound of ► *sarcosine* and ► *oleic acid.* Antistatic, surfactant and foaming agent in cosmetics.

TEA-Oleyl Sulfate

Can be vegetable/synthetic or animal. Chemically altered ► *oleyl alcohol.* Emulsifier, surfactant and foaming agent in cosmetics.

TEA-Palm Kernel Sarcosinate

Vegetable/synthetic/animal or vegetable/synthetic/microbiological. Altered palm kernel ► *fatty acids* and ► *sarcosine.* Antistatic, surfactant and foaming agent in cosmetics.

TEA-Palmitate

Mostly vegetable/synthetic, can also be partly animal. Chemically altered ► *palmitic acid.* Emulsifier, surfactant and cleansing agent in cosmetics.

TEA-Stearate
Can be vegetable/synthetic or animal. Chemically altered ► *stearic acid*. Emulsifier, surfactant and cleansing agent in cosmetics.

TEA-Tallate
Synthetic/vegetable. Chemically altered ► *fatty acids* from ► *tallol*. Emulsifier, surfactant and cleansing agent in cosmetics.

TEA-Undecylenoyl Hydrolyzed Collagen
From killed animals. Chemically/enzymatically altered ► *collagen*. Antidandruff agent, antistatic, surfactant and skin conditioner in cosmetics.

Testes (Lysat.) Bovis ► *Organ Extracts*

Testicular Extract
From killed animals. Extract from mammal testicles. Skin conditioner in cosmetics.

Testosterone
From living/killed animals or synthetic. A ► *steroid* that plays an important part as a male sexual hormone (androgen) in vertebrates, including humans. Is produced in the testicles, in women and children in small quantities in the adrenal glands. Can be obtained from testicles, is industrially produced from ► *cholesterol*. In pharmaceutical drugs, e.g. for treating hormonal disorders. Used for doping in athletics and bodybuilding.

Theobroma Cacao Butter ► *Cocoa butter*

Thermally Oxidized Soybean Oil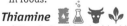
Interacted with Mono- and Diglycerides of Fatty Acids
(E 479b)
Mostly vegetable, can also be partly animal. Soybean oil chemically altered by reaction with ► *fatty acids* at high temperatures. Emulsifier, foam inhibitor and anticaking agent in foods.

Thiamine
(Vitamin B₁. Thiaminchlorid)
Can be synthetic or microbiological, can theoretically also be animal or vegetable. A water-soluble ► *vitamin* particularly important for the nervous system. Is produced by microorganisms, plants and fungi. Occurs especially in whole grain products, pulses, nuts and yeasts, also in animal tissues. Usually obtained synthetically or using bacterial cultures. Used as an active agent (► *thiamine hydrochloride* or ► *thiamine nitrate*) in cosmetics and medicines.

Thiamine HCl ► *Thiamine Hydrochloride*

Thiamine Hydrochloride
(Thiamine HCl)
Can be synthetic or microbiological, can theoretically also be animal or vegetable. Salt of ► *thiamine*. Skin conditioner in cosmetics. In medication for treating vitamin B deficiency, in food supplements and animal food.

T

Thiamine Nitrate
Can be synthetic or microbiological, theoretically also animal or vegetable. Salt of ► *thiamine*. Skin conditioner in cosmetics. In medication for treating vitamin B deficiency, in food supplements and animal food.

Thckener ► *Gelling Agents*

Threonine
(L-threonine)
Mostly microbiological, can also be animal or vegetable. An essential ► *amino acid*. Constituent of animal and vegetable ► *proteins*. Can be obtained from bacterial cultures, but also from degraded proteins, either animal or vegetable. Antistatic and hair conditioner in cosmetics. In infusion solutions for parenteral nutrition. In animal feed.

Thunnus Extract
From killed animals. Extract of whole tunas from commercial fishing. Emollient in cosmetics.

Thymol
Can be vegetable or synthetic. Constituent of essential oils, for instance in thyme (► *thymus [2]*). Also obtainable from petroleum products. Hair dye, denaturant and masking agent in cosmetics. Disinfectant and refreshing ingredient in mouthwashes and toothpastes. Used for treating skin disorders in both human and veterinary medicine.

Thymus (1)
(Sweetbread)
From killed animals. Internal organ that plays a part in the development of the immune system in adolescent mammals. Most often from slaughtered calves, but also from lambs. Used as a food and as a source of ► *thymus extract* and ► *thymus hydrolysate*.

Thymus (2)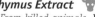
(Thyme)
Vegetable. A plant genus containing species valued for their essential oils and used as medicinal and culinary herbs. Used in cosmetics as a tonic and for its refreshing fragrance (*Thymus serpillum* extract, *Thymus vulgaris* extract, *Thymus vulgaris* oil). Listed here due to possible confusion with the animal organ of the same name (► *thymus [1]*).

Thymus Extract
From killed animals. Extracts or chemically/enzymatically altered ► *proteins* from the ► *thymus (1)* of mammals. Skin conditioner in cosmetics.

Thymus Hydrolysate
From killed animals. Chemically/enzymatically altered ► *proteins* from the ► *thymus (1)* of mammals. Skin conditioner in cosmetics.

Thymus Serpillum Extract. Thymus Vulgaris Extract. Thymus Vulgaris Oil
► *Thymus (2)*

Thymus Suis ► *Organ Extracts*

Thyroxine
(Levothyroxine. L-thyroxine. T₄. Tetraiodothyronine)
Can be animal, microbiological or vegetable. A thyroid hormone that plays an important role in regulating metabolic processes throughout the entire body. Industrial production from ▶ *tyrosine*. In medication for treating hypothyroidism and for preventing or treating thyroid diseases.

TIPA-Stearate
Can be vegetable/synthetic or animal. Chemically altered ▶ *stearic acid*. Emulsifier, surfactant and cleansing agent in cosmetics.

Tocophereth-n
Mostly vegetable/synthetic, can also be partly animal. ▶ *PEG* compounds of ▶ *vitamin E*. Surfactants and skin conditioners in cosmetics.

Tocopherol. Tocopherol-Rich Extract ▶ *Vitamin E*

Tocopherol Acetate ▶ *Tocopheryl Acetate*

Tocopherol Nicotinate ▶ *Vitamin E*

Tocopherol Linoleate ▶ *Vitamin E*

Tocopherol Succinate ▶ *Tocopheryl Succinate*

Tocophersolan
Mostly vegetable/synthetic, can also be partly animal. ▶ *PEG* compound of ▶ *Vitamin E* and ▶ *succinic acid*. Antioxidant in cosmetics.

Tocopheryl Acetate
(Tocopherol acetate. Vitamin E acetate)
Synthetic. Compound of ▶ *vitamin E* and acetic acid, and ▶ *provitamin* of vitamin E. Obtained from petroleum derivatives. In vitamin supplements and medication. Antioxidant in cosmetics.

Tocopheryl Linoleate ▶ *Vitamin E*

Tocopheryl Linoleate/Oleate
Can be vegetable/synthetic or animal. Compound of ▶ *vitamin E*, ▶ *linoleic acid* and ▶ *oleic acid*. Antioxidant and skin conditioner in cosmetics.

Tocopheryl Nicotinate ▶ *Vitamin E*

Tocopheryl Succinate
(Tocopherol succinate. Vitamin E succinate)
Mostly vegetable, can also be partly animal or synthetic. Compound of ▶ *vitamin E* and succinic acid. Antioxidant in cosmetics. In dietary supplements.

Tortoiseshell
From killed animals. The upper ▶ *horn* plates of the shells of turtles, especially Hawksbill sea turtles. Obtained by heating the living animals in boiling wateror over fire until the shell softens and can be removed. In accessories such as spectacle frames, combs,

hair clips, bracelets, etc., as well as in arts and crafts. Trade in tortoiseshell is banned under the Convention on International Trade in Endangered Species (CITES).

Trachea Hydrolysate
From killed animals. Chemically/enzymatically altered ► *proteins* from the windpipes of mammals. Skin conditioner in cosmetics.

Train Oil
(Whale oil)
From killed animals. Liquid ► *wax* or oil from the body ► *fat* of whales (also see ► *spermaceti*). Used earlier as lamp oil, candle wax, in soaps and in foods. No longer in use due to the moratorium on commercial whaling implemented by the International Whaling Commission in 1986. The term "train oil" can refer not only to whale oil but also oil from other marine mammals, and in German the corresponding term "Tran" refers to all ► *marine oils*.

Triacetin
(E 1518. Glycerin triacetate. Glycerol triacetate. Glyceryl triacetate)
Mostly vegetable, can also be from killed animals. Acetic acid compound of ► *glycerol*. Antimicrobial agent, film forming agent, solvent, plasticizer and hair dye in cosmetics. Carrier substance in foods (only permitted for chewing gum and ► *flavourings*). Plasticizer for lacquers and adhesives, including adhesives in cigarette filters.

Triarachidin
Can be vegetable or animal. Compound of ► *glycerol* and ► *arachidic acid*. Emollient, emulsifier and skin conditioner in cosmetics.

Tricalcium Phosphate ► *Calcium Phosphate*

Tricaprin
(Glycerol tricaprate. Glycerol decanoate)
Mostly vegetable, can also be animal. ► *Triglyceride* of ► *capric acid*. Emollient, solvent and skin conditioner in cosmetics.

Tricaprylin
(Glycerintricaprylat. Glycerol trioctanoate. Tricaprylat)
Mostly vegetable, can also be animal. ► *Triglyceride* of ► *caprylic acid*. Emollient, solvent and skin conditioner in cosmetics.

Tricaprylyl Citrate
Can be vegetable/microbiological or partly animal. Citric acid compound of ► *glycerol* and ► *caprylic acid*. Emollient in cosmetics.

Triceteareth-4 Phosphate
Can be synthetic/vegetable/mineral or animal. ► *PEG* compound of ► *glycerol* and ► *cetostearyl alcohol*. Surfactant in cosmetics.

Triceteth-5 Phosphate
Can be synthetic/vegetable/mineral or partly animal. ► *PEG* compound of ► *glycerol* and ► *cetyl alcohol*. Surfactant in cosmetics.

T

Tricetyl Phosphate

Can be synthetic/vegetable/mineral or partly animal. Compound of ► *glycerol* and ► *cetyl alcohol*. Film forming agent and plasticizer in cosmetics.

Tricetylmonium Chloride

Can be vegetable/synthetic or partly animal. Ammonium compound of ► *glycerol* and ► *cetyl alcohol*. Antistatic and hair conditioner in cosmetics.

Trideceth-2 Carboxamide MEA

Can be vegetable/synthetic or partly animal. ► *PEG* compound of ► *decyl alcohol*. Viscosity controlling agent and foam booster in cosmetics.

Trideceth-n Phosphate

Can be synthetic/vegetable/mineral or partly animal. ► *PEG* and phosphate compounds of ► *glycerol* and ► *decyl alcohol*. Trideceth-3 phosphate and trideceth-10 phosphate are used as emulsifiers in cosmetics, trideceth-6 phosphate as a surfactant.

Trideceth-n

Can be vegetable/synthetic or partly animal. ► *PEG* compounds of ► *glycerol* and ► *decyl alcohol*. Emulsifiers in cosmetics. Trideceth-6, trideceth-8 and trideceth-12 are also used as surfactants, trideceth-20 and trideceth-50 also as cleansing agents, trideceth-21 only as a surfactant and cleansing agent.

Trideceth-n Carboxylic Acid

Can be vegetable/synthetic or partly animal. Compounds of ► *glycerol* and ► *decyl alcohol*. Surfactants, cleansing substances and foaming agents in cosmetics.

Tridecyl Alcohol

Can be vegetable or partly animal. Compound of ► *glycerol* and ► *decyl alcohol*. Emollient, refatting agent, emulsion stabilizer and viscosity controlling agent in cosmetics.

Tridecyl Behenate

Can be vegetable or partly animal. Compound of ► *glycerol*, ► *decyl alcohol* and behenic acid. Emollient and skin conditioner in cosmetics.

Tridecyl Cocoate

Can be vegetable or partly animal. Compound of ► *glycerol*, ► *decyl alcohol* and coconut ► *fatty acids*. Emollient and skin conditioner in cosmetics.

Tridecyl Erucate

Can be vegetable or partly animal. Compound of ► *glycerol*, ► *decyl alcohol* and vegetable erucic acid. Emollient in cosmetics.

Tridecyl Ethylhexanoate

Can be vegetable or partly animal. Compound of ► *glycerol*, ► *decyl alcohol* and ► *caproic acid*. Emollient and skin conditioner in cosmetics.

Tridecyl Isononanoate

Can be vegetable or partly animal. Compound of ► *glycerol*, ► *decyl alcohol* and vegetable nonanoic acid. Emollient and skin conditioner in cosmetics.

Tridecyl Myristate
Can be vegetable or partly animal. Compound of ► *glycerol*, ► *decyl alcohol* and ► *myristic acid*. Emollient and skin conditioner in cosmetics.

Tridecyl Neopentanoate
Can be vegetable or partly animal. Compound of ► *glycerol*, ► *decyl alcohol* and vegetable valeric acid. Binding agent, emollient and skin conditioner in cosmetics.

Tridecyl Salicylate
Mostly synthetic/vegetable, can also be partly animal. Compound of ► *glycerol*, ► *decyl alcohol* and salicylic acid. Antistatic and skin conditioner in cosmetics.

Tridecyl Stearate
Tridecyl Stearoyl Stearate
Can be vegetable or animal. Compounds of ► *glycerol*, ► *decyl alcohol* and ► *stearic acid*. Emollients and skin conditioners in cosmetics.

Tridecyl Trimellitate
Can be vegetable/mineral or partly animal. Compound of ► *glycerol*, ► *decyl alcohol* and mellitic acid (mineral). Emollient and skin conditioner in cosmetics.

Tridecylbenzenesulfonic Acid
Can be vegetable/synthetic or partly animal. Compound of ► *glycerol*, ► *decyl alcohol* and synthetic benzenesulfonic acid. Surfactant, foaming and cleansing agent in cosmetics.

Triethonium Hydrolyzed Collagen Ethosulfate
From killed animals. Chemically/enzymatically altered ► *collagen* (from ► *leather*). Antistatic, hair and skin conditioner in cosmetics.

Triglycerides
(Triacylglycerides. Triacylglycerols. Glycerol triesters)
Can be animal or vegetable. Compounds of ► *glycerol* with three ► *fatty acid* molecules, either as simple triglycerides (three identical fatty acids) or mixed triglycerides (different fatty acids). Main constituents of natural ► *fats*. Also classified according to the constituent fatty acids or their chain length. Within this context ► *medium-chain triglycerides* have a special status. Examples of triglycerides: ► *tricaprin*, ► *tricaprylin*, ► *trilaurin*, ► *trilinolein*, ► *triolein*, ► *tripalmitin*, ► *triricinolein*, ► *tristearin*.

Trihydroxymethoxystearin
Can be vegetable/synthetic or animal. Hydrocarbon compound of ► *stearic acid*. Emollient and skin conditioner in cosmetics.

Trihydroxystearin
Can be vegetable/synthetic or animal. Hydrocarbon compound of ► *glycerol* and ► *stearic acid*. Emollient, skin conditioner, solvent and viscosity controlling agent in cosmetics.

Triiodothyronine
(T₃. Levotharonine. L-thyronine)
Can be animal, microbiological or vegetable. A thyroid hormone that plays an important

role in regulating metabolic processes throughout the entire body. Produced via transformation of ► *thyroxine*. In medication for treating hypothyroidism and for preventing/treating thyroid diseases.

Triisocetyl Citrate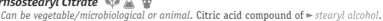
Can be vegetable/microbiological or partly animal. Citric acid compound of ► *glycerol* and ► *cetyl alcohol*. Emollient and skin conditioner in cosmetics.

Triisopalmitin
Can be vegetable or partly animal. Compound of ► *glycerol* and ► *palmitic acid*. Emollient in cosmetics.

Triisopropyl Trilinoleate
Can be vegetable/synthetic or partly animal. Hydrocarbon compound of ► *glycerol* and ► *linoleic acid*. Emollient and skin conditioner in cosmetics.

Triisostearin
Can be vegetable or animal. Compound of ► *glycerol* and ► *stearic acid*. Emollient, skin conditioner, solvent and viscosity controlling agent in cosmetics.

Triisostearin PEG-6 Esters
Can be vegetable/synthetic or animal. ► *PEG* compound of ► *glycerol* and ► *stearic acid*. Emollient and skin conditioner in cosmetics.

Triisostearyl Citrate
Can be vegetable/microbiological or animal. Citric acid compound of ► *stearyl alcohol*. Emollient and skin conditioner in cosmetics.

Triisostearyl Trilinoleate
Can be vegetable or animal. Compound of ► *glycerol*, ► *stearyl alcohol* and ► *linoleic acid*. Emollient and skin conditioner and viscosity controlling agent in cosmetics.

Trilactin
Can be vegetable/microbiological or partly animal. Compound of ► *glycerol* and ► *lactic acid*. Humectant and moisturizer in cosmetics.

Trilaneth-4-Phosphate
From living or killed animals. Chemically altered ► *lanolin*. Viscosity controlling agent in cosmetics.

Trilinoleic Acid
Can be vegetable or partly animal. Compound of ► *glycerol* and ► *linoleic acid*. Emollient, skin conditioner, refatting substance and viscosity controlling agent in cosmetics.

Trilinolein
Can be vegetable or partly animal. ► *Triglyceride* of ► *linoleic acid*. Emollient, refatting substance, solvent and viscosity controlling agent in cosmetics.

Trilinolenin
Can be vegetable or partly animal. ► *Triglyceride* of ► *linolenic acid*. Emollient and refatting substance in cosmetics.

Trimethylolpropane Tricaprylate/Tricaprate
Can be vegetable/synthetic or partly animal. Hydrocarbon compound of ► *capric acid*, ► *caproic acid* and ► *caprylic acid*. Emollient, skin conditioner in cosmetics.

Trimethylolpropane Triisostearate
Can be vegetable/synthetic or animal. Hydrocarbon compound of ► *stearic acid*. Emollient, skin conditioner in cosmetics.

Trimethylolpropane Tristearate
Can be vegetable/synthetic or animal. Hydrocarbon compound of ► *stearic acid*. Emollient in cosmetics.

Trioctyldodecyl Borate
Mostly mineral/synthetic/vegetable, can also be partly animal. Boric acid compound of ► *octyl dodecanol*. Emollient in cosmetics.

Trioctyldodecyl Citrate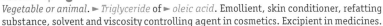
Mostly synthetic/vegetable/microbiological, can also be partly animal. Citric acid compound of ► *octyl dodecanol*. Emollient and skin conditioner in cosmetics.

Triolein
Vegetable or animal. ► *Triglyceride* of ► *oleic acid*. Emollient, skin conditioner, refatting substance, solvent and viscosity controlling agent in cosmetics. Excipient in medicines.

Triolein PEG-6 Esters
Can be vegetable/synthetic or animal. ► *PEG* compound of ► *glycerol* and ► *oleic acid*. Emollient, skin conditioner and surfactant in cosmetics.

Trioleth-8 Phosphate
Can be vegetable/synthetic or animal. Polymer compound of ► *oleyl alcohol*. Emulsifier in cosmetics.

Trioleyl Citrate
Can be vegetable/microbiological or animal. Citric acid compound of ► *glycerol* and ► *oleyl alcohol*. Emollient and plasticizer in cosmetics.

Trioleyl Phosphate
Can be mineral/vegetable or animal. Compound of ► *glycerol* and ► *oleyl alcohol*. Emollient, skin conditioner and plasticizer in cosmetics.

Tripalmitin
Mostly vegetable, can also be animal. ► *Triglyceride* of ► *palmitic acid*. Emollient, skin conditioner, refatting substance, solvent and viscosity controlling agent in cosmetics.

Tripalmitolein
Can be vegetable or animal. ► *Triglyceride* of ► *palmitoleic acid*. Emollient, refatting substance in cosmetics.

Triricinolein
Can be vegetable or partly animal. ► *Triglyceride* of vegetable ricinoleic acid. Emollient and refatting substance in cosmetics.

T

Tristearin

Can be from killed animals or vegetable. ► *Triglyceride* of ► *stearic acid*. Main constituent of ► *tallow*. Obtained either from tallow or palm oil. Emollient, skin conditioner, refatting agent, solvent and viscosity controlling agent in cosmetics. Excipient in medicinal creams.

Tristearyl Citrate

Can be vegetable/microbiological or animal. Citric acid compound of ► *glycerol* and ► *stearyl alcohol*. Emollient, skin conditioner in cosmetics.

Tristearyl PG-Phosphate Dimonium Chloride

Can be vegetable/synthetic or animal. Ammonium and phosphoric acid compound of ► *glycerol* and ► *stearyl alcohol*. Antistatic and hair conditioner in cosmetics.

Tristearyl Phosphate

Can be mineral/vegetable or animal. Phosphoric acid compound of ► *glycerol* and ► *stearyl alcohol*. Surfactant in cosmetics.

Trypsine

From killed animals. An ► *enzyme* produced in the pancreas that breaks down ► *protein* in the small intestine (► *protease*). Obtained from the pancreases of pigs or cattle. Constituent of ► *pancreatin*. Used in cell cultures.

Tryptophan
(L-tryptophan)

Can be synthetic, vegetable, microbiological or animal. An essential ► *amino acid*. Is involved in ► *protein* synthesis in the body and is transformed into the neurotransmitters serotonin and ► *melatonin* as well as vitamin B_3 (► *niacin*). Present in many foods, especially in ► *lactalbumin* in ► *milk* and ► *cheese*. Also in animal tissues, ► *eggs*, peas, nuts and potatoes. Industrially produced via biosynthesis from ► *serine*, petroleum products or vegetable sugars. Antistatic in cosmetics. In nutritional supplements and as additive in animal food.

Tuberculin

Microbiological. ► *Protein* preparation from cultures of *Mycobacterium bovis* (bovine tuberculosis pathogen) or *Mycobacterium avium* (avian tuberculosis pathogen) incubated in synthetic fluid media, then killed and purified. In skin tests for diagnosing exposure to tuberculosis bacteria.

Tuberculinum Bovinum (Nosode)

From killed animals. Preparation from the infected lymph nodes of slaughtered cattle suffering from tuberculosis. In ► *homeopathic medicines*.

Turtle Oil
(Sea turtle oil)

From killed animals. ► *Fat* obtained from the muscles and genitals of sea turtles. In soaps, skin creams and other cosmetics. Trade in turtle oil is banned under the Convention on International Trade in Endangered Species (CITES).

Tyrian Purple

From killed animals. Purple dye obtained from the hypobranchial glands of certain sea snails. Was used especially in ancient times for dyeing expensive fabrics. As only a very small amount of the dye can be obtained from one snail, it is still very expensive. It is now used very rarely, e.g. in religious robes or as a pigment used in painting or conservation/restoration.

Tyrosine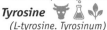

(L-tyrosine. Tyrosinum)

From killed or living animals, microbiological or vegetable. Nonessential ► *amino acid*, occurs in many animal ► *proteins*. Is involved in the production of neurotransmitters and skin pigments (► *melanin*). Can be obtained from substances rich in ► *casein* or ► *keratin*. Can also be obtained from vegetable proteins or yeast cultures. Used as a performance-enhancing nutritional supplement. Active agent in antidepressive medication. Antistatic, tanning agent, hair and skin conditioner in cosmetics.

T

U

Ubiquinone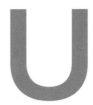
(Coenzyme Q₁₀. CoQ₁₀. CoQ. Q-10)
Microbiological or synthetic, can theoretically also be animal. Biologically active substance that in combination with ► *enzymes* plays an important part in metabolism and energy balance. Occurs naturally in all organisms, especially in animal fatty tissue and fat-rich plants. Three methods are used for industrial production: yeast fermentation, bacterial fermentation and chemical synthesis. Antioxidant and skin conditioner in cosmetics. Used as a dietary supplement (its benefit is debated).

Udder Extract
From killed animals. Extract from mammals' udders. Skin conditioner in cosmetics.

Umbilical Extract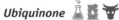
From living or killed animals. Extract from the umbilical cords of mammals. Skin conditioner in cosmetics.

Undecylenoyl Collagen Amino Acids
From killed animals. Chemically altered ► *amino acids* from ► *collagen*. Antistatic and cleansing agent in cosmetics.

Undecylenoyl Hydrolyzed Collagen
From killed animals. Chemically/enzymatically altered ► *collagen*. Antistatic, hair and skin conditioner, and cleansing agent in cosmetics.

Unsaturated Fatty Acids
Mostly vegetable, but can also be animal. Collective term for ► *fatty acids* that possess one (monounsaturated fatty acids) or more (polyunsaturated fatty acids) "double-bonds" (two neighbouring carbon atoms are doubly bonded with each other). Monounsaturated fatty acids occur most commonly in vegetable oils, but also in animal fats such as ► *fish oil*, ► *tallow* and ► *butterfat*. The most important of the monounsaturated fatty acids is ► *oleic acid*. ► *Omega-3 fatty acids* make up a special group of the polyunsaturated fatty acids. Additional examples are ► *arachidonic acid* and ► *linoleic acid*.

Urea
(Carbamide. E 927b)
Synthetic, can theoretically also be from animals. A nitrogen compound and metabolic

end product excreted by animals in urine. Occurs naturally in urine and other animal body fluids. Industrial mass production from ammonia and carbon dioxide. Antistatic, humectant and skin conditioner in cosmetics. Ingredient in ointments (heals wounds, softens calluses). Additive in cigarettes. Stabilizer in chewing gum. In propellants, plastics, detergents, fertilizers, printing inks and textile dyes.

Urea Peroxide
Synthetic. Compound of ▶ *urea*. Oxidant in cosmetics.

Urea/Melamine/Formaldehyde Resin
Synthetic. Compound of ▶ *urea* and ▶ *melamine resin*. Viscosity controlling agent in cosmetics.

Urease
Vegetable. An ▶ *enzyme* that breaks down ▶ *urea*. Occurs in yeasts, bacteria and plants. Produced from beans (e.g. soy). Viscosity controlling agent in cosmetics.

Uric Acid
Synthetic, can theoretically also be from animals. A nitrogen compound and metabolic end product excreted by animals with the urine. Occurs naturally in urine and other animal body fluids. Industrially produced synthetically. Buffering agent and skin conditioner in cosmetics.

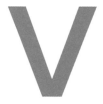

V

VA/Crotonates/Vinyl Neodecanoate Copolymer
VA/Isobutyl Maleate/Vinyl Neodecanoate Copolymer

Mostly vegetable/synthetic, can also be partly animal. Synthetic polymer compounds of ► *capric acid*. Antistatic, film forming agent and hair fixative in cosmetics.

Vaccine

From living or killed animals. A medicinal preparation comprising mostly ► *proteins* or genetic material from killed or weakened disease pathogens (bacteria or viruses). For the classical production of vaccines, fertilized chicken ► *eggs* are used. Millions of these each year are infected with the pathogen against which the vaccine is to be employed (one egg per vaccine dose). The pathogen grows over a period of several days. Then the eggs are destroyed and the pathogen is extracted and processed to a serum. Each vaccine dose thus means the death of one chicken embryo. A newer method of vaccine production employs cell cultures instead of eggs. These cultures are of animal origin, e.g. tissue samples from dog kidneys, whereby they can be reproduced as needed, and once the cell line is established, additional tissue samples are not necessary, so that the "consumption" of animal substances is a fraction of that involved in the classical method. At present there are no vaccines entirely free of animal substances.

Valine

Can be vegetable/microbiological or synthetic. An essential ► *amino acid*. Occurs naturally in animal and vegetable ► *proteins*. Obtained from petroleum products or biotechnologically from vegetable substances with the aid of microorganisms. Antistatic and skin conditioner in cosmetics. In infusion solutions.

Vasa (Lysat.) Bovis ► *Organ Extracts*

Vellum ► *Parchment*

Venom

From living or killed animals. Term for toxins from biting or stinging animals (e.g. insects, snakes or spiders) that contain species-specific ► *proteins* and ► *enzymes*. Obtained for medical drugs, cosmetic ingredients or ► *homeopathic medicines*. Some examples: ► *batroxobin*, ► *bee venom*, ► *lachesis*, ► *phospholipase A₂*. Some antihypertensive drugs are emulations of snake venoms (e.g. ► *captopril*, ► *lisinopril*), but are in fact synthetic.

Vipera Berus

From living animals. Venom of the common adder. In ► *homeopathic medicines.*

Vitamins

Can be animal, vegetable, microbiological or synthetic. Collective term for organic compounds required by the body not as a source of energy, but rather for other vital functions, blood formation, bone formation, cell division and hormone balance. The body is unable to produce these substances itself, therefore they must be supplied via nutrition (partly as ► *provitamins*). There are fat-soluble and water-soluble vitamins (see the following entries).

Vitamin A

Can be synthetic or animal. Collective term for fat-soluble ► *vitamins* that play an important part in the formation and growth of various tissues as well as in process of sight. Formed in the human body from provitamin A (► *carotene*). The most important A vitamin is ► *retinol* (vitamin A_1).

Vitamin A₁ ► Retinol

Vitamin B

Can be vegetable, animal or microbiological. Collective term for water-soluble ► *vitamins* that play an important part in cell metabolism. B vitamins do not make up a uniform group of substances, but differ in structure and function. Some substances previously considered B vitamins (e.g. vitamin B_4, vitamin B_{13}) are now no longer regarded as such. The eight substances that are now identified as B vitamins are: ► *vitamin B_1*, ► *vitamin B_2*, ► *vitamin B_3*, vitamin B_5 (► *pantothenic acid*), ► *vitamin B_6*, vitamin B_7 (► *biotin*), vitamin B_9 (► *folic acid*) and ► *vitamin B_{12}*.

Vitamin B₁ ► Thiamine

Vitamin B₂ ► Riboflavin

Vitamin B₃ ► Niacine

Vitamin B₅ ► Pantothenic Acid

Vitamin B₆

(Pyridoxine [Pyridoxine-5'-phosphate. Pyridoxine hydrochloride. Pyridoxine HCl]. Pyridoxal [Pyridoxal-5'phosphate]. Pyridoxamin [Pyridoxamin-5'phosphate])
Synthetic or microbiological. Collective term for a group of water-soluble ► *vitamins* that play an important part in metabolism (especially of ► *amino acids*). Occur in small amounts in almost all vegetable and animal tissues. Industrial production from petroleum derivatives or ► *alanine*. Pyridoxine is used as an antistatic, hair and skin conditioner in cosmetics, and pyridoxal-5'-phosphate as a skin conditioner. Used in medicine for treating vitamin B_6 deficiency (very rare, caused by drug side effects, alcohol abuse or pregnancy).

Vitamin B₇ ► Biotin

Vitamin B₉ ► Folic Acid

Vitamin B₁₂

(Cobalamin. Antipernicious anaemia factor. Extrinsic factor)

Microbiological or animal. Collective term for a group of cobalt compounds that play an important part in blood formation and nerve functions, and are involved in the metabolism of all cells. Vitamin B_{12} is produced only by microorganisms (e.g. in the digestive tracts of animals or in the earth) and is present in ► *meat*, ► *milk* and ► *eggs*. Is not contained in plants, but can be found in fermented vegetable foods (unreliable source). Is produced industrially using bacterial cultures. Cyanocobalamin, hydroxocobalamin or methylcobalamin are used as active agents in medication (for treating vitamin B_{12} deficiency and cyanide poisoning), food supplements for boosting physical and mental performance, and fortified foods. Skin conditioner in cosmetics.

Vitamin B₁₃ ► *Orotic Acid*

Vitamin C

(Ascorbic acid. E 300)

Vegetable or microbiological. Water-soluble ► *vitamin.* Occurs in many plants. Industrial synthesis from sugars or with genetically modified organisms. Antioxidant in foods and cosmetics. Skin protecting substance in cosmetics. Active agent in medicines and food supplements.

Vitamin D

(Calciferol)

Can be animal, vegetable or synthetic. Collective term for fat-soluble substances that belong to the ► *steroids.* Strictly speaking, vitamin D is not a ► *vitamin,* as the human body is able to synthesize provitamin D_3 (► *7-Dehydrocholesterol*) from ► *cholesterol* and convert it into active vitamin D (calcitriol) in skin exposed to sufficient sunlight using the ultraviolet rays in the sunlight. It would be more correct to speak of a hormone and its precursors. Calcitriol plays a central role in the body's calcium status, e.g. in cell nuclei, blood, and the formation and maintenance of bone substance. The most important D vitamins for humans are cholecalciferol (► *vitamin D₃*) and ergocalciferol (► *vitamin D₂*).

Vitamin D₂

(Ergocalciferol. "vegetable vitamin D")

Vegetable. Variant of ► *vitamin D* produced via conversion of ► *ergosterol* by exposure of the skin to sunlight. Industrial production via UV irradiation of ergosterol. In medicines, food supplements and fortified foods.

Vitamin D₃

(Cholecalciferol. Colecalciferol. "animal vitamin D")

From living/killed animals, can also be synthetic. Variant of ► *vitamin D* produced in the skin from ► *cholesterol* via exposure to sunlight. Industrial production from ► *cholesterol* or ► *lanolin.* In medicines, food supplements and fortified foods (in most margarines).

Vitamin E

(Tocopherol. Tocopheryl acetate. Tocopheryl linoleate. Tocopheryl nicotinate. E 306 [Tocopherol-rich extracts]. E 307 [Alpha-tocopherol]. E 308 [Gamma-tocopherol]. E 309 [Delta-tocopherol])

V

Can be vegetable, animal or synthetic. Collective term for a group of fat-soluble substances that play an important role in the body as antioxidants. Occur naturally especially in vegetable oils, but also in ▶ *butter* and ▶ *fish oil*. Obtained primarily from vegetable oils, but also from ▶ *fish liver oil* or petroleum derivatives. Tocopheryl acetate is always synthetic. In vitamin pills, food supplements and fortified foods. Also used in foods as antioxidants. Skin conditioner and antioxidant in cosmetics.

Vitamin F

Obsolete term for essential ▶ *fatty acids*, especially ▶ *linoleic acid* and *linolenic acid*.

Vitamin H ▶ Biotin.

Vitamin K

(Phylloquinone. Phytomenadione. Phytonadione [vitamin K_1]. Menaquinone [vitamin K_2]. Menadione [vitamin K_3])

Synthetic, can theoretically also be vegetable, microbiological or animal. Collective term for fat-soluble vitamins important for regulating blood clotting, bone metabolism and cell growth. Two forms occur naturally: vitamin K_1 (also called phylloquinone, phytomenadione or phytonadione) especially in green leafy vegetables; vitamin K_2 (menaquinone) is produced by bacteria, e.g. in the large intestine, and is also found in animal tissues, ▶ *milk* and ▶ *eggs*. Other forms (e.g. menadione, referred to as vitamin K_3) are exclusively synthetic. All forms are obtained industrially from petroleum derivatives. Vitamin K_1 is used for standard prevention of bleeding in newborn infants and for treating and preventing bleeding due to adult vitamin K deficiency, for instance in the case of intestinal disorders or overdosed anticoagulant medication (e.g. warfarin). Also used as a skin conditioner in cosmetics. Vitamin K_3 is used as a masking agent in cosmetics.

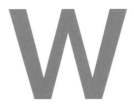

Wax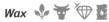

Can be vegetable, animal, mineral or synthetic. Term for substances from various sources that share the following properties: hard to brittle, varying from coarse to finely crystalline, malleable at 20 °C, melting point above 45 °C. Consistency and solubility vary considerably depending on temperature, polishable under light pressure. In the narrower sense, compounds of ► *fatty acids* and ► *fatty alcohols*. Examples of animal waxes: ► *beeswax*, ► *shellac cera*, ► *lanolin*, ► *spermaceti*. Examples of vegetable waxes: carnauba wax, candellila wax, Japan wax. Examples of mineral waxes: ► *ceresin*, ► *montan wax*, ozokerite. Examples of synthetic waxes (from petroleum products): paraffins, microcrystalline waxes. Skin and hair conditioners in cosmetics. Bulking agent, glazing agent and anticaking agent in foods. Also in candles and art materials (oil pastels, crayons and modelling wax). In all kinds of polishes, impregnators and coatings (e.g. furniture polish, floor wax, wood treating agents, wax for sport equipment, car polish, shoe polish, impregnators for textiles and papers).

Whale Oil ► *Train Oil*

Wheatgermamidopropyl Dimethylamine Hydrolyzed Collagen

From killed animals. Chemically altered ► *collagen*. Antistatic, skin and hair conditioner in cosmetics.

Wheatgermamidopropyl Dimethylamine Lactate

Can be vegetable or partly animal. Compound of ► *lactic acid* and substances from wheat germ. Surfactant in cosmetics.

Whey

(Milk plasma)

From living and killed animals (► milk). The watery part of ► *milk* that remains after removing the ► *casein* and most of the ► *butterfat*. Byproduct of cheese production. Food ingredient (► *whey powder*). Skin conditioner in natural cosmetics. Generally allowed for use in organic farming. Source of ► *milk serum*. Fire retardant in ecological wood chip insulation. In detergents. Nutrient medium for ► *lactic acid bacteria*.

Whey Powder

From living and killed animals (► milk). Dried ► *whey*, consists mainly of ► *lactose* and

► *whey protein*. Ingredient in margarines, baked goods, confectionery and savoury snacks. In infant formulas, food supplements and diet products. In animal feed.

Whey Protein

From living and killed animals (► milk). The ► *proteins* in ► *whey*, comprising mostly ► *lactoglobulin* and ► *albumin*, also immunoglobulins. In nutritional supplements and bodybuilding formulas.

Wild Honey

From living or killed animals. ► *Honey* made by ► *bees* from ► *honeydew* from various trees. Used as food.

Wine

Vegetable, is often treated with animal substances. Alcoholic beverage made by fermenting grapes. Is often "fined," i.e. purified of undesired clouding substances, using minerals (e.g. bentonite, diatomcaeous earth/kieselgur) vegetable extracts (e.g. tannins, agar agar) or animal substances (e.g. egg white [see ► *albumen*],► *isinglass*, ► *gelatin* or ► *casein*). These fining agents are not subject to mandatory labelling, and the use of animal substances is widespread, so that wine must be regarded as not vegan unless stated otherwise. Used mainly as a recreational beverage, sometimes also in ritual or religious contexts, and also as a cooking ingredient in some foods.

Wool

Mostly from living, but also from killed animals. The ► *hair* of sheep, in a broader sense also the hair of other mammals, such as angora and cashmere goats, camels, alpacas, vicuñas and angora rabbits. Depending on the species, the wool is shorn, combed out or plucked, or obtained from the skins of killed animals. Used in large quantities as a raw material for diverse textiles, including clothing, shoe linings, blankets and carpets, and as filling in mattresses, upholstery, furniture, etc. Is woven, spun or worked to ► *felt*. Also used as ecological insulating material and industrial material.

Wool Alcohol ► *Acetylated Lanolin Alcohol*

Wool Felt ► *Felt*

Wool Grease ► *Lanolin*

Wool Wax ► *Lanolin*

Wool Wax Alcohol(s) ► *Lanolin Alcohol*

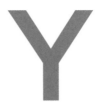

Yak Wool
(Yak hair)

From living or killed animals. Woolly hair of a bovine species native to Central Asia. Obtained by combing and shearing as well as from the skins of killed yaks. In clothing, mattresses, blankets, cushions, brushes.

Yeast Palmitate

Mostly microbiological/vegetable, can also be partly animal. Reaction product of ► *palmitic acid* and baker's yeast. Skin conditioner in cosmetics.

Yellow Wax ► Beeswax

Yogurt

From living and killed animals (► milk). ► *Milk* that has been fermented using ► *yogurt cultures*, usually cows' milk, but also from sheep or goats. Can also be made using soy milk, however according to food regulations only fermented animal milk may be sold as "yogurt." Used as food and food ingredient. hair conditioner and skin protective substance in cosmetics.

Yogurt Cultures

Microbiological, can be grown on animal culture media. ► *Lactic acid bacteria* that metabolize ► *sugar* to ► *lactic acid* and are used for making ► *yogurt*, especially *Lactobacillus acidophilus*, *Lactobacillus bulgaricus,* and *Streptococcus thermophilus.* The culture media can be animal (dairy products) or vegetable sugars.

Yogurt Filtrate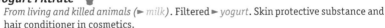

From living and killed animals (► milk). Filtered ► *yogurt.* Skin protective substance and hair conditioner in cosmetics.

Yolk ► Egg Yolk

Z

Zea Mays Silk Extract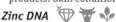
Vegetable. Extract from maize (corn) blossoms. Not to be confused with animal ► *silk* products. Skin conditioner in cosmetics.

Zinc DNA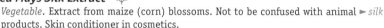
Mineral/animal or mineral/vegetable. Zinc compound of ► *DNA.* Skin conditioner in cosmetics.

Zinc Glutamate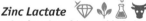
Mostly mineral/vegetable, can theoretically also be partly animal. Zinc salt of ► *glutamic acid.* Deodorant and skin conditioner in cosmetics.

Zinc Hydrolyzed Collagen
From killed animals. Chemically/enzymatically altered ► *collagen.* Antistatic, skin and hair conditioner in cosmetics.

Zinc Lactate
Can be mineral/vegetable/microbiological or partly animal. Zinc salt of ► *lactic acid.* Deodorant in cosmetics.

Zinc Laurate
Mineral/vegetable, can theoretically be partly animal. Zinc salt of ► *lauric acid.* Deodorant in cosmetics.

Zinc Myristate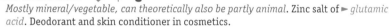
Mostly mineral/vegetable, can also be partly animal. Zinc salt of ► *myristic acid.* Opacifier, viscosity controlling agent and anticaking agent in cosmetics.

Zinc Neodecanoate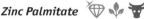
Mostly vegetable/mineral, can also be partly animal. Zinc salt of ► *capric acid.* Opacifier and viscosity controlling agent in cosmetics.

Zinc Orotate ► *Orotic Acid*

Zinc Palmitate
Mostly mineral/vegetable, can also be partly animal. Zinc salt of ► *palmitic acid.* Deodorant in cosmetics.

Z

Zinc Stearate

Can be mineral/animal or mineral/vegetable. Zinc salt of ► *stearic acid*. Colourant and anticaking agent in cosmetics.

Zwitterionic Surfactants ► *Amphoteric Surfactants*

VEGANISSIMO A to Z

Part 2

Product Labelling

- *Food*
- *Supplements/Natural health products*
- *Pharmaceutical drugs*
- *Cosmetics*
- *Household cleaning products*
- *Textiles*
- *Footwear*
- *Seals, logos and labels*

About Product Labeling

In light of the number of ingredients that may be either of animal origin or vegan, the information provided by manufacturers regarding their products is of the greatest importance—especially in the case of products containing a number of ingredients. The widespread use of processing aids that are not subject to mandatory labeling or of ingredients that may have been tested on animals underlines this importance.

While allergens in foods are subject to mandatory labelling and must be declared, there are no comparable statutory provisions for labelling vegetarian or even vegan products.

Warning notices regarding possible traces of allergenic animal substances can be helpful, for example when consumers choose a pragmatic approach, i.e. to draw a line between trace amounts resulting from production methods (cross-contamination) and actual ingredients, but they don't necessarily make buying decisions much easier.

Some producers choose to provide additional information, such as "vegetable" or "vegan" to clarify in those cases where ingredients might also be of animal origin. This may pertain to single ingredients or complete products. This is, however, not legally defined in Canada; the reliability of such claims depends on whether the producer is prepared to disclose more information than is legally required.

What is most dependable and helpful are labels and seals that clearly and unequivocally identify products as being vegan (see page 256). Products that bear such labels can be purchased without first having to examine the ingredients list at length or to send individual queries to producers, as long as the labels themselves entail verifiable, clear, unequivocal and uniform standards.

That said, there is not one definitive label, bur rather a number of logos administered by various organizations according to their own criteria.

On the following pages we will introduce you to statutory labelling requirements and various product labels, and consider to what extent they can provide sufficient and reliable information as to whether a product is actually vegan or not in light of individual consumers' personal standards. However, due to the scope and complexity of the subject matter, the information provided here can only provide an overview and cannot be regarded as exhaustive.

The following pages deal with foods that are not necessarily animal but may be either vegetable, mineral or animal. The object is to demonstrate how labelling can be used to ascertain whether a potentially vegan product is actually vegan or not. To this end, not all aspects of food labelling are covered, but rather those that are actually relevant for such an assessment. Aspects such as nutrition facts, alcohol content or meat labelling regulations are therefore not taken into consideration.

Labels on prepackaged foods must contain an ingredients list, in which the ingredients are shown in descending order of their proportion of the prepackaged product or as a percentage of the product. The order or percentage must be that of the ingredients before they are combined to make the product.

Ingredients are named according to their specific or common names. Certain components or classes of ingredients, such as ingredients made up of other ingredients or subject to compositional standards, may be named according to the class of ingredients they belong to, e.g. certain fats or oils (see the following section), baking powder, breads, breadcrumbs, wheat flours, cheeses, milk, whey and whey products, carbonated, chlorinated or fluorinated water, vinegars or pickles.

Fat

Labelling of prepackaged foods (except those intended for children under two years of age) must include the amount of fat in grams per serving of stated size and percentage of the daily value per serving, as well as the energy value from fat in Calories per serving.

Vegetable fats and oils must be obtained entirely from the botanical source after which they are named. With the exception of olive oil, they may contain certain additives (e.g. emulsifiers or preservatives), as long as these are declared on the label. Mixed vegetable oils may be labelled either singly or as *vegetable oil*.

Animal fats, oils or tallow must be named according to the animal or meat from which they are obtained, e.g. *chicken fat*, *cod liver oil* or *beef tallow*. *Lard*, *leaf lard* and *suet* do not require the name of the animal or meat, or the addition of *fat*, *oil* or *tallow*. Mixed marine oils may simply be called *marine oil*.

The following legally defined fats and oils are or may be of animal origin.

Butter: food prepared from milk or milk products with not less than 80 percent milk fat. It may contain bacterial cultures, salt or food colour.

Margarine: plastic (i.e. semisolid) or fluid emulsion of water in fats and/or oil that are not derived from milk and may have been hydrogenated, with not less than 80 percent fat and/or oil. Margarine may contain skim milk powder, buttermilk (liquid or powder), whey solids, modified whey solids, protein, lecithin, mono- and diglycerides and sorbitan tristearate.

Calorie-reduced margarine: margarine with less than 40 percent fat and/or oil and 50 percent of the calories that would be normally present if the product were not calorie-reduced.

Lard: rendered fat from hogs.

Leaf lard: lard from the internal fat of hog abdomens.

Shortening: semisolid food (except for butter or lard) prepared from fats, oils or a combination of fats and oils (can be either vegetable or animal).

Suet: fat from the kidney region of cattle.

When the aforementioned fats and oils are ingredients of another product, their components are not required to be shown on a label. The components of vegetable or animal fats or oils used as ingredients, as well as hydrogenated, modified or interesterified vegetable or animal fats or oils comprising less than 15 percent of prepackaged products, also do need not be declared.

Dairy products

Milk and dairy products are subject to mandatory labelling as allergens (see page 244), so that foods containing them are always recognizable as such and need no further explanation. Labelling regulations for milk and dairy products themselves also need not be dealt with in any detail, as such products are obviously of animal origin, therefore not vegan.

It is, however worth taking a brief look at the legally defined names exclusively reserved for animal milk and dairy products: *butter, cream, cream cheese, yogurt, cheese, ice cream, milk, milk fat (butter fat), whey, sour cream.*

Successful lobbying by the dairy industry probably means that this situation is also likely to stay that way in the forseeable future. By the way, it is such lobbying that led to margarine being banned in many parts of Canada for a long time, and until 2008 margarine sold in Quebec was not allowed to be coloured yellow, as that colour was reserved by law for butter only.

Flavouring

Food flavouring must either be declared as *flavour* or with an exact description of the flavour. Flavours derived from single sources are named according to the name of the plant or animal source plus the word *flavour*. Flavours derived from plants or animals, e.g. via distillation, dehydration, fermentation, heating etc, but without the use of chemical or enzymatic processing may be described as *natural flavour*. Those obtained in whole or in part by chemical synthesis must be declared as *artificial flavour*, *imitation flavour* or *simulated flavour*.

However, the exact sources of flavouring preparations do not necessarily have to be stated, nor do the individual components of flavouring preparations used as ingredients in foods have to be named, so that it is often not discernible whether they are vegetable or animal. In many cases the use of the word *flavour* is sufficient.

Only when a flavour can cause an allergic reaction (see page 244) must the actual substance be declared, so that at least some animal flavours can be identified. Many producers do, however, voluntarily declare vegetable or animal flavours as such.

Enzymes

Enzymes are substances capable of catalyzing specific biochemical reactions, without themselves becoming part of these reactions. They can be obtained from plants, animals or microorganisms, or products thereof, and are used for the production, processing, preparation, treatment, packaging, transport or storage of a variety of foods and beverages to fulfil a technological purpose.

The Canadian Food and Drug Regulations define which enzymes may be used as food additives and from which sources they may be obtained. They are subject to the same labelling requirements as other food additives, i.e. they need not be declared when used as processing aids that are no longer present in the final product. This means that enzymes of animal origin (e.g. lipase, pancreatin, pepsin or trypsin) used in food production need not necessarily be declared, so that seemingly vegan foods may in fact not be.

The only way to be entirely certain that foods do not contain animal enzymes is to ask the producer or look out for products that are explicitly vegan (e.g. vegan logos, see pages 256–258) or organic (organic products may only contain enzymes of microbiological origin).

Food additives

A food additive is any chemical substance that is added to food during preparation or storage and either becomes a part of the food or affects its characteristics for the purpose of achieving a particular technical effect, for example to enhance the appearance, texture, or keeping qualities of a food or serve as an essential aid in the processing of food.

Under the Canadian Food and Drug Regulations, food additives do not include:
- food ingredients such as salt, sugar, starch
- vitamins, minerals, amino acids
- spices, seasonings, flavouring preparations (including flavour enhancers)
- agricultural chemicals
- veterinary drugs
- food packaging materials

Only food additives listed in the Tables of Division 16 in the Food and Drug Regulations (currently 429 in total) are permitted to be used in food.

Some substances used in food are considered to be food processing aids, not food additives, and are not subject to mandatory labelling. This is the case when they are no longer present in the final product, except for "negligible" residues, and do not affect its characteristics.

The mandatory labelling requirements for food additives allow us to at least recognize which foods may contain nonvegan additives. Absolute certainty, however, is not possible, in part because not all substances are required to be declared (see the previous paragraph), but also because the sources of additives are not usually declared in detail and may vary.

Food additives may also be listed on some imported goods using the International Numbering System (INS) that assigns unique numbers to food additives. These are used for example in Europe as "E numbers," e.g. E 155, E 160a or E 160f. Some of the substances assigned such numbers are not food additives according to Canadian law, for instance flavour enhancers.

Some of the substances used as food additives are chemically manufactured, some with the aid of microorganisms and others using raw materials from vegetable sources.

Additives can also be produced using animal substances, however only a few of these cannot also be derived from vegetable or mineral sources.

The fact that animal substances are often used as undeclared industrial processing aids nonetheless remains a problem that we unfortunately cannot address in any detail within the framework of this book; we can only establish whether a substance as such is animal or not.

The following food additives are always of animal origin:
- beeswax
- (bovine) rennet
- cochineal (carmine)
- gelatin
- lanolin
- pancreas extract
- pancreatin
- pepsin
- shellac
- spermaceti wax
- trypsin

The following food additives are most often of animal origin:
- L-cystine
- L-cysteine (hydrochloride)

The following additives can be of animal origin:
- glycerol, either from animal or vegetable fats
- lecithin, usually derived from soy, also from eggs or sunflower seeds
- lysozyme, can be from eggs, also produced microbiologically
- lactic acid, can be from dairy products or fermented vegetable sugars

The production of many food additives involves fatty acids obtained chemically or mechanically from edible fats. These can be animal fats (for instance, lard, tallow or butterfat), but producers often choose to use vegetable fats—especially soy, rapeseed or corn oil. This may be for cost reasons, or also in response to consumer wishes, as animal fats are often perceived as being detrimental to health.

However, even if fatty acids of animal origin are now used less often for manufacturing food additives, there is no guarantee that this is actually true in any given case. The only way to be absolutely sure is to ask the producer or to look out for products labelled as 100 percent vegetable or vegan (see pages 256–259).

Some examples of food additives produced from fatty acids:
- fatty acid esters of ascorbic acid (ascorbyl palmitate, ascorbyl stearate)
- polysorbates (e.g. polysorbate 60, polysorbate 80)
- sodium, potassium, calcium and magnesium salts of fatty acids (e.g. potassium stearate, sodium palmitate, calcium stearate)
- mono- and diglycerides of fatty acids and their esters
- sucrose esters of fatty acids
- polyglycerol esters of fatty acids
- propylene glycol esters of fatty acids
- sorbitan fatty acid esters (e.g. sorbitan monostearate, sorbitan trioleate)

Additives have the following functions (also see the glossary, pages 291–294):
- antioxidants
- anticaking agents
- antifoaming agents
- bleaching, maturing, and dough conditioning agents
- colouring agents
- carriers or extraction solvents
- emulsifiers
- emulsifying salts
- firming agents
- food enzymes
- gelling agents
- glazing and polishing agents
- humectants
- preservatives
- pressure-dispensing agents
- pH-adjusting agents
- release agents
- sequestering agents
- starch-modifying agents
- stabilizers
- sweeteners
- thickening agents
- texture-modifying agents
- whipping agents
- miscellaneous agents
- yeast foods

Allergens

As foods that can cause allergies, the following substances must always be declared regardless of their amounts (animal substances are denoted with *):

- almonds, Brazil nuts, cashews, hazelnuts, macadamia nuts, pecans, pine nuts, pistachios or walnuts
- peanuts
- sesame seeds
- wheat and triticale
- eggs*
- milk*
- soybeans
- crustaceans*
- shellfish*
- fish*
- mustard seeds
- gluten protein, modified gluten protein, or gluten protein fractions from barley, oats, rye, triticale or wheat (or a hybridized strain of any of these cereals)
- sulphites

This makes it possible to always ascertain at least some animal ingredients beyond all doubt, regardless of their quantities.

A declaration of substances that are not ingredients but may be contained in trace amounts for technological reasons (for instance because other foods containing allergens are processed using the same equipment), is currently not required. However, producers may voluntarily do so to avoid legal liability.

In Canada, dietary supplements are classified not as food, but rather as "natural health products" (NHPs). These include vitamins, minerals, amino acids, fatty acids and other substances derived from plants or animals. The labels must include a list of the medicinal ingredients with their proper names and quantities per dose, preferably in descending order of quantity, as well as a description of their sources (specific plants or animals, or parts thereof). The label must also contain a list of the non-medicinal ingredients, under their common names and in any order. Medicinal and non-medicinal ingredients must each be clearly identified as such. Also required are statements of the recommended use, recommended dosage and health warnings. Nutritional information is not permitted.

NHPs can quite often be of animal origin, e.g. omega-3 fatty acids from fish oil, or fat-soluble vitamins or other substances from animal tissue, however labelling requirements ensure a high degree of certainty as to whether natural health products are vegan or not, so that it is easy to avoid nonvegan products. Specific logos or seals can be of additional assistance (see pages 256–263).

Some health products may not be NHPs, but rather non-prescription drugs, for instance when they also contain medicinal ingredients that are not of natural origin (see the next page).

The labels of nonprescription drugs intended for human consumption must contain a quantitative list of the medicinal ingredients by their proper or common names and a list of all nonmedicinal ingredients in alphabetical order or in descending order of their proportion in the drug, preceded by words that clearly distinguish them from the medicinal ingredients.

In the case of flavour, fragrance or pharmaceutical ink, the expressions *flavour/saveur*, *fragrance/parfum* and *pharmaceutical ink/encre pharmaceutique*, respectively, may be included in the list to indicate that such ingredients have been added to the drug, instead of listing those ingredients or combinations of them individually. The labels must also contain directions for use and dosage recommendations.

A declaration of the sources of medicinal or non-medicinal ingredients, e.g. animal or vegetable, is neither required nor commonplace, although some manufacturers respond to consumer wishes and voluntarily provide such information, e.g. on their websites.

Unfortunately, labels of prescription drugs or drugs administered under the supervision of a medical practitioner are not required to contain a statement of the non-medicinal ingredients and must only state the medicinal ingredients as described above. In these cases it is necessary to confer with the practitioner as to the exact composition of the drug in question.

The term "cosmetics" encompasses both beauty and personal care products and is often synonymous with personal hygiene. Canadian law defines cosmetics as "any substance or mixture of substances manufactured, sold or represented for use in cleansing, improving or altering the complexion, skin, hair or teeth, and includes deodorants and perfumes."

A personal care product can be defined as a substance or mixture of substances which is generally recognized by the public for use in daily cleansing or grooming. Depending on the ingredients and the claims of a product, a personal care product can be regulated as a cosmetic or a drug (see the previous page).

A beauty product or grooming aid is usually a cosmetic, but is legally classified as a drug if it makes any claims to modify body functions or prevent/treat disease.

Cosmetics include:

- skin care products (creams, emulsions, lotions, gels, oils)
- facial masks
- make-up (fluids, pastes, powders) and make-up removers
- lip care and beauty products
- facial and body powders
- cleansing and deodorizing soaps
- perfumes, eau de toilette, etc.
- bath and shower products (salts, foams, oils, gels)
- depilatory products
- deodorants and antiperspirants
- hair dyes
- hair curling/waving and straightening products, hair fixatives
- hair cleansing products (lotions, powders, shampoos)
- hair conditioners (lotions, creams, oils)
- shaving products (shaving creams, aftershaves, etc.)
- dental and oral care products
- nail care and beauty products
- genital hygiene products
- sunscreens, sunblocks, etc.
- tanning products
- skin whitening products
- antiwrinkle agents

Cosmetic ingredients must be declared according to the International Nomenclature of Cosmetic Ingredients (INCI). A list of ingredients must appear on the outer label of a cosmetic (or on an attached tag, tape or card or an accompanying leaflet), with each ingredient listed only by its INCI name. Certain defined ingredients may instead be listed according to their English or French common names, e.g. *Goat milk* or *Lait de chèvre* instead of *Caprae Lac*, or *Tallow* or *Suif* instead of *Adeps Bovis*. An ingredient that has no INCI name must be listed by its chemical name.

The ingredients must be listed in descending order of predominance, in their concentration by weight. Ingredients that are present at a concentration of 1 percent or less and all colouring agents, regardless of their concentration, may be listed in random order after the ingredients that are present at a concentration of more than 1 percent.

In the case of fragrance and flavour, the words *parfum* and *aroma*, respectively, may be inserted at the end of the list of ingredients to indicate that such ingredients have been added to the cosmetic to produce or to mask a particular odour or flavour.

As cosmetic ingredients must be listed according to their INCI or trivial names, we have decided for the most part not to include brand names for substances in this book.

Cosmetic ingredients with INCI names are also classified according to their functions (also see the following page). The ingredients list in this book therefore includes both the names and the functions of the ingredients listed.

List of Cosmetic Ingredient Functions According to INCI

- abrasive
- anticaking
- antidandruff
- antimicrobial
- antiperspirant
- antiseborrheic
- astringent
- bleaching
- bulking
- cleansing
- denaturant
- depilatory
- emollient
- emulsion stabilizing
- foaming
- gel forming
- hair dyeing
- hair waving or straightening
- hydrotrope
- nail conditioning
- moisturizing
- oral care
- pearlescent
- preservative
- reducing
- refreshing
- skin protecting
- solvent
- stabilizing
- tanning
- UV absorber
- viscosity controlling

- absorbent
- anticorrosive
- antifoaming
- antioxidant
- antiplaque
- antistatisc
- binding
- buffering
- chelating
- cosmetic colourant
- deodorant
- detangling
- emulsifying
- film forming
- foam boosting
- hair conditioning
- hair fixing
- humectant
- keratolytic
- masking
- opacifying
- oxidizing
- plasticizer
- propellant
- refatting
- skin conditioning
- smoothing
- soothing
- surfactant
- tonic
- UV filter

You can find explanations of those terms that are not self-explanatory in the glossary on pages 291–294.

Household Cleaning Products

The term "household cleaning products" covers a wide range of products, including dish soaps, laundry detergents, fabric softeners, bleaches, toilet cleaners, polishes, surface cleaners, etc.

Curiously, none of these products is required by law to carry an ingredients list, the only statutory labelling requirements being safety and first aid advice for any hazardous chemicals contained. This means that consumers basically have no idea what they are buying unless the producer voluntarily discloses the product's contents.

That said, there is a growing awareness of consumers' desire to make informed decisions and many manufacturers therefore do in fact disclose the contents of their products.

North American industry organizations have even developed a voluntary ingredient communication initiative for the product categories "air care," "automotive care," "cleaning," and "polishes and floor maintenance products." The guidelines provide for product labels that include a list of all ingredients, with those present at a concentration greater than one percent listed in descending order of predominance. The ingredients are to be identified using one or more of the following naming systems: International Nomenclature of Cosmetic Ingredients (INCI), International Union of Pure and Applied Chemistry (IUPAC), Chemical Abstract Service (CAS), common chemical name.

A product labelled in accordance with these guidelines allows a fairly accurate assessment as to whether a product is vegan or not, insofar as substances that are either always or never of animal origin can be clearly identified. In the case of substances that may or may not be animal, only certification seals or logos (see pages 256–263), or corresponding statements made by the manufacturer, can provide absolute certainty.

Canadian law requires that consumer textile articles be labelled with regard to their textile fibre content. The provisions are quite comprehensive and require fairly detailed declaration of the various fibres, so consumers can be relatively sure of what they are buying. However, the complete composition of textile articles must not always be declared, as the following information shows.

According to Canadian law, any consumer textile article, or any textile fibre, yarn or fabric used or to be used in a consumer textile article, is a "textile fibre product" and must be labelled as such.

Textile labels must show the generic name of each textile fibre comprising 5 percent or more by mass of the total fibre mass of the article, including their percentage by mass of the total fibre mass of the article. Fibres that either singly or together make up less than 5 percent may be declared as *other fibres*.

Natural fibres for which no generic name has been prescribed are to be declared according to the the names by which they are commonly known in Canada.

The label disclosing the textile fibre content must be attached to the article or its packaging or otherwise displayed in a clearly visible manner.

Textile fibre means any natural or manufactured matter that is capable of being made into a yarn or fabric, including human hair, kapok, feathers and down and animal hair or fur that has been removed from an animal skin.

Fabric means any material woven, knitted, crocheted, knotted, braided, felted, bonded, laminated or otherwise produced from, or in combination with, a textile fibre.

On the following pages are lists of textile fibres according to their origin (animal, vegetable, chemical and other), as defined by Canadian law or common usage.

Animal textile fibres

Textile fibres obtained from sheep or lambs are labelled as **wool.**

Textile fibres from Angora goats can be labelled as **wool**, **mohair**, **mohair wool** or **Angora goat hair**.

Textile fibres from cashmere goats can be labelled as **wool**, **Cashmere**, **Kashmir wool** or **Kashmir goat hair**.

Textile fibres from the following animals can be labelled either as **wool**, as the name of the animal or as the name of the animal together with the words **wool** or **hair**: **alpaca**, **vicuna**, **camel** or **llama**.

The hair or fur removed from the skin of other animals is labelled using the name of the animal together with the words **hair**, **fibre** or simply as **fur fibre**, e.g. **angora rabbit hair** or **angora rabbit fibre**.

The undercoating of waterfowl, including goose, duck or swan, consisting of light fluffy filaments (barbs) growing from a quill point but without a quill shaft is labelled as **down**.

The individual external horny structure that forms the body covering of birds and consists of a quill point, quill shaft and vanes, with or without an aftershaft, is labelled as **feather**.

Fibres other than those described above are labelled using the name by which they are commonly known in Canada, e.g. **silk**. Also see *protein* on the following page.

Vegetable textile fibres

Abaca	fibres from the leaf sheaths of abacá plants (Manila hemp)
Coconut/Coir	fibres from the fruit of coconuts
Cotton	fibres from the seeds of cotton plants
Flax/Linen	bast fibres from the stalks of flax plants
Hemp	bast fibres from the stalks of hemp plants
Jute	bast fibres from the stalks of corchorus plants
Kapok	fibres from the seed pods of the kapok tree
Ramie	bast fibres from plants of the nettle family
Rubber	elastic fibres from sap of rubber trees (can also be synthetic)
Sisal	fibres from the leaves of the sisal agave

Chemical and other textile fibres

Acetate	cellulose fibres, 74%–92% acetylated
Acrylic	long chain synthetic polymer, more than 85% acrylonitrile
Anidex	long chain synthetic polymer
Aramid	synthetic polymer fibres (e.g. *Kevlar*)
Azlon	see *protein* (next page)

Chlorofibre	long chain synthetic polymer, more than 50% vinyl chloride
Cupro	cellulose treated with copper and ammonium
Elastane	see *spandex* (below)
Fluorofibre	fibres made from fluorocarbon monomers
Glass	glass fibres
Lastol	elastic olefin fibres
Lyocell	fibres from dissolved, extruded and spun cellulose
Metallic	plastic-coated metal or plastic/other core covered with metal
Modacrylic	long chain synthetic polymer, 35%–85% acrylonitrile
Modal	chemically treated cellulose fibres
Nitrile	long chain polymer, more than 85% vinylidene dinitrile
Nylon (polyamide)	synthetic fluorocarbon fibres
Olefin	see *polyolefin* (below)
Paper	paper fibres
PLA	see *polylactic acid* (below)
Polyamide	see *nylon* (above)
Polyester	synthetic polymer fibres
Polyethylene	long chain synthetic polymer fibres, at least 85% ethylene
Polylactic acid (PLA)	fibre composed of at least 85% lactic acid ester derived from naturally occurring sugars
Polyolefin (olefin)	long chain synthetic polymer fibres, at least 85% olefin
Polypropylene	long chain synthetic polymer fibres, at least 85% propylene
Polyurethane	long chain synthetic polymer (urethane) fibres
Polyvinyl chloride	long chain synthetic polymer, more than 85% vinyl chloride
Protein (azlon)	chemically treated (regenerated) fibres from animal proteins (e.g. keratin, silk protein, milk protein)
PVC	see *polyvinyl chloride* (above)
Rayon	a variety of forms of chemically treated cellulose; includes *cupro*, *viscose*, *modal* and *lyocell* (see previous entries)
Rubber	elastic natural (see previous page) or synthetic fibres
Spandex (elastane)	elastic fibres, at least 85% polyurethane
Triacetate	cellulose fibres, more than 92% acetylated
Vinal/Vinylal	long chain synthetic polyvinyl fibres
Vinyon	see *polyvinyl chloride* (above)
Viscose	dissolved and spun cellulose fibres

Exemptions from labelling requirements

Articles intended for one-time use only are exempt from mandatory textile labelling, as well as the following articles that have a textile fibre product incorporated in them:

- overshoes, boots, shoes, indoor slippers, footwear liners and insoles
- handbags, luggage, carrying cases and brushes
- toys, ornaments, pictures, lamp shades, tapestries, wall hangings, wall coverings, room dividers, screens, book covers, book marks, gift wrap, flags and pennants
- sports and games equipment other than sport garments
- lawn and beach furniture, including lawn and beach umbrellas and parasols and hammocks
- playpens, crib-pens, strollers, jumpers, walkers and car seats for infants or children
- labels, adhesive tapes and sheets, cleaning cloths and wipers, therapeutic devices and heating pads
- pet accessories
- musical instruments and accessories
- belts, suspenders, arm bands, garters, sanitary belts and bandages
- consumer textile articles in which any textile fibres contained serve only as findings (trims, buttons, hooks, embellishments, etc.)
- consumer textile articles in which any textile fibres contained serve only as filling or stuffing
- straw or felt headwear, padding or helmets worn in sports, curler head covers, hair nets and shower caps
- carpet underpadding
- non-fibrous materials that do not have a fabric support, including films and foams
- household twine, string, craft ribbon not intended to be used in the construction of other textile articles subject to labelling requirements, baler twine, binder twine and gift wrap ribbon.

In Canada, there are no legal provisions for declaring the composition of shoes, boots, etc., as textile labelling requirements exclude footwear. The only labelling requirements apply to protective foorwear with regard to their resistance against hazards such as impact, chainsaw cuts, punctures, electric shock, etc.

By comparison, all shoes in the European Union must be labelled with regard to the composition of their uppers, lining and sock, and outer sole, stating whether these are leather, coated leather, textile or other (synthetic) materials (see the pictograms below). In the United States, footwear must at least be labelled in such a way that it is recognizable whether upper, lining and sock, and outer sole are in fact leather, imitation/simulated leather, or processed leather.

Even though footwear need not be labelled with respect to composition in Canada, much of the footwear available is imported, so it is likely that you will see labelling using the pictograms shown on this page or statements as to whether the materials are man-made or genuine leather, or a combination of symbols and statements. Canadian manufacturers may also make such statements voluntarily.

Failing that, you will have to keep your eyes open for shoes explicitly labelled as "vegan," "vegetarian," "animal-free" or "cruelty-free."

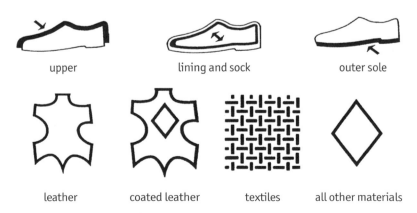

| upper | lining and sock | outer sole |

| leather | coated leather | textiles | all other materials |

General remarks on logos and labels

The logos presented here are a selection of the product labels most relevant to Canada. With the help of these labels and the advice in this book, you can be fairly certain about the origin of the ingredients in the goods you buy, despite otherwise seemingly confusing labelling.

The logos are presented in the order of their relevance from a vegan point of view: first vegan and vegetarian logos, then logos for products not tested on animals, and then organic and GMO-free logos.

Some of the logos are more relevant to Europe than to Canada; however, we have included them for completeness' sake. You may see them on imported products, and they may also become more common in the future.

The more logos or seals a product has, the more certain you can be about its contents, as the product has been assessed by two or more organizations.

Nonetheless, we would like to point out that the logos are allocated based on information provided by the producers, which means that errors cannot entirely be ruled out.

Besides that, the "vegan" logos do not categorically rule out traces of animal substances, for instance when vegan and nonvegan products are made using the same equipment. There can only be absolute certainty if vegan products are made using equipment specifically reserved for such products.

Vegan Trademark

Perhaps the best known label for vegan products is the trademark and certification logo issued by the UK-based Vegan Society. It is used for labelling vegan foods, cosmetics, clothing and commodities.

Producers who wish their products to carry the Vegan Trademark must register their products with the Vegan Society. They must submit a complete list of all the ingredients used in the product, including those not subject to mandatory labelling. They must also declare all the substances used in any form during production, not only those present in the final product.

Both the product itself and the production process must be free of animal substances and may not involve animal testing. All stages of development and production, including all the individual ingredients, must be free of animal substances, byproducts or derivatives. All stages of development and production, including all the individual ingredients, may not involve any form of animal testing, whether by the producer or commissioned third parties.

If products contain genetically modified organisms, these must be declared and may not contain any genetic material of animal origin.

Vegan foods produced using the same equipment or in the same facilities as animal products may not be produced at the same time. Surfaces and utensils must be cleaned thoroughly before the production of vegan foods, in order to minimize contaminating them with traces of animal substances. Separate utensils are strongly recommended.

Products that pass the Vegan Society standards may be sold and advertised using the logo and the statement "Registered with the Vegan Society."

Certified Vegan

The Certified Vegan logo is a registered trademark of Vegan Action, a United States nonprofit organization dedicated to educating the public about veganism and assisting vegan-friendly businesses.

The logo is applied to foods, clothing, cosmetics and other items that contain no animal products and are not tested on animals.

Both the product itself and the production process must be free of animal substances and may not involve animal testing. All stages of development and production, including all the individual ingredients, must be free of animal substances, byproducts or derivatives.

Products containing genetically modified organisms that may have involved animal genes or animal-derived substances in their development or production must be labelled as such.

Products may be produced using machinery used for processing animal products. Companies must give assurance that the machinery is cleaned thoroughly between nonvegan and vegan batches.

Sugar refined though bone char may not carry the label. Any companies that use sugar in their products must send a statement from the sugar supplier guaranteeing that they do not use animal products in the production of the sugar.

V Label

The V Label is the registered trademark of the European Vegetarian Union (EVU) used for designating vegetarian or vegan foods. It is not yet used on Canadian products, but should soon be; it can already be seen on imported products.

The label contains the word "vegetarian" in English or another European language, and a statement assigning the product to one of four categories: *Ovo-lacto-vegetarian* (with milk and eggs), *Lacto-vegetarian* (with milk, no eggs), *Ovo-vegetarian* (with eggs, no milk) or *Vegan* (see the illustration).

A producer wishing to use the V Label must disclose the product's complete composition. All the ingredients must be vegetarian, i.e. the product may not contain or have been processed with any substances from dead animals, royal jelly or battery eggs.

Products in the categories *Ovo-lacto-vegetarian*, *Lacto-vegetarian* and *Ovo-vegetarian* may contain honey. Milk products must not have been processed with animal rennet. Products labelled as *Vegan* must not contain or have been processed with any animal substances.

Genetically modified products cannot qualify for the label.

Vegetarian Society Approved

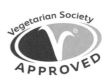

The label Vegetarian Society Approved is a registered trademark of the UK-based Vegetarian Society used for labelling foods, cosmetics, clothing and commodities. It is not currently used on products made in Canada but may be seen on imported products.

Products must not contain substances from slaughtered animals. They may contain substances from living animals, but eggs must be free-range. They also must not contain genetically modified substances. Neither the ingredients nor the final product may be tested on animals in accordance with the criteria of the Leaping Bunny logo (see the next page).

If products are made using the same equipment as nonvegetarian products, all machines, utensils, surfaces and clothing items must be thoroughly cleaned before production and packaging of the vegetarian products. The producer must ensure that vegetarian and nonvegetarian products cannot be confused.

"Caring Consumer"

The U.S.-based organization PETA (People for the Ethical Treatment of Animals) lists companies that don't test on animals and also licenses the Caring Consumer logo for cruelty-free cosmetics, personal care products, household products, and companion animal food.

A company wishing to be certified "cruelty-free" must confirm that it neither conducts nor commissions animal testing of any cosmetics and/or household products or of ingredients used in formulations of such products. It must also require that manufacturers of any finished product it sells or distributes does not conduct or commission animal testing of the cosmetics and/or household products, including formulations and ingredients of such products.

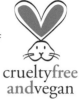

A company can be certified "cruelty-free and vegan" if its products do not contain any animal ingredients or products derived from any animal matter.

PETA also has a searchable database of cruelty-free and vegan companies: *www.peta.org/living/beauty-and-personal-care/companies/default.aspx*

Corporate Standard of Compassion for Animals ("Leaping Bunny")

The Leaping Bunny is an internationally recognized logo for cosmetics and household products not tested on animals.

The Corporate Standard of Compassion for Animals—also known as the Humane Cosmetics Standard (HCS) or Humane Household Products Standard (HHPS)—was developed by an international coalition of animal protection groups and is administered by the Coalition for Consumer Information on Cosmetics (CCIC) and the European Coalition to End Animal Experiments (ECEAE).

Products that have been licensed to carry the logo, and their individual ingredients, must not have been tested on animals since the deadline for compliance declared by the manufacturer. The use of substances supplied by third-party companies who test on animals or commission such tests is also not permitted.

However, the products may contain ingredients from killed or living animals, although the ECEAE does encourage the use of vegan products and highlights in its publications companies that are certified both HCS/HPPS and vegan.

BDIH seal

The BDIH seal for certified natural cosmetics is issued by the German Association of Industrial Companies and Trading Firms (BDIH) for pharmaceuticals, healthcare products, food supplements and personal hygiene products, also represented by the International Organic and Natural Cosmetics Corporation (IONC).

Certified products may not have been tested on animals, neither during development nor as a final product. This includes tests conducted by third parties.

Raw materials not commercially available before January 1, 1998 may only be used if they have not been tested on animals (except for tests conducted by third parties without being commissioned to do so by the producer).

The use of substances from dead vertebrates (e.g. emu oil, mink oil, marmot oil or other animal fats, collagen) is not allowed. Raw materials derived from dead invertebrates (e.g. chitin, silk protein or shellac) are permitted, however.

Substances produced by living animals (e.g. beeswax, honey and milk) are permitted. When substances can be derived from both animals and plants, the vegetable variant must be used in accordance with a white list compiled by the BDIH.

The BDIH seal is not currently used in Canada, but may be seen on some imported products.

NaTrue label

The NaTrue label certifies cosmetics in three categories: natural cosmetics, partly organic natural cosmetics and organic cosmetics. The criteria include strict regulations allowing only natural, nature-derived and nature-identical substances.

The regulations concerning the use of animal substances correspond to those of the BDIH seal.

The NaTrue label is not used in Canada, but may be seen on imported products.

"Choose Cruelty Free"

Choose Cruelty Free (CCF) is an Australian-based nonprofit organization that accredits manufacturers of cosmetics and household products not tested on animals.

NOT TESTED ON ANIMALS

In order to qualify, a manufacturer must either have never tested its products or their ingredients on animals or have not tested them on animals within a period of five years immediately preceding the date of application for accreditation. This includes tests performed by someone else on behalf of the manufacturer.

CCF will not accredit a manufacturer if any of its products contains any ingredients that are derived from an animal killed specifically for that ingredient or that are commercially significant slaughterhouse byproducts. It also will not accredit a company if an ingredient is forcibly extracted from a live animal in a manner that occasioned pain or discomfort, is derived from any wildlife, or is a byproduct of the fur industry.

A company's products need not be vegan for it to be accredited, although CCF does highlight manufacturers of vegan products on its website.

Canada Organic

The official Canadian organic logo certifies products with an organic content that is greater than 95 percent according to Canadian requirements for organic products.

The use of the organic logo is voluntary.

Products with between 70 percent and 95 percent organic ingredients may be labelled as containing organic ingredients, but may not carry the logo.

The logo does not guarantee that a product is vegan or even vegetarian. The Organic Production Systems standards merely stipulate that "livestock" living conditions and handling be "humane" and suited to the general needs of the animals. Substances from both living and slaughtered animals can be certified organic.

The organic logo does, however, ensure that there are no hidden animal fats in the form of food additives (except for glycerol, which is permitted and may be derived from animal or vegetable fats).

Imported products must meet the requirements of the Canada Organic Regime. Should imported products bear the logo, the statement *Product of* or *Imported from*, immediately followed by the name of the country of origin, must appear in close proximity to the logo or the designations.

In accordance with bilateral agreements, products certified organic in either the United States or the European Union qualify as organic in Canada and do not need extra certification. They may be advertised and sold in Canada using the Canada Organic logo as well as the USDA or EU organic logos (see next page).

USDA Organic

Products sold in the United States claiming organic status, whether domestic or imported, are required to adhere to the National Organic Program (NOP) administered by the United States Department of Agriculture (USDA).

The USDA organic seal certifies products with an organic content that is greater than 95 percent.

The use of the USDA organic seal is voluntary. Like the Canadian logo, it can be used for labelling both vegetable and animal products.

EU organic logo

Since July 1, 2010, all packaged organic products made in the European Union and certified according to the EU Regulation on organic production and labelling of organic products must carry the new logo. The origin of the ingredients must also be stated (EU and/or non-EU).

The EU organic logo, like the Canadian logo, can be used for labelling both vegetable and animal products.

Organic logos issued by national authorities in European countries may be used alongside the EU logo.

Ecocert

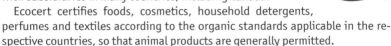

Ecocert is a French-based organic certification organization with subsidiaries in many countries, including Canada.

Ecocert certifies foods, cosmetics, household detergents, perfumes and textiles according to the organic standards applicable in the respective countries, so that animal products are generally permitted.

In the case of cosmetic products, Ecocert does not allow ingredients from dead animals (except for shellac—this substance is classified as "produced by animals").

Substances produced by animals (e.g. dairy products, honey, beeswax and lanolin) are permitted.

Global Organic Textile Standard (GOTS)

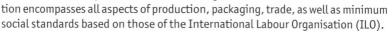

The GOTS seal for organically grown natural fibres was introduced in 2008. Textiles containing 70–94 percent organic fibres are labelled "made with x% organic materials." Products with more than 95 percent are labelled "organic." The certification encompasses all aspects of production, packaging, trade, as well as minimum social standards based on those of the International Labour Organisation (ILO).

The GOTS seal does certify both vegetable and animal textiles, but it helps to not only identify more ecological products, but also to distinguish organic cotton from conventional cotton, which is also highly problematic from a vegan point of view (also see page 281).

Natural Products Association Natural Seal

The Natural Products Association is a United States nonprofit organization that certifies personal care and home care products made using natural and sustainable ingredients.

Products labelled as "natural" must contain at least 95 percent ingredients from natural sources, except for certain synthetic substances deemed safe for humans and the environment.

Companies must avoid animal testing except where required by law, but substances from living mammals and killed invertebrates are permitted, so the Natural Seal cannot provide reliable information as to whether a product is vegan.

GMO-free products

Labelling products as free of genetically modified organisms (GMOs) does not entail any statement as to whether a product is vegan, but we include the topic for completeness' sake.

Unfortunately there is no mandatory labelling for GMOs in North America, so the only way to avoid GMOs is to buy organic products or products with voluntary labelling, for instance the Non-GMO Project seal shown here. The Non-GMO Project verifies GMO-free products as well as assisting producers in avoiding and reducing the risk of GMO contamination.

VEGANISSIMO A to Z

Part 3

Vegan Alternatives to Animal Ingredients

- *Food*
- *Dietary supplements*
- *Pharmaceutical drugs*
- *"Pet" food*
- *Cosmetic products*
- *Household cleaning products*
- *Clothing and accessories*
- *Footwear*
- *Brushes and brooms*
- *Interior decoration, household items*
- *Sport and leisure*
- *Arts and crafts*
- *Photography and printing*
- *Musical instruments*
- *Electronics and technology*

Vegan Alternatives to Animal Ingredients

As we already described in the introduction to this book, we had to find a way of addressing the subject of alternatives outside the bounds of the A to Z list.

There were two main reasons for this—one pragmatic, the other more philosophical. On the one hand it became apparent that it was simply impractical to name one or more alternatives for as many as 2,500 animal substances, many with a number of possible sources or uses.

On the other hand, the question of alternatives to animal ingredients leads down the wrong path; after all, the task at hand is actually to identify vegan commodities in their own right and not to lead a "proxy" life. It is simply the omnipresence of animal products in a society based on animal products that forces us to look for "alternatives."

Therefore, although we decided not to abandon the term "alternatives," we decided not to deal with these only along the lines of the animal ingredients, but to focus on which products vegan consumers will actually look for. We have correspondingly broken down the vegan alternatives into the following categories:

- Food
- Dietary supplements
- Pharmaceutical drugs
- "Pet" food
- Cosmetic products
- Household cleaning products
- Clothing and accessories
- Footwear
- Brushes and brooms
- Interior decoration, household items
- Sport and leisure
- Photography and printing
- Arts and crafts
- Musical instruments
- Electronics and technology

Within each of these categories we have sought to address the most important questions and point out the most important vegan products, without any pretense of completeness. Rather, our major objective is to raise awareness of the possibilities of a vegan way of life.

We want the following pages to be understood as guidance and not as the answer to all questions. We have endeavoured to both provide substantiated and well-researched information and to present it in clear and understandable language. At the same time, we realize that statements that are at least partly based on personal experience will always tend to be subjective.

The decision to live a vegan life is by nature a personal one, based on subjective motives that need not always be the same. Such a decision is also not abstract, but must be lived; therefore a certain subjectivity at this point may be not only inevitable but also necessary.

Food

"So what are you actually allowed you eat?"

What vegan hasn't been asked that question (much too often)? Usually the question is still well-meaning and simply fails to recognize both that being vegan is voluntary and that there is a huge range of fresh, tasty and affordable vegan foods, whether fruit, vegetables, legumes or cereals, and diverse ways of preparing these.

However, as soon as you are dealing with prepackaged or convenience products, there is some truth in the question, as the omnipresence of animal ingredients, especially dairy products, can make shopping very challenging.

Nonetheless, there are foods that are explicitly vegan, including those intended to be alternatives (some say "surrogates" or "substitutes") to products that are not even remotely vegan, such as meat and cheese.

We would like to do some imaginary shopping with you and take a look at the vegan products that are available in the supermarkets, health food stores and mail order or online shops. We will cover basic foods, beverages, desserts, and alternatives to meats and sausages, dairy products and other foods of animal origin.

Bread and pastries

Bread is one of the products you would expect to be vegan, as the basic recipe consists of water, flour, yeast and salt.

However, bread is often made using bread improvers, which often enough are not vegan, e.g. cysteine or fatty acid glycerides. Unfortunately such baking aids need not even be declared. Some breads also have dairy products added, especially white breads and toasting breads. Some sourdough breads may also contain honey.

Those breads most likely to be vegan are whole food or organic breads, as these do not contain such dough improvers, although other nonvegan ingredients may still be used. Therefore you must still pay close attention to the labelling or, if you have the time and inclination, bake your own bread.

If sweet pastries, croissants, etc. happen not to contain butter, they often contain baking margarine instead, which is also used for greasing baking trays. This compound ingredient may seem to be vegan, but it can just as easily contain animal fats.

When it comes down to it, if you don't want to risk consuming any undeclared animal baking aids you may just have to find a baker you can trust or do your own baking.

Butter

Butter is used for spreading on bread and as a baking and cooking ingredient. In both cases vegetable margarine is a good alternative, as long as it contains no dairy components (e.g. whey or yogurt) and no animal vitamin D_3. Such margarines are available in supermarkets and health food stores, and some of them are even explicitly labelled as vegan.

Pasta

Pasta, just like bread, is basically vegan, containing flour or semolina and water. However, eggs are often also added. Fortunately this is always included in the ingredients list and is often emphasized by the manufacturers as a an indicator of quality. This makes it quite easy to dodge such products.

Italian-style pasta made using durum wheat is often vegan, besides generally being some of the best and often also the cheapest pasta. Sometimes other ingredients are added, for example as colourings or flavours. These are usually vegetable (e.g. spinach, turmeric, tomato), but can also be animal, such as sepia (cuttlefish ink) in black pasta.

Filled pastas, such as tortelloni or ravioli, are also available as vegan varieties in health food stores, for instance with spinach, tomato, vegetables, tofu or mushrooms. One should just be careful with regard to dairy, as some meat-free pasta products do contain cheese.

When ordering in restaurants, you should always make sure that the pasta used is in fact vegan, as eggs are also regarded as an indicator of quality in housemade pasta, as is the use of melted butter.

Meat

There is a wide range of meat-like vegan products currently available, whether sausages, cold cuts, steaks, nuggets, mince, goulash, etc. These are usually based on soy protein/tofu, and/or wheat protein (also known as seitan). Such products often emulate the flavour, texture and appearance of conventional meat products.

While they may not be necessary from a purely nutritional point of view and some people (both vegans and nonvegans) reject them as "surrogate" or "pseudo" meat, when it comes down to it, it is simply a matter of taste, and they do have a place within the spectrum of vegan foods.

Some caution must be exercised to make sure that such products are really vegan, however, as there are also vegetarian alternatives to meat that contain egg white or dairy products.

Emulsifier lecithin

It is hard to imagine industrially produced foods without lecithin, which is why it makes sense to take a closer look at it as an individual ingredient, even if it is not a consumer product in its own right but an additive. Lecithin can be animal (from egg yolk), but is usually made from soy, sometimes also from sunflower seeds. If you want to be on the safe side, make sure the ingredients list clearly states that it is soy or sunflower lecithin.

Fats/oils

In addition to butter, other animal fats are processed in conventional foods, usually as lard, tallow or fish oil, whether as a baking or cooking ingredient or for preparing foods (frying, deep frying). Alternatives to solid animal fats are coconut and palm fats (or hydrogenated or esterified vegetable fats). There is also a diverse range of vegetable oils from seeds, nuts and fruits, the best known being sunflower seed, rapeseed and corn oils.

Animal fats in convenience products are often not obviously recognizable, hiding behind long names ending in "fatty acids." Some manufacturers make a point of declaring the fatty acids they use as "vegetable" in the ingredients list, but this is not required. If you want to be on the safe side, keep to organic products or stay away from convenience products not explicitly labelled as vegan.

Eggs

Eggs are not only eaten as food in their own right but also fulfil a number of functions as an ingredient in conventional foods (flavour, as a binding agent or thickener, and for texture) that cannot always be achieved by vegan alternatives due to the specific characteristics of the egg protein. What is most difficult to emulate is egg white foam, making some cakes and sweets much more difficult (e.g. meringue or sponge).

Vegetable binding agents and thickeners can be used instead of egg white, for instance guar gum, locust bean gum (carob gum), starch from a variety of plants, soy flour, xanthan gum, and algae products such as carrageenan, agar-agar and calcium alginate. These are increasingly used in industrially produced foods (including those with no claim to being vegan, but made for "normal" consumers), making it easier to do away with eggs. These alternatives can also be used at home, whether individually or as "egg replacers" (a combination of various binding agents), available for instance in health food stores.

Good alternatives to eggs in baking recipes are mashed ripe bananas or flax seed (add boiling water, soak and purée) .

A good alternative to eggs as a cooking ingredient is tofu (especially the softer silken tofu), with or without one of the aforementioned vegan binding agents.

Milk

Fortunately, animal milk is one of the "products" for which a wide range of vegan alternatives is available almost everywhere, first and foremost as soy milk, but also rice, spelt, oat, nut or hemp milks. Such plant milks are now available in practically every supermarket, discount stores or health food shops, whether unsweetened or sweetened, plain or in a variety of different flavours, organic or fortified with vitamins and minerals.

Soy milk and other plant milks can be used the same way you would use animal milk, whether as a beverage, in breakfast cereals, or for cooking and baking.

Strictly speaking, plant milk may not legally be sold as "milk" (thanks to the animal product lobby), which is why it is often labelled with slightly modified spelling, e.g. "soymilk" instead of "soy milk," or for instance as "soy drink."

Cream

Cream, like eggs, is an animal product whose characteristics significantly depend on the proteins it contains, and for a long time there were no good alternatives. Today, however, a number of different products can be used as coffee cream, whipped topping, or cooking and baking ingredients, so that even vegan cream cakes are possible. These products can be based on soy, rice, cereals or nuts, and are available in health food stores and from vegan mail order companies, and also in some conventional supermarkets.

You can also use coconut milk instead of cream as a cooking ingredient, although the typical coconut flavour doesn't appeal to everybody.

Cheese

Cheese owes its typical characteristics most of all to the milk protein casein, which does not exist in a vegetable form. There are alternatives, however. For instance, you can flavour sauces with brewer's yeast. You can also use nut pastes, tofu and a variety of spices to replace cheese.

And finally, there are in fact ready-to-use vegan alternatives to cheese, usually based on soy, whether in slices, blocks, or as soft cheeses (cream cheese or cottage cheese). These are most easily available in health food and organic stores and some supermarkets, as well as from vegan mail order retailers.

Savoury spreads, pesto, etc.

It almost seems strange to refer to spreads as "alternatives," as this is where vegan cuisine is unparalleled. Nonetheless, there are two reasons to take a closer look. First of all, the range of products is so varied that it can help to make vegan food even more diverse, also because they can be used in all sorts of ways, not just on bread. Spreads with their diversity can especially help fledgling vegans get started. Second, there are also many nonvegan spreads, so that it is worth spotlighting the difference. These nonvegan spreads often contain yogurt or other dairy products, sometimes also eggs or even meat. If you're not careful, the supposedly vegan product you just bought could turn out not to be.

Vegan spreads are usually based on one of three main ingredients: tofu, sunflower seeds or yeast. Depending on the product, additional ingredients can include herbs, spices, fruit or vegetables. Spreads can also consist mainly of various kinds of vegetables.

Besides being used for sandwiches, spreads can also be used instead of cream or cheese for making sauces, as ingredients for dressings and as dips. They can also be used instead of cheese and/or eggs in gratinéed dishes, stuffed dishes, casseroles, etc.

Other spreads of interest to vegans are the spicy spreads based on concentrated yeast or yeast extract, usually fortified with B vitamins. These are for instance Vegex from the United States, Cenovis from Switzerland or Marmite and Vegemite from the United Kingdom, Australia and New Zealand.

Sweet spreads

Alongside jams and jellies, chocolate and nougat spreads are perhaps the most popular sweet spreads. Most of them contain dairy products, even some dark chocolate spreads. However, health food and organic stores and some supermarkets also stock vegan chocolate and nougat spreads. Other vegan sweet spreads include carob spreads, nut pastes and fruit spreads, jams and jellies, as long as they do not contain honey. With regard to the sugar such spreads contain, see below.

Honey

Replacing honey as a sweetener is relatively easy. Besides sugar there are various syrups that can be used on bread and in desserts, e.g. agave syrup, maple syrup, caramel syrup, sugar beet syrup, fruit syrups (apple, pear) and invert sugar syrup. In the case of products based on sugar there is still the risk that the sugar was refined using animal char.

Sugar

Refined sugar may have been purified using activated carbon of animal origin ("animal charcoal" or "bone char"), if it was obtained from sugar cane. Beet sugar does not require this kind of processing and should therefore normally be vegan. As it is not immediately possible to recognize where refined sugar comes from and how it has been processed, the following section deals with available alternatives.

In addition to the controversial artificial sweeteners (e.g. aspartame and saccharin) there is raw cane sugar, available in different grades, from whole cane sugar (dried sugar cane juice) through dark muscovado to natural brown sugar (demerara or turbinado). These sugars are made by crystallizing and/or centrifuging the sugar cane juice more or less in order to remove or keep the molasses and other substances as desired.

Other alternatives are fructose and the aforementioned alternatives to honey, as well as stevia, a natural sweetener obtained from the leaves of the stevia plant, approved as a food additive in a number of countries including the United States and the European Union. Stevia has not yet been approved as a sweetener in Canada, but whole leaves or powder are available for personal culinary use.

Savoury sauces

Many commercially available sauces contain animal substances, but there are also vegan sauces. White sauces (dressings, hollandaise, etc.) are rarely vegan, as they usually contain dairy products. Some sauces (especially the cheaper ones) may be vegan at least as far as the ingredients list goes, e.g. garlic sauces, and grill and barbecue sauces. Sauces explicitly labelled as vegan are most readily available in health food and organic stores, and from vegan mail order companies. Vegan sauces are also very easy to make, for instance using different spreads, soy yogurt (see below), vegan cream, vegetable stock, brewer's yeast, herbs and spices.

Sweet sauces

Conventional sweet sauces (vanilla, chocolate, caramel, etc.) can contain dairy products. You can, however, find some sauces in health food stores and supermarkets that at least according to the ingredients list are vegan.

Yogurt

Many health food stores and supermarkets now stock vegan alternatives to yogurt, sometimes also called "soygurt." These contain the same yogurt cultures as conventional yogurt, but some producers do state that they grow them on vegan culture mediums. Soy yogurt is available both as plain and fruit yogurt.

Mayonnaise

Conventional mayonnaise is an emulsion of oil and vinegar, with egg yolk as an emulsifier, but there are also vegan versions, for instance based on soy or with pea protein as a binding agent. They are most easily available in health food stores or from vegan mail order companies. The same applies to remoulade. You can also make your own mayonnaise by blending vegetable oil, soy milk and vinegar.

Puddings and desserts

You can make vegan pudding using standard pudding powder and plant milk (soy, oat, rice, etc.). However, pay attention to the ingredients list—not every pudding powder is actually vegan. There are also ready-made soy desserts in a variety of flavours, available in many supermarkets, as well as in health food stores and vegan online shops.

Other ready-made desserts often contain gelatin, dairy products or egg, although sometimes vegetable binding agents or soy are used instead. Here you will have to pay close attention to the ingredients list or buy only products labelled as vegan (from health food stores and vegan online shops).

Ice cream

You can find vegan ice cream either as dairy-free sorbets or as soy ice cream. Sorbets are available in ice cream parlours, health food stores or supermarkets, and soy ice cream is most readily available in health food or organic stores, sometimes also in ice cream parlours. When ordering in ice cream parlours it is wise to ask about the ingredients, as some fruit varieties sometimes are made using dairy (i.e. sherbet instead of sorbet).

A great alternative is to make your own ice cream, for instance with an ice cream maker. Ingredients can include fruit, syrups, soy cream and soy yogurt. There are also ready-made dry vegan ice cream mixes that only need water or soy milk added, available in health food stores or from mail order retailers.

Gelling agents and thickeners

Many industrially produced foods contain gelling agents and/or thickeners from a variety of sources. One reason we specifically mention this here is because they are sometimes the subject of misunderstandings. Sometimes the expression "vegetable gelatin" is used, or the term "gelling agent" is equated with "gelatin." In fact, most gelling agents and thickeners are of vegetable origin, e.g. agar-agar, locust bean gum, pectin, sodium alginate or xanthan gum. Only gelatin is always animal and never vegetable.

Beverages (including alcohol)

When it comes to beverages, the devil really is in the details, because a beverage may appear to be vegan going by the ingredients list, but in fact have been treated with animal substances. Substances used as processing aids are not subject to mandatory labelling requirements if they are no longer present in the final product except for "negligible" residues and do not affect its characteristics.

Clear fruit juices may have been "fined" (cleared of clouding substances) for instance with gelatin, egg white or activated carbon. As this is not usually stated on the label, your only options are to either directly ask the producer or stick to naturally cloudy juice (not from concentrate).

Apart from those beverages that obviously contain milk, there are others (e.g. soft drinks, mixed drinks) that may be partly animal, e.g. with honey or cochineal. Industrially produced drinks may contain sugar processed with animal charcoal. Some food additives used may also be of animal origin (see page 241).

Beer can also be fined using animal substances, such as gelatin, isinglass, casein or egg white. Beer brewed in Germany is normally not fined, but may contain some potentially animal additives (lactic acid, caramel colouring). Beer that is brewed according to the German *Reinheitsgebot* ("Purity Law") and correspondingly labelled is always free of any additives, and is therefore always vegan. Otherwise you will have to look out for beers that are labelled as suitable for vegans.

Wine is almost always fined, and usually animal fining agents are used (isinglass, gelatin, casein or egg white). This is often not declared, so that often only directly asking the producer can provide the desired information. Vegan wines are available from online retailers, as well as in some supermarkets and liquor stores. An internet search for vegan wine will lead you to wine growers who produce at least some vegan wines (using mineral, but also vegetable fining agents) and label them as suitable for vegans.

Stronger alcoholic beverages can often be nonvegan. Liqueurs in particular can contain animal ingredients, including cream, honey, eggs or carmine. Animal ingredients are sometimes named and sometimes not—for instance when they're part of compound ingredients or used as processing aids. The sugar often contained may have been refined using animal charcoal. Some liquors, e.g. sake and some brands of vodka, can also be treated with animal substances. To be entirely sure you will need to read the label carefully or ask the producer.

The website _www.barnivore.com_ has a good list of vegan and nonvegan beers, wines and liquors.

In the case of cocktails/mixed drinks (e.g. in bars or at parties), expect them to contain animal products unless you actually know otherwise. In addition to the nonvegan beers, wines, spirits and liqueurs already mentioned, mixed drinks will often have other animal ingredients added, whether dairy products, eggs or honey, or for instance Worcester sauce containing anchovies. To be on the safe side, state beforehand that you want a vegan beverage.

Convenience foods

Prepared or convenience foods play an increasingly prominent role in modern life, whether they be soups, pasta, microwave meals or ready-to-eat desserts. In order to achieve the desired characteristics, food producers often employ a whole arsenal of ingredients and additives, many of which are or can be non-vegan. There is, however, an increasing number of explicitly vegan convenience foods, for instance the alternatives to meat or the soy-based desserts already mentioned. If a product is not labelled as vegan (for instance with one of the logos named from page 256 on), you will have to read the ingredients list—which is exactly where this book comes in handy. The simpler and healthier option is to fall back on unprocessed foods as far as possible or to prepare your own meals.

Dietary supplements

Dietary supplements (which by the way are made for the meat-eating majority of our society, not for vegetarians or vegans!) often contain animal ingredients, especially fatty acids and vitamins from animal fat tissues, e.g. fish liver or tallow. The source is generally stated specifically, but not out of any sense of duty, but rather because in the case of supplements the animal source is often regarded as a guarantee for the quality of the nutrients contained.

The best "alternative" to food supplements is a diverse diet that provides all the nutrients you need on its own. The health benefits of many dietary supplements are medically questionable anyway, and if genuine deficiencies should arise, they are more a case for your medical practitioner than for the drugstore.

One exception is vitamin B_{12}, of which vegan foods contain none or very little if they are not artificially fortified. The question as to whether the human body is able to provide itself with sufficient vitamin B_{12} via its own bowel bacteria is debated, and environmental organisms ("contamination") as a possible source would also seem uncertain in the light of our sanitized modern way of life. If you don't use fortified foods, it is advisable to take a vitamin B_{12} supplement, available as vegan drops, drinks and capsules, for instance in drugstores or by mail order.

Another possible exception is vitamin D. Normally the human body is able to meet its own needs as long as the skin is exposed to sufficient sunlight. However, in most of North America (and all of Canada), the sunlight is too weak during the winter months to guarantee an adequate production of vitamin D. This affects vegans and nonvegans alike, by the way. In addition, many people spend too little time outdoors even in the summer, so vitamin D production may in fact be insufficient throughout the whole year. Therefore, if you are unable to build up enough vitamin D during the summer to last the whole year, it might be a good idea to take a vitamin D supplement. However, you will need to be careful that it does not contain animal vitamin D_3. There are vegan supplements with vitamin D_2, which is biotechnologically obtained from a precursor present in fungi, although this variant is said not to be as easily accessible for our bodies. However, there are now also vegan vitamin D supplements available that contain vitamin D_3 (the variant produced in our bodies and best suited to our needs) from non-animal sources.

Pharmaceutical drugs

It can be especially difficult for vegans to make decisions about taking medical drugs, because—unlike in other areas of life—it is no longer simply about how you choose to lead your life, but about your own health, in the worst case even a question of life or death.

There are a lot of drugs that can contain animal substances, and there are even some that always do. Sometimes the active ingredients are animal, but more often the excipients (nonmedicinal ingredients such as carriers, stabilizers or bulking agents) are, especially in tablets. Perhaps the most commonly used substance is lactose, used as a carrier and bulking agent. Alternatives are starch, cellulose and other binding agents; many tablets are now lactose-free. Other substances used are gelatin (especially in capsules, but also in pills and tablets), cochineal (carmine) and shellac, as well as substances based on fatty acids, especially magnesium stearate (binding agent in tablets), which can be either of animal or vegetable origin.

Examples of potentially animal active ingredients include insulin (can come from cattle or pigs, however now these variants are normally only used for people who have used such insulins for many years and would experience problems adjusting to nonanimal insulin), anticoagulants (especially heparin), amino acid infusions (drip feeds), hormone preparations (e.g. calcitonin) and vitamin products (e.g. vitamin D). Finding vegan alternatives to such products can sometimes be very difficult, or even entirely unsuccessful.

Heparin, for instance, is obtained from the internal organs of slaughtered pigs and is used as subcutaneous injections after surgery and accidents, and for bed-ridden patients, in order to prevent life-threatening blood clots (thromboses). There are also animal-free alternatives, such as the synthetic anticoagulant fon-daparinux or genetically engineered hirudin, but these are normally only used when there are medical reasons for not using heparin, which is still the standard therapy.

Since deciding whether or not to use a specific drug can depend on many fac-tors, even without considering where its substances come from, and such a deci-sion normally can only be made in consultation with a medical practitioner, we cannot deal with the subject in any greater depth. The statements made here are intended simply to point out problematic issues. The search for vegan medicine and any decision for or against certain drugs should be discussed by doctor and patient case by case.

In the case of nonprescription drugs (cold medicine, ointments, etc.), the tips in this section and the entries in this book's ingredients list can help you find suitable vegan medicine based on the legally required ingredient declaration.

"Pet" food

There are few topics that can polarize as much as the question of whether do-mestic animals ("pets"), whose diet normally partly or completely consists of the flesh of other killed animals, can or even should be fed vegan food. For some people, animal rights considerations make it unacceptable to support the kill-ing of animals by feeding domestic animals conventional animal food, whereas others denounce feeding normally carnivorous animals with vegan food as being inappropriate to the animals' biological needs. Sometimes even a kind of role reversal can take place, with consumers of animal products (meat-eaters) accus-ing ethically (animal-rights) motivated vegans of endangering the well-being of animals.

We have consciously decided not to address the question of whether "keep-ing" domestic animals is at all reconcilable with a vegan way of life. We assume that the animals are simply there (for whatever reasons), and will deal only with the practical question, whether and how they can be fed vegan food from a biological point of view.

We will also not address animals' natural hunting behaviour and treat this too as a given.

We unequivocally reject keeping animals in terrariums, aquariums or cages. For this reason we deliberately will not discuss foods for any such animals.

For the main part this section is about cats and dogs, as other mammals typically kept at home can normally be fed an entirely vegetable diet without any difficulties. It is, however, worth pointing out that some food for small animals does contain animal fat (e.g. lard in food balls).

Dogs generally can be fed vegan food without any problems, as all the nutrients they require are also available in vegetable foods. There are, however, also special vegan dog foods. Feeding cats a vegan diet is not possible without further ado, as they cannot synthesize the (for them essential) amino acid taurine themselves and normally have to ingest it with their food (prey). Feeding cats a vegan diet is only possible as long as vegan cat foods fortified with sufficient synthetic taurine are used. There are vegan complete foods for both cats and dogs, suited to their respective needs (e.g. by mail order).

Prepared meat "substitutes" intended for human consumption are not suitable for animals and may even be dangerous.

Cosmetic products

The biggest problem involved in evaluating cosmetic ingredients is the fact that there is a barely imaginable number of approved and theoretically usable substances for any conceivable function (surfactants, skin conditioners, soothing agents, plasticizers, etc.). The complete CTFA/INCI ingredients list covers several hundred letter-size pages!

We originally intended to name the most important vegan ingredients for each cosmetic function. However, it soon became apparent that naming useful vegan alternatives for each animal ingredient was almost impossible, especially since that would have meant listing as many as fifty possible alternatives for a single ingredient, which wouldn't have left the reader any wiser.

At the same time, it is important to note that some ingredients are normally of vegetable origin, but principally can also be of animal origin, depending on production methods and current technical developments. The substances used in any given case depend on the producer's criteria. Organic or conventional agriculture? Native or imported? Vegetable, animal or synthetic? As natural as possible? As effective as possible? As cheap as possible?

In addition to that, cosmetic products usually consist of several ingredients, so that judging a single product only according to the ingredients list and looking for alternatives can end up being an almost hopeless endeavour.

For these reasons, distinct labelling of final products is the easiest and surest way—and probably also the only practicable way— of recognizing vegan cosmetics. For this reason we refer you to the section "Seals, logos and labels" (pages 256–263).

Household cleaning products

In the absence of legally binding labelling requirements for household cleaning products, it would be impossible to judge whether a product contains ingredients of animal origin.

Fortunately, the voluntary labelling guidelines developed by North American industry organizations (see page 250) provide for labelling along the lines of cosmetics labelling. As the number of ingredients in a household cleaning product tends to be less than in cosmetic products, this can make recognizing vegan products somewhat easier than with cosmetics.

That said, you can only be really sure by buying products labelled as vegan, for example with a vegan logo or detailed declaration that includes the origin of the individual ingredients, or by directly asking the producers. Some producers (for instance organic producers) do in fact go further than required by the guidelines and provide additional information on their labels, such as "vegetable alcohol" or "sugar surfactants."

Clothing and accessories

Most clothing items are made from cotton, a purely vegetable fibre. However, conventional cotton is grown in monocultures that are highly susceptible to pests. These pests are combated using massive amounts of highly toxic pesticides, with devastating and even lethal effects on the environment, humans and other animals, so that conventionally grown cotton is not only ecologically harmful, but also strictly speaking not even vegan.

An alternative is organically grown cotton. This is still a niche product, but its share of the market is on the rise.

Some items of clothing are made partly or completely of animal products, especially shoes, jackets, sweaters, belts, gloves, scarves, ties and blouses. The animal materials used are usually skins ("leather"), wool, hair, and silk.

Buttons and accessories can also be made from from seashells, mother of pearl, bone, horn and antlers.

Alternatives to animal hair or wool are vegetable and synthetic fibres. You can find lists of these fibres on pages 252–253.

Footwear

Perhaps the hardest part of finding vegan clothing is the search for leather-free footwear. Leather is still generally seen as standing for quality, whereas shoes made from synthetic materials are often (unfortunately not always wrongly) regarded as being inferior "plastic." Therefore shoe shops still stock relatively few leather-free shoes. Those shoes that are leather-free are often made of fabric and do not offer real protection in cold or wet weather.

There is, however, an increasing number of synthetic leather shoes in shoe shops, department stores and clothing chain stores. One advantage of these shoes is the often low price, although their range and quality can vary considerably. Also, although the leather is synthetic, it is not always possible to know with certainty that such shoes are vegan, because the adhesives used, for instance, could theoretically be made using animal bones or skins. On the other hand, synthetic adhesives are so ubiquitous and inexpensive that you can rely on the cheap shoes really being free of animal adhesives. Unfortunately, the lack of mandatory labelling for footwear (see page 255) makes it hard to be absolutely sure with regard to the remaining materials.

The best option is to buy unequivocally vegan shoes. By now there is an excellent range of vegan shoes made using quality synthetic materials. These come from a number of companies around the world (in Europe, Australia and North America) who make them (or have them made) using cruelty-free materials, and who also pay attention to fair working conditions and ecological considerations. The comfort and quality of such shoes are in no way inferior to conventional leather shoes, and they are generally no more expensive than comparable leather shoes. Vegan shoes are available from vegan mail order companies and even in vegan retail stores in larger cities.

Brushes and brooms

You can find many products in the house that at least traditionally have been made using animal hair or bristles: brooms, scrubbing brushes, shoe brushes, paint brushes, hairbrushes, make-up brushes, shaving brushes, etc. They can be made using pig bristles, or the hair of badgers, martens, weasels or squirrels.

Good alternatives are brushes with synthetic hairs or bristles, which have already largely replaced the traditional bristles in modern households, or vegetable fibres such as coconut or sisal. Painting brushes with animal hair are still commonly used, but there are also quality brushes with synthetic hair (for instance nylon). Shaving brushes are still usually made with badger hair, but shaving brushes with synthetic hair are also available.

Interior decoration and household items

A household can contain many animal substances. For example, blankets, sheets and covers can contain wool, silk and hair (for instance from camels, llamas and goats), and quilts, pillows, mattresses and seating may be stuffed with feathers, down and wool.

The best alternative for bedclothes in general is cotton, with the reservation regarding pesticides already stated in the section "Clothing and accessories." When buying blankets, sheets and covers you can choose between a variety of vegetable and synthetic fibres instead of wool, hair or silk, whether as woven fabric or fleece (also see pages 252–253).

A cheap and widespread alternative to pillows and cushions with animal fillings are those filled with synthetic hollow fibres. You can also buy quilted blankets with plant fibres, for instance kapok (also known as vegetable down), the hollow fibre from the seeds of the tropical kapok tree. Kapok is used for making a light fleece with excellent insulating properties and is also especially suitable for allergy sufferers. There are also quilts and pillows available that are filled with cotton or foam flocks.

Mattresses are available in a variety of vegetable and synthetic materials, also with different combinations for different properties such as warmth, elasticity and firmness. Some of the materials used are rubber/latex, kapok, coconut fibres, grasses, straw, cotton and a range of synthetic foam materials.

Both the covers and the padding of seating furniture can be animal, whether leather/hide, wool or hair. Alternatives are the same as with mattresses.

Carpets and mats often contain wool, sometimes also silk. Alternatives are carpets with plant fibres (e.g. sisal, coir [coconut] or seagrass) or synthetic pile.

Wooden furniture can contain animal substances both in the joints (e.g. casein, bone or hide glue) and the surface treatment (shellac or beeswax in varnishes, waxes and sealants). Alternatives are furniture with screw joints or synthetic glues, as well as vegetable or synthetic waxes, oils and varnishes.

Animal materials are also used in general furnishing, decorative and utility objects, for instance silk, wool, leather or capiz shells in lamp shades; silk in curtains; or bone, horn or mother of pearl in handles, buttons and all kinds of ornaments. Alternatives are various kinds of synthetic materials and woods, as well as vegetable and synthetic fibres.

Fine tableware can be made of bone china, porcelain that contains bone ash. This is characterized by its particularly pure white and high translucency. Alternatives are earthenware and porcelain, provided the porcelain is solely mineral in origin. The latter is often recognizable by its slightly creamy white.

General cleaning and polishing utensils, such as chamois leather, dusters and cloths, can be made of real leather, animal hair (especially wool) or feathers. Inexpensive alternatives consist of synthetic fibres, such as in microfibre cloth.

Sport and leisure

Equipment for sport and leisure encompasses some areas that have already been covered, especially clothing and footwear. In the case of some sports, however, it's not just a matter of clothing in general but also specific protective clothing, which can be made of or include leather.

Beyond that, there are the objects typical to each type of sport, such as balls and bats. Some sports, such as football, soccer, rugby, handball, baseball, hockey and cricket, use leather balls, although they are sometimes replaced by synthetic balls.

In sports that use bats and rackets, leather (e.g. handles), gut strings (e.g. tennis and badminton rackets) and feathers (e.g. the shuttlecock in badminton) may be used.

Archery traditionally uses a number of animal materials. The bowstring can be real sinews or gut; the arrows can have real feathers; and the quiver, arm guards and fingertabs can be leather. The bow itself can partly be made of horn.

In many cases, animal materials in sports equipment have been partly or completely replaced by a variety of high-tech materials (e.g. microfibres, polymers, fibreglass or carbon fibres). However, certain animal materials (e.g. gut) are still often regarded as superior and therefore preferred, especially in top-level sports.

In most cases it is possible to find alternatives, although in the case of team sports convincing both sides to switch to vegan gear probably won't be easy.

The sports named here are only a few examples from the diverse world of sport. There are also some kinds of "sport" that are absolutely not vegan, such as equestrian sports and greyhound racing. Here there can be no alternative other than boycotting them.

Arts and crafts

Arts and crafts have traditionally involved the use of animal substances. This is often still the case, although the number of quality vegan alternatives is rising.

Paintbrushes are most commonly animal (see "Brushes and brooms" on page 283), but painting surfaces are also still often treated with animal substances, e.g. rabbit-skin glue, bone glue or casein on canvases.

Paper used for drawings, paintings and prints can also often contain animal glue as a binding agent or surface treatment.

Varnishes for oil paintings can contain shellac or beeswax.

Artists' colours can also have added beeswax (oil paints or wax crayons) or honey (watercolour). Tempera painting uses egg yolks or casein as emulsifiers for the paint mixtures.

Some paint pigments used to be obtained from animals, e.g. carmine red from scale insects or Tyrian purple from sea snails. These pigments are now rarely used in artists' paints. Industrially produced pigments are either mineral, vegetable or synthetic. Ink can however still contain real cuttlefish ink (sepia) and shellac.

Shellac is also used as a fixative for pastel and pencil drawings.

Printmaking (etching) can involve the use of shellac or tallow in the printing plates' acid-resistant ground. Also, rollers and so-called tampons with leather surfaces are used to transfer the ink to the paper.

Sometimes real sponges are used for watercolour painting. Man-made sponges, for instance made out of cellulose, are available as an alternative.

Finely woven silk is used as a painting surface. Silk was also formerly used in silkscreen printing, but nylon gauze is now used instead. Silk is still used in textile art, as is wool, for making felt and in knitwear and weaving.

Adhesives commonly used in arts and crafts often contain animal glue, and varnishes, waxes and paints can also contain shellac or beeswax. Synthetic adhesives and varnishes are available as suitable alternatives.

In addition to the brushes already mentioned, some rollers have animal hide. Leather is used both as a material and in tools and equipment (straps and belts, bags, handles, polishing surfaces). Alternatives are textiles with vegetable or synthetic fibres, e.g. microfibres, synthetic fleeces and fabrics.

Materials traditionally used in sculpting and carving are not only wood and stone, but also horn, bone and ivory. An alternative is "vegetable ivory," from the seeds of ivory-nut palm trees. A material commonly used for modelling is beeswax.

Although so many animal materials are used, contemporary artists nonetheless have a wide range of nonanimal materials and utensils to choose from, whether brushes and rollers with synthetic fibres; primers, paints, solvents and varnishes based on vegetable and/or synthetic oils and resins; or papers without animal glues.

Photography and printing

Up to the present day, gelatin is part of the colour-carrying layer in photographic negatives and photographic papers, making vegan photography very difficult, especially if you want prints of your photos. Digital photography has asserted itself in recent years, but photo prints are still printed on paper that contains gelatin—both in commercial printing services and at home.

One alternative is printing on "normal" paper, which is admittedly less pleasing, or the use of digital photo frames, although the screens themselves potentially could contain animal substances (see page 287).

Another possibility is the use of quality artists' papers without a layer containing gelatin, whereby these could also contain animal glue. In the end, the only way to be sure is to ask the paper manufacturer.

Musical instruments

For instruments that are still traditionally made, animal materials are often integral components and even responsible for the respective instruments' typical characteristics.

This makes it especially difficult to find alternatives to at least some musical instruments.

Good examples are the bowed string instruments (violin, viola, cello and double bass). The components are made of wood stuck together using hide glues, the varnish often contains shellac and/or propolis, and the bows are strung with horsehair. As far as we know, no traditionally made bowed string instruments are made without animal substances.

Rather expensive acoustic alternatives to traditionally made bowed string instruments are high-quality carbon fibre instruments. Alternatives that are less expensive include electric instruments in various price categories and made from a variety of materials such as fibreglass, carbon fibres or wood. Instead of horsehair, synthetic fibres can be used as bow strings.

In addition to animal glues and varnishes, plucked string instruments (e.g. guitar, lute, mandolin, harp) are made using gut strings, bone (saddle), horn (bridge) and leather (strap).

Alternatives are acoustic instruments made without animals glues (as far as this is ascertainable), with straps made of synthetic leather or vegan textiles, and with synthetic varnish, strings, saddles and bridges. Other alternatives are electric instruments made from different materials such as fibreglass, carbon fibres, metal or solid wood.

The skins of some percussion instruments (drums) are made from animal skins, however modern percussion instruments normally use synthetic skins.

Traditionally, white piano keys were made of ivory. The keys of modern instruments are normally made of synthetic materials, especially since trading in ivory is almost entirely banned. Only the keys of very expensive instruments may be made of legal ivory.

Ornamental parts of instruments in general can be made of horn, bone, leather and mother of pearl.

Electronics and technology

Animal substances can even be present in all kinds of technical appliances or be used for their production. For instance, the liquid crystals in LCD screens and displays (televisions, computers, cell phones, information screens, digital picture frames, etc.) may be based on cholesterol.

Gelatin is often used in metal processing in order to improve the quality of the metal structure. This can for instance be the case with cadmium in batteries or copper in circuits. Even the zinc in galvanized steel (e.g. in the casings of household appliances) can be processed with the help of gelatin. Bone ash may also be used in metal processing.

These are just two examples of how substances of animal origin pervade our modern society. In fact, substances such as gelatin, but also animal fats in the form of emulsifiers and surfactants, are employed in many other technical applications to which we owe the comforts of our way of life—whether they be the metals already mentioned or foams, plastics, etc.

At present it is extremely difficult—if not impossible—to find alternatives, but perhaps the following remarks may be helpful.

Closing remarks

Especially the aforementioned appliances and seemingly innocuous objects that surround us in everyday life quickly bring us to the limits of our ability to make decisions, because these are concealed technical production processes that we as consumers can hardly be aware of or understand, and that are very rarely declared in any way.

However, this does not mean that we have no influence on this state of affairs, because we can in fact make a considerable difference in two ways.

First, we can be conscious consumers. We don't need a new cell phone every year or the newest television set, even if we can afford them. Functioning appliances don't need to be replaced just because they are a bit older. If we have to use products that might contain (or have been made using) animal substances, and if we are not able to find alternatives, then we can at least keep the consumption down. Our conscious consumption can change the demand.

Second, "hidden" animal substances are part of a macroeconomic exploitation of animals. The more animal body parts, body fluids and excretions are used, the more profitable are the breeding, keeping and killing of animals overall. Conversely, every reduction in the demand for obviously animal "products" means that the exploitation becomes less profitable overall, until at some stage it may become necessary to search for alternatives to animal substances. Thus we can even indirectly influence the profitability of products we don't even use ourselves.

Our overall behaviour decides whether animals are exploited for our purposes. Each decision for a vegan alternative makes a difference that contributes to reducing or even completely preventing the suffering of sentient living beings.

VEGANISSIMO A to Z

Part 4

References and Resources

- *Glossary*
- *Bibliography*
- *Online resources*
- *Canadian legislation*

Abrasive Removes materials from various body surfaces or aids mechanical tooth cleaning or improves gloss.

Absorbent Takes up water- and/or oil-soluble dissolved or finely dispersed substances.

Anticaking agent Allows free flow of solid particles and thus avoids agglomeration of powders into lumps or hard masses. Used in moulding processes as release agent to avoid adhesion of mould and parts or to permanently separate parts.

Anticorrosive Prevents corrosion of the packaging.

Antifoaming agent Suppresses foaming during or after production.

Antimicrobial Helps control the growth of micro-organisms. *Also see "Preservative."*

Antioxidant Inhibits reactions promoted by oxygen and preserves by retarding deterioration, rancidity, or discolouration due to oxidation. *Also see "Preservative."*

Antidandruff Helps control dandruff.

Antiperspirant Reduces sweating.

Antiseborrheic Helps control sebum production (oily skin secretion).

Antistatic Reduces static electricity by neutralizing electrical charge on a surface (e.g. hair).

Astringent Contracts the skin.

Binding agent Provides cohesion in cosmetics that contain powdery substances.

Bleach, bleaching agent Lightens the shade of hair or skin, lighten or decolour textiles.

Bleaching, maturing, and dough conditioning agents Act on flour to produce a product of consistent quality and colour. Bleaching and maturing agents hasten the oxidation and aging processes. Dough conditioners improve the handling properties of the dough and reduce mixing time, resulting in better texture, volume, and crumb evenness.

Buffering agent Stabilizes the acidity of cosmetics. *In foods also "pH-adjusting agent."*

Bulking agent Reduces bulk density of cosmetics, increases the volume of mixed substances without altering their main properties.

Carriers or extraction solvents Substances used to dissolve, dilute, disperse or otherwise physically modify food additives, flavours, enzymes, nutrients or other substances without changing their function (and without exerting a technological effect itself), or to enable the extraction of substances from food.

Chelating agent Reacts and forms complexes with metal ions which could affect the stability and/or appearance of cosmetics. *Also known as "sequestering agent."*

Cleansing substance Helps to keep the body surface clean.

Colourant/Colouring agent Colour that gives foods or cosmetics an appetizing/attractive appearance.

Denaturant Renders cosmetics unpalatable, so that they cannot be eaten or drunk.

Deodorant Reduces or masks unpleasant body odours.

Depilatory Removes unwanted body hair.

Derivative A substance that is obtained from another substance or is formed from that substance via chemical processes.

Detangling Reduces or eliminates hair intertwining due to hair surface alteration or damage and thus helps combing.

Dietetic foods Foods for a defined group of persons and special dietary requirements, with a distinct difference to foods for general consumption, e.g. solid food for infants or food for persons with metabolic disorders.

Emollient Softens and smoothes the skin.

Emulsifier Promotes the formation of finely dispersed mixtures (emulsions) of normally immiscible liquids by altering their interfacial tension.

Emulsifying salt Rearranges cheese proteins in the manufacture of processed cheese, in order to prevent fat separation.

Emulsion Finely dispersed mixture of two normally unblendable liquids (e.g. water and oil).

Essential Denomination for substances that the body cannot produce and must therefore be supplied with the diet, e.g. certain amino acids, fatty acids, minerals and vitamins.

Excipient A substance that in itself is inactive, but has the function of supporting an active agent or facilitating its application, for instance as a bulking agent, carrier (see above) or coating substance in pharmaceutical drugs.

Film forming agent Produces, upon application, a continuous film on skin, hair or nails.

Fining The removal of undesired opacifying substances (floating particles, organic compounds such as carbohydrates or proteins) from wine or other beverages. Fining agents (e.g. activated carbon, silicates or animal proteins) bind the opacifying substances to their surface and precipitate with them to the bottom of the vessel.

Firming agent Food additive that maintains the texture of various foods, such as processed or prepared fruits, vegetables and fish products, which would otherwise go soft as a result of heat treatment during processing.

Flavour enhancer Enhances the flavour of foods without adding a flavour of its own.

Foam boosting agent Improves the quality of the foam produced by a system by increasing one or more of the following properties: volume, texture and/or stability.

Foaming agent Traps numerous small bubbles of air or other gas within a small volume of liquid by modifying the surface tension of the liquid. Ensures that foamed foods (such as cream or pudding) remain appetizing, light and fluffy, and palatable for longer periods.

Food enzyme Enzyme used to promote desirable chemical reactions in food.

Gel forming agent Gives the consistency of a gel (a semisolid preparation with some elasticity) to a liquid preparation.

Gelling agent Food additive used to thicken and stabilize various foods. Provides the foods with texture through formation of a gel. Some stabilizers and thickening agents are gelling agents.

Glazing and polishing agents Food additives that give foods a shiny appearance or protective coating, preventing loss of aroma, flavour or humidity, and extending shelf life.

Hair conditioner Leaves the hair easy to comb, supple, soft and shiny and/or imparts volume, lightness, gloss, etc.

Hair fixing agent Permits physical control of hairstyle.

Hair waving or straightening substance Modifies the chemical structure of the hair, allowing it to be set in the style required.

Humectant Holds and retains moisture in the skin or cosmetic product, or in foods.

Hydrogenation Process by which organic substances are exposed to and saturated by the gas hydrogen. Most commonly used in the food industry for converting liquid vegetable oils into solid or semisolid fats, for instance in margarine.

Hydrolysis Splitting of chemical compounds under the influence of water, usually in the presence of a catalyst (such as an acid) or an enzyme.

Hydrotrope Enhances the solubility of a substance that is only slightly soluble in water.

Keratolytic Helps eliminate the dead cells of the *stratum corneum* (outer skin layer).

Masking agent Reduces or inhibits the basic odour or taste of the product.

Minerals Naturally occurring inorganic nutrients, e.g. calcium, potassium, magnesium and sodium.

Miscellaneous agents Include a variety of food additives, e.g. carbonating agents in soft drinks, plasticizing agents (*see "Plasticizer"*), clarifying agents in beer (*see "Fining"*), deodorizing agents in fats and oils, foaming agents in beverages, and tableting aids.

Moisturizer Increases the water content of the skin and helps keep it soft and smooth.

Opacifier Reduces transparency or translucency of cosmetics.

Oral care Provides cosmetic effects to the mouth, e.g. cleansing, deodorizing, protecting.

Oxidizing agent Changes the chemical nature of another substance by adding oxygen or removing hydrogen.

Pearlescent Imparts a nacreous (pearl-like) appearance to cosmetics.

pH-adjusting agent Food additive that changes or maintains the desired pH value (acidity or alkalinity) of a foodstuff. *In cosmetics also known as a "buffering agent."*

Plasticizer Softens and makes supple another substance that otherwise could not be easily deformed, spread or worked out.

Polishing agent see "Glazing agent."

Preservative Used to prevent or delay spoilage in food, caused by microbial growth or enzymatic and chemical actions. *Also see "Antimicrobial" and "Antioxidant."*

Pressure-dispensing agent Acts as propellant to dispense foods such as whipped toppings from aerosol containers.

Raising agent Substance that incorporates gas bubbles (usually carbon dioxide) in dough, thus raising and leavening it.

Reducing agent Changes the chemical nature of another substance by adding hydrogen or removing oxygen.

Refatting agent Replenishes the lipids of the hair or of the top layers of the skin.

Release agent Helps food separate from surfaces during or after manufacturing.

Sequestering agent Combines with metallic elements in food, thereby preventing their taking part in reactions leading to colour or flavour deterioration.

Skin conditioner Maintains the skin in good condition.

Skin protecting substance Helps to avoid harmful effects to the skin from external factors.

Smoothing agent Used to achieve an even skin surface by decreasing the skin's roughness or irregularities.

Solvent Dissolves other substances.

Soothing agent Helps relieve discomfort of the skin or of the scalp.

Stabilizer Improves ingredients or formulation stability and shelf life.

Starch-modifying agent Alters the property of starch in order to enable it to withstand heat processing and freezing and thus maintain the appearance and consistency of foods.

Surfactant Lowers the surface tension of liquids, aids the even distribution of cosmetic products. In laundry detergents, surfactants raise the solubility of fat and dirt particles.

Sweetener Additive (other than conventional nutritive sweeteners such as sucrose, fructose, or glucose) that imparts a sweet taste to foods or is used as a tabletop sweetener.

Tanning agent Darkens the skin with or without exposure to ultraviolet light.

Texture-modifying agent Contributes to or maintain desirable consistency in foods.

Thickening agent Substance used to adjust the consistency of processed products. Binds water and increases the viscosity of mixtures without substantially modifying their other properties. Provides body, increases stability, and improves suspending action.

Tonic Produces a feeling of well-being on skin and hair.

UV absorber Protects the cosmetic product from the effects of ultraviolet light.

UV filter Filters certain ultraviolet rays in order to protect the skin or the hair from harmful effects of these rays.

Viscosity Measure of the thickness of a fluid. The greater the viscosity, the greater the thickness.

Viscosity controller Increases or decreases the viscosity *(see above)* of cosmetics.

Viscous Having a high viscosity *(see above)*.

Wetting agent Surfactant *(see above)* used to achieve a better distribution of liquids on surfaces or materials.

Whipping agent Assists in the production and maintenance of stable whipped products.

Yeast foods Substances that serve as nutrients for yeasts such as those used in the manufacture of beer and in the making of bread.

Bibliography

Allen, Sam. *Classic Finishing Techniques*. Hannover: New York: Sterling, 1995.

Bährle-Rapp, Marina. *Springer Lexikon Kosmetik und Körperpflege*. Heidelberg: Springer Medizin Verlag, 2007.

Baltes, Werner. *Lebensmittelchemie*. Berlin/Heidelberg: Springer, 2007.

Beament, James: *The Violin Explained: Components, Mechanism, and Sound*. Oxford: Oxford University Press, 2000.

Belitz, Hans-Dieter, Werner Grosch, and Peter Schieberle. *Food Chemistry*. Berlin/Heidelberg: Springer, 2009.

Blaschek, Wolfgang. *Hagers Handbuch der Pharmazeutischen Praxis, Folgeband 8, Stoffe E–O*. Berlin: Springer, 1993.

Brockmann, Walter, Paul L. Geiß, Jürgen Klingen, and Bernhard Schröder. *Klebtechnik: Klebstoffe, Anwendungen und Verfahren*. Weinheim: Wiley-VCH, 2005.

Bundesverband Deutscher Industrie- und Handelsunternehmen for Arzneimittel, Reformwaren, Nahrungsergänzungsmittel und Körperpflegemittel (BDIH). *Be Natural*. Mannheim: BDIH, 2010.

Burczyk, Frank, and Aggy Gianni. *Kosmetiklexikon Inhaltsstoffe von A–Z*. Munich: Ehrenwirth, 1999.

Canadian General Standards Board. *Organic Production Systems General Principles and Management Standards*. Gatineau: Canadian General Standards Board, 2006.

Chou, Chung Chi. *Handbook of Sugar Refining: A Manual for the Design and Operation of Sugar Refining Facilities*. New York: John Wiley & Sons, 2000.

Coalition for Consumer Information on Cosmetics. *The Corporate Standard of Compassion for Animals*. Philadelphia: Coalition for Consumer Information on Cosmetics, 2009.

Demeter-International e. V. *Production Standards for the Use of Demeter, Biodynamic and Related Trademarks*. Darmstadt: Demeter-International e. V., 2011.

Eisenbrand, Gerhard, and Peter Schreier. *RÖMPP Lexikon Lebensmittelchemie*. Stuttgart: Thieme, 2006.

Eising, Susi, Martina Görlach, and Odette Teubner. *Das große Buch der Meeresfrüchte*. Munich: Gräfe und Unzer, 2005.

Elmadfa, Ibrahim, Erich Muskat, and Doris Fritzsche. *GU Kompass E-Nummern und Zusatzstoffe*. Munich: Gräfe und Unzer, 2009.

Goffer, Zvi. *Archaeological Chemistry*. Hoboken: John Wiley & Sons, 2007.

Hamer, Frank, and Janet Hamer. *The Potter's Dictionary of Materials and Techniques*. Philadelphia: University of Pennsylvania Press, 2004.

Health Canada. *Food Additive Dictionary*. Ottawa: Health Canada, 2006.

Health Canada. *Guide to Cosmetic Ingredient Labelling*. Ottawa: Health Canada, 2009.

Health Canada. *Labelling Guidance Document*. Ottawa: Health Canada, 2006.

Hess Natur-Textilien GmbH. *Hess Natur Catalog Fall/Winter 2012*. Butzbach: Hess Natur-Textilien GmbH, 2012.

Industrieverband Körperpflege- und Waschmittel e. V. (IKW). *Das NaTrue-Siegel - Bio- und Naturkosmetik, der Sie vertrauen können*. Frankfurt am Main: IKW, 2009.

Industrieverband Körperpflege- und Waschmittel e. V. (IKW). *Faktenblatt Wasch- und Reinigungsmittel*. Frankfurt am Main: IKW, 2007.

Industrieverband Körperpflege- und Waschmittel e. V. (IKW). *Kosmetika - Inhaltsstoffe - Funktionen*. Frankfurt am Main: IKW, 2005.

Johannes Gerstaecker Verlag. *Gerstaecker Hauptkatalog 2012/2013*. Eitorf: Johannes Gerstaecker Verlag, 2012.

Kremer Pigments Inc. *Kremer Pigments Catalog*. New York: Kremer Pigments Inc., 2009.

Kugler, Eduard. *Geigenbau - die Faszination*. Norderstedt: Books on Demand, 2008.

Meindertsma, Christien. *PIG 05049*. Rotterdam: FLOCKS, 2007.

Minoggio, Markus. *Was der Körper wirklich braucht: Über Nahrungsergänzungsmittel, Vitamine und Pseudoprodukte*. Vienna: Goldegg, 2008.

Müssig, Jörg. *Industrial Applications of Natural Fibres: Structure, Properties and Technical Applications*. Chichester, UK: Wiley, 2010.

ÖKO-TEST-Verlag GmbH: *Ökotest Kompass E-Nummern*. Frankfurt am Main: ÖKO-TEST-Verlag GmbH, 2009.

ÖKO-TEST-Verlag GmbH. *Ökotest Kosmetik-Liste*. Frankfurt am Main: ÖKO-TEST-Verlag GmbH, 2010.

Peden, James A. *Vegetarian Cats and Dogs*. Troy, MT: Harbingers of a New Age, 1999/2011.

Phillips, Clive J. C. *Principles of Cattle Production*. Wallingford, UK: CABI, 2010.

Pötzsch, Bernd, and Katharina Madlener. *Gerinnungskonsil: Rationelle Diagnostik und Therapie von Gerinnungsstörungen*. Stuttgart: Thieme, 2002.

Rote Liste Service GmbH. *Rote Liste 2012*. Frankfurt am Main: Rote Liste Service GmbH, 2012.

Salmang, Hermann, and Horst Scholze. *Keramik*. Berlin: Springer, 2006.

Schartl, Manfred, Manfred Gessler, and Arnold von Eckardstein. *Biochemie und Molekularbiologie des Menschen*. Munich: Urban & Fischer, 2009.

Silva, H. M., C. J. Wilcox, A. H. Spurlock, F. G. Martin, and R. B. Becker. "Factors Affecting Age at First Parturition, Life Span, and Vital Statistics of Florida Dairy Cows." *Journal of Dairy Science* Vol. 69 (2) (1986): 470–476.

Southgate, Paul C., and John S. Lucas. *The Pearl Oyster*. New York: Elsevier, 2008.

Ternes, Waldemar, Alfred Täufel, Liselotte Tunger, and Martin Zobel. *Lebensmittellexikon*. Hamburg: Behr's Verlag, 2005.

Teut, Michael, Jörn Dahler, Christina Lucae, and Ulrich Koch. *Kursbuch Homöopathie*. Munich: Urban & Fischer, 2008.

Vandamme, Erick J. (ed.). *Biotechnology of Vitamins, Pigments and Growth Factors*. New York: Elsevier Applied Science, 1989.

Völker, Ursula (ed.), and Katrin Brückner (ed.). *Von der Faser zum Stoff. Textile Werkstoff- und Warenkunde*. Hamburg: Büchner, 2009.

von Bruchhausen, Franz (ed.). *Hagers Handbuch der Pharmazeutischen Praxis, Folgeband 2, Drogen A - K/Folgeband 3, Drogen L–Z*. Berlin: Springer, 1998.

Wagner, Monika, Dietmar Rübel, and Sebastian Hackenschmidt. *Lexikon des künstlerischen Materials: Werkstoffe der modernen Kunst von Abfall bis Zinn*. Munich: C. H. Beck, 2010.

Walter de Gruyter GmbH. *Pschyrembel Klinisches Wörterbuch*, 263rd edition. Berlin: Walter de Gruyter GmbH, 2012.

Wassermann, Ludwig. *Was sind Backmittel?*. Bonn: Wissensforum Backwaren e. V., 2009.

Weiß, Jürgen, Wilhelm Pabst, Karl E. Strack, and Susanne Granz. *Tierproduktion*. Stuttgart: Parey, 2005.

Winter, Ruth. *A Consumer's Dictionary of Food Additives*. New York: Three Rivers Press, 2009.

Woltman, Scott J., Gregory D. Jay, and Gregory P. Crawford. *Liquid Crystals: Frontiers in Biomedical Applications*. World Scientific Pub Co., 2007.

The following list is not intended to be either exhaustive or representative, but rather to present some of the internet resources referred to while researching this book. The addresses belong to government agencies, interest groups and private companies. Naming the addresses expressly does not entail any endorsement of the contents of the respective websites. The owners of the domains are solely responsible for the contents of the websites. Some of the websites named are German, however many of these also have an English version or can be automatically translated.

www.aegmis.de
www.aerzte-gegen-tierversuche.de
www.afdc.energy.gov
www.akema.it
www.albertschweitzerfoundation.org
www.alpaka.info
www.angora.de
www.artes-biotechnology.com
www.backmittelinstitut.de
www.barnivore.com
www.bdih.de
www.biopure.com
www.biotechnologie.de
www.biotest.com
www.bmelv.de
www.borealisgroup.com
www.britannica.com
www.ccspa.org
www.ceralan.fi
www.chemgapedia.de
www.chemicalland21.com
www.chemie.de
www.choosecrueltyfree.org.au
www.codexalimentarius.net
www.cognis.com
www.competitionbureau.gc.ca
www.cosmeticanalysis.com

www.cosmeticsinfo.org
www.cosmos-standard.org
www.demeter.net
www.dfo-mpo.gc.ca
www.dhu.de
www.diamant-zucker.de
www.diamo-violins.de
http://earthlings.com
http://ec.europa.eu
www.ecocert.com
http://europa.eu
www.fachinfo.de
www.fao.org
www.farmsanctuary.org
www.findadhesives.com
www.food-detektiv.de
www.freepatentsonline.com
www.gerstaecker.de
www.gfe-ev.de
www.global-standard.org
www.gmo-compass.org
www.gocrueltyfree.org
www.govtrack.us
www.greenpeace.org
www.hc-sc.gc.ca
www.heel.ca
www.igb.fraunhofer.de

www.ihd-dresden.de
http://ijt.sagepub.com
www.ikw.org
www.imperial-oel-import.de
www.impfen.de
www.incredibow.com
www.indianshellac.com
www.inspection.gc.ca
www.ionc.de
www.kentdisplays.com
www.kremerpigments.com
www.lactic-acid.com
www.lamee.de
www.lanolin.com
www.leapingbunny.org
www.lecithinguide.com
http://leginfo.legislature.ca.gov
www.lookchem.com
www.ltz.de
www.lubrizol.com
www.malacsoc.org.uk
www.manufactum.com
www.margarine-institut.de
http://mediastorm.com/publication/
    black-market
www.merckgroup.com
www.merriam-webster.com
www.ncbi.nlm.nih.gov
www.natrue.org
www.nongmoproject.org
www.novartis-vaccines.com
www.npainfo.org
www.oekotest.de
http://onlinelibrary.wiley.com
www.organicbiologique.ca

www.organicguide.com
www.orthomol.de
www.osti.gov
www.percoba.com
www.peta.org
www.pharmafoods.co.jp
www.pharma.us.novartis.com
www.phw-gruppe.de
www.rivella.ch
www.roeper.de
www.rote-liste.de
www.sanofi.ca
www.sekowa.de
www.sigmaaldrich.com
www.stopforcefeeding.com
www.suedzucker.de
www.thefreelibrary.com
www.tierrechte.de
http://usa.weleda.com
www.usda.gov
http://us.hessnatur.com
www.vegan.org
www.vegansociety.com
www.vier-pfoten.org
http://vitamind.ucr.edu
www.wala.de
www.wiesenhof-online.de
www.wiesenhof-pilzland.de
http://de.wikipedia.org
http://en.wikipedia.org
www.wissenschaft-online.de
www.wissensforum-backwaren.de
www.wissen.spiegel.de
www.wool.com

Consumer Chemicals and Containers Regulations, 2001; SOR/2001-269;
current to November 14, 2011; last amended on June 20, 2011

Consumer Packaging and Labelling Act; R.S.C., 1985, c. C-38;
current to October 31, 2011

Consumer Packaging and Labelling Regulations; C.R.C., c. 417;
current to October 31, 2011

Cosmetic Regulations; C.R.C., c. 869;
current to October 31, 2011; last amended on June 14, 2007

Fisheries Act; R.S.C., 1985, c. F-14;
current to November 25, 2012; last amended on June 29, 2012

Food and Drugs Act; R.S.C., 1985, c. F-27;
current to October 31, 2011; last amended on June 16, 2008

Food and Drug Regulations; C.R.C., c. 870;
current to November 14, 2011; last amended on October 27, 2011

Marine Mammal Regulations; SOR/93-56;
current to November 25, 2012; last amended on February 10, 2011

Natural Health Products Regulations; SOR/2003-196;
current to November 14, 2011; last amended on June 1, 2008

Organic Products Regulations, 2009; SOR/2009-176;
current to October 31, 2011; last amended on June 30, 2009

Textile Labelling Act; R.S.C., 1985, c. T-10;
current to November 14, 2011

Textile Labelling and Advertising Regulations; C.R.C., c. 1551;
current to November 14, 2011; last amended on March 25, 2010

Canadian legislation online:

Consolidated Acts and regulations of Canada

English: http://laws-lois.justice.gc.ca/eng
French: http://laws-lois.justice.gc.ca/fra